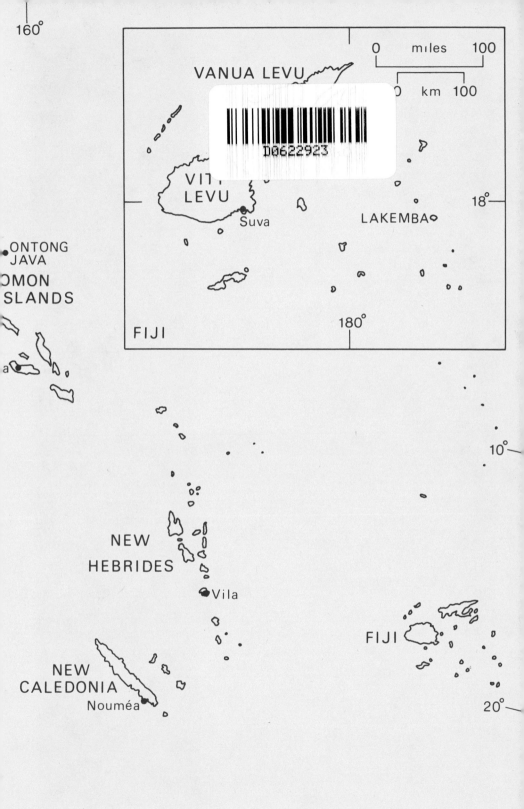

160°

VANUA LEVU

0   miles   100

0   km   100

18°

VIT
LEVU

Suva

LAKEMBA

ONTONG
JAVA

OMON
SLANDS

FIJI

180°

10°

NEW

HEBRIDES

Vila

FIJI

NEW
CALEDONIA

Nouméa

20°

170°   180°

Subsistence and Survival

Rural Ecology in the Pacific

Subsistence and Survival

Rural Ecology in the Pacific

Edited by

TIMOTHY P. BAYLISS-SMITH

*Department of Geography,
University of Cambridge, England*

and

RICHARD G. FEACHEM

*Ross Institute of Tropical Hygiene,
London, England*

1977

ACADEMIC PRESS

LONDON · NEW YORK · SAN FRANCISCO

A Subsidiary of Harcourt Brace Jovanovich, Publishers

ACADEMIC PRESS INC. (LONDON) LTD
24–28 Oval Road,
London NW1

United States Edition published by
ACADEMIC PRESS INC.
111 Fifth Avenue,
New York, New York 10003

Library of Congress Catalog Card Number: 77–77365
ISBN: 0–12–083250–x

Text set in 11/12 pt. Monophoto Baskerville
Printed in Great Britain by
William Clowes & Sons Limited
London, Beccles and Colchester

Notes on Contributors

Timothy P. Bayliss-Smith, Ph.D. (Cantab), *Department of Geography, University of Cambridge, Downing Place, Cambridge CB2 3EN, England.*

Assistant Lecturer in Geography at the University of Cambridge and Fellow of St. John's College, Cambridge. His research has centred around the ecology and use of resources by village populations. He has done fieldwork in the Solomon Islands and more recently in Fiji, where he participated in an inter-disciplinary project within the Man and the Biosphere programme organized by UNESCO.

William C. Clarke, Ph.D. (Berkeley), *Department of Geography, University of Papua and New Guinea, Box 4820, University Post Office, Papua, New Guinea.*

Professor of Geography, University of Papua New Guinea. Formerly Senior Research Fellow in Human Geography, Research School of Pacific Studies, Australian National University. His principal research interests are traditional tropical agriculture and ethnobotany. He has carried out extensive fieldwork in the Highlands of Papua New Guinea and is currently involved in studies of arboriculture and taro cultivation.

Mark D. Dornstreich, Ph.D. (Columbia), *120 Cherry Valley Road, Princeton, New Jersey 08540, U.S.A.*

Formerly Assistant Professor of Anthropology at Livingston College, Rutgers University. He has done anthropological and ecological fieldwork in New Guinea centering around the subjects of subsistence and ethnobotany. He is currently researching on the ecological and social implications of different systems of food production.

Richard G. A. Feachem, Ph.D. (N.S.W.), *Ross Institute of Tropical Hygiene, London School of Hygiene and Tropical Medicine, Keppel Street, London WC1E 7HT, England.*

Lecturer in Tropical Public Health Engineering in the Ross Institute of Tropical Hygiene, London School of Hygiene and Tropical Medicine. Formerly in the Department of Civil Engineering at the University of Birmingham. His research has concentrated particularly on various aspects of water supply and excreta disposal in low-income communities in developing countries. He has recently directed a multi-disciplinary investigation of village water supplies in Lesotho.

Richard W. Hornabrook, M.D. (N.Z.), F.R.A.C.P., *27 Orchard Street, Wadestown, Wellington, New Zealand.*

Neurologist at Wellington Hospital, New Zealand. Formerly Director of the Papua New Guinea Institute of Medical Research. His research interests are in the fields of clinical neurology, neuroepidemiology and human biology. He has a general interest in man in tropical forest ecosystems. He has been involved in most aspects of biological research in various areas of Papua New Guinea.

Harley I. Manner, M.A. (Hawaii), *Department of Geology and Geography, Bucknell University, Lewisburg, Pennsylvania 17837, U.S.A.*

Assistant Professor of Geography, in the Department of Geology and Geography at Bucknell University, Lewisburg, Pennsylvania. Major research interests include man–land interactions, biogeography, tropical agroecosystems and the processes of agricultural intensification in New Guinea.

Margaret McArthur, Ph.D. (A.N.U.), *4051 Black Point Road, Honolulu, Hawaii 96816, U.S.A.*

Formerly Senior Lecturer in Anthropology, University of Sydney. After participating in nutrition surveys in Papua New Guinea and among Australian Aborigines in 1947–48, she studied anthropology in London, and subsequently carried out inter-disciplinary research for several United Nations organizations in South East Asia and Africa. Currently she is preparing a critical assessment of research on human biology in Papua New Guinea.

Bonnie, J. McCay, Ph.D. (Columbia), *Department of Human Ecology and Social Science, Cook College, Rutgers University of New Jersey, P.O. Box 231, New Brunswick, New Jersey 08903, U.S.A.*

Assistant Professor of Anthropology in the Department of Human Ecology and Social Sciences, Cook College, Rutgers University. Her principal research interests are the anthropology and ecology of common property resource systems and "appropriate technology" development. She carried out fieldwork in north-eastern Newfoundland, Canada, and is currently involved in a study of a coastal area of New Jersey.

George E. B. Morren, Ph.D. (Columbia), *Department of Human Ecology and Social Sciences, Cook College, Rutgers University of New Jersey, P.O. Box 231, New Brunswick, New Jersey 08903, U.S.A.*

Assistant Professor of Anthropology and Ecology in the Department of Human Ecology and Social Science, Cook College, Rutgers University. He has worked on a variety of ecological and ethnological problems including the interactions of people and terrestrial mammals, settlement pattern and movement, agriculture, and the ecological functions of social and ritual behaviour. Research has been in the Upper Sepik region of Papua New Guinea. Currently he is interested in developing multi-disciplinary approaches to assessing the environmental and human impacts of change in complex societies.

Peter F. Sinnett, M.D. (Sydney), M.R.A.C.P., *22 Roebuck Street, Red Hill, A.C.T. 2603, Australia.*

Formerly Professor of Human Biology, University of Papua New Guinea and Senior Research Fellow of the National Heart Foundation of Australia. He has worked mainly on nutrition in relation to cardio-vascular disease, with fieldwork in Papua New Guinea. Currently he is studying the electrocardiographic characteristics of Papua New Guinea populations as part of the International Biological Programme.

Jeremy M. B. Smith, Ph.D. (A.N.U.), *Department of Geography, University of New England, Armidale, New South Wales 2351, Australia.*

Lecturer in Biogeography at the Department of Geography, University of New England. Interests centre largely around ecological and bio-geographical problems of high tropical mountains, especially the origins and migrations of their floras, with fieldwork in Borneo and New Guinea.

Andrew P. Vayda, Ph.D. (Columbia), *Department of Human Ecology and Social Science, Cook College, Rutgers University of New Jersey, P.O. Box 231, New Brunswick, New Jersey 08903, U.S.A.*

Professor of Anthropology and Ecology, Department of Human Ecology and Social Sciences, Cook College, Rutgers University. Editor-in-chief of "Human Ecology: An Interdisciplinary Journal". He has researched in human ecology in Polynesia, Melanesia (New Guinea) and insular South East Asia. Currently he is involved in research and teaching programmes concerned with environmental problems in developing countries.

Roy Wagner, Ph.D. (Chicago), *Department of Anthropology, University of Virginia, Charlottesville 22903, U.S.A.*

Professor and Chairman of the Department of Anthropology, University of Virginia. Formerly Associate Professor of Anthropology, Northwestern University. He has worked mainly on the symbology of sociality and ritual in Highlands of New Guinea. His current interests include the semiotics of human moral and cosmological conceptualization, the implications of meaning for demography, and myth as symbolic construction.

Preface

This book spans a wide range of material. The geographical range of our contributions extends from the glaciated uplands of Papua New Guinea, through the montane forests and grasslands of the Highlands, into the coastal jungles, and across to the smaller islands and atolls of the South West Pacific. The subject matter includes the ecology of man's environment, man's use and perception of biological resources, and the physiology and health of the human organism itself. Using traditional labels, the contributors include anthropologists, geographers, human biologists, a nutritionist, a botanist and a public health engineer.

Despite this diversity — but, in a sense, because of it — there is a common theme which runs through the book, and it is one that is reflected in our subtitle "Rural Ecology in the Pacific". The ecology of man is a subject now recognized as being of importance. All too often, it is argued, a narrow and specialized approach to problems has led to a situation where the investigator "cannot see the wood for the trees" — and, in particular, fails to take account of the interrelatedness of man and nature.

On the other hand, the concept of human ecology is of such daunting breadth that until recent years few workers in the human sciences have felt confident enough to reach out to embrace it. Dealing successfully with the complexity of man's relationship to his environment is a delicate balancing act which requires a firm base. It has been the traditional specialist disciplines of anthropology, biology and so on that have supplied this firm foundation, and which in turn produce the different emphases (cultural, environmental, physiological, nutritional, and so on) that distinguish the chapters in this book. An explicit awareness of the interrelation of man and environment nevertheless persists, and it provides one unifying theme for the book.

A second source of unity is the geographical region that has supplied the "laboratory" for the research that is reported and reviewed in these pages: the Melanesian area of the South West Pacific. In this case it has been the diversity of human habitats, cultures and populations in this region that has attracted researchers, and which has

provided valuable conditions of comparability between the many
different communities and ecosystems. The substantial body of data
that has been accumulated for Melanesia on matters relating to man's
ecology is a second source of strength for those who wish to adopt a
broad, inter-disciplinary approach to problems of human subsistence
and survival.

This body of data on human ecology in the Pacific, to which this
book is an addition, forms a most important resource for the governments of the newly independent countries of the region. The editors
reject the current wave of apology for expatriate research in the
Pacific and would stress rather the invaluable base of information about
villages and villagers which has been painstakingly built up over the
last two decades. This information is a unique resource for the development planner and policy maker as well as for the agricultural extension
officer and medical practitioner. We would hope that for every one
student or academic that reads this book there will be ten others who
are more actively employed in developing countries in making decisions
or acting upon them.

The fact that the authors of this book have, in some ways, a shared
overview of reality and a common region of interest does not mean that
they are necessarily in agreement with each other over particular
issues. Since they approach their subject matter from different angles,
it is inevitable that different explanations will sometimes be proposed.
It would perhaps be surprising if any consensus view were to emerge,
when an explicitly integrative approach to the man–environment
dichotomy, though often proposed, has been only recently attempted.
The editors will be well satisfied if this book is seen as pointing the way
towards a better view of a specific reality, and towards a sounder basis
for specific policy. In addition, however, there are wider issues of
human subsistence and survival that are raised in these pages and it is
towards these issues that future research must ultimately be directed.

In the preparation of this book we gratefully acknowledge help
given by staff of the Department of Geography, University of Cambridge, and the Department of Civil Engineering, University of
Birmingham. At Cambridge we would like to thank Michael Young
and Arthur Shelley for the maps and diagrams, and R. Coe for his work
on the photographs. At Birmingham, Wendy Dorman was responsible
for much of the typescript, and Stuart Edwards helped with photo-
graphy. We are especially grateful to Jennifer Bardsley of Academic
Press Ltd. in London for her patient, sympathetic and highly professional help.

April 1977   Timothy P. Bayliss-Smith
                                          Richard G. Feachem

Contents

1. Human Ecology: Theory and Practice

2. Environments and the Human Organism

3. Environmental Change and Human Activity

4. Environmental Exploitation and Human Subsistence

5. Environment and Man: Policy, Perception and Prospect

List of Maps

Part 1

Human Ecology: Theory and Practice

Chapter I

The Human Ecologist as Superman?

RICHARD G. A. FEACHEM

*London School of Hygiene and Tropical Medicine,
London, England*

I. INTRODUCTION

As I write this chapter the manuscript of the book lies on the deck in front of me. Glancing through the many pages of typescript, I wonder what it all signifies. Who will read it apart from fellow academics and students? Will it be of any real value to the people of the rural tropics, or will it merely serve to preserve and promote the discipline and thereby reduce the chances that the authors of the various chapters will be unemployed? Will the findings embodied here materially effect the life and well being of any Pacific islanders? Because of this research will anything be done that would have been left undone, or will any project be abandoned that would otherwise have been executed? Looking back at recent publications comparable to this (Brookfield, 1973; Ward, 1972) I am not hopeful about the answers to these questions. Yet I remain unshakeably convinced that there exists in these studies a potential for practical application and that they, and others like them, provide for Melanesia a background of information on human ecology which is second to none. This information could play a crucial role in the formulation and execution of development policies which would promote rural welfare, in addition to achieving national economic goals.

Such an act of faith is necessary when one considers the apparaent foolishness of the things we do. Leafing through the manuscript I can visualize Manner cutting down huge trees and, no doubt watched by incredulous indigenes, weighing them; I see Bayliss-Smith rushing up and down a beach on Ontong Java counting and weighing fish as the canoes come in; I see myself wading around in streams looking for bacteria while being accused of looking for gold; I see Hornabrook putting people in polythene bags; I see Dornstreich, deep in the forest, harassing *Phalanger maculatus*; and I wonder at Wagner arguing in language so abstract that his friends at Karimui will surely never understand his true meaning.

II. FIELDWORK

These images highlight a theme of this volume—namely fieldwork. All contributors have undertaken long periods of intensive investigation in relatively limited geographical areas (see Map 1) and have generally acted as participant observers. Although it is not academically fashionable to stress the rigours of such an approach, and most contributors are too modest to do this anyway, it is nonetheless true that many of the studies reported here are based on extremely arduous fieldwork of a particularly tedious and painstaking kind. This has been brought about by the combination of the classic social anthropologist's method, of living in the community being studied, and the modern ecologist's approach to data collection and the need for precision and experimental rigour. It is this devotion to fieldwork which is the *sine qua non* of good human ecology in the rural tropics and Melanesia has been the site of a substantial proportion of the numerate fieldwork conducted in recent years.

III. THE INDIVIDUAL OR THE TEAM?

Scientists embarking upon research into aspects of human ecology in the rural tropics are faced with an important dilemma which is well illustrated by the studies reported here. Research in human ecology essentially necessitates a high level of multi-disciplinary activity and researchers must collect and analyse data which are conventionally the province of many different disciplines, each with its own traditions and methodologies. The dilemma, therefore, is whether to tackle one's selected research topic individually or whether to undertake a multi-

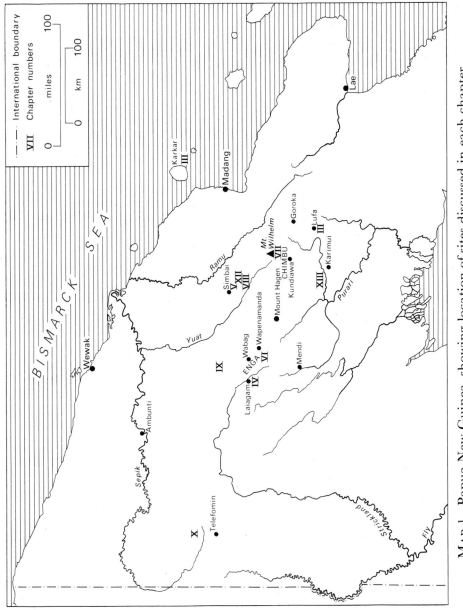

MAP 1. Papua New Guinea, showing location of sites discussed in each chapter.

disciplinary team investigation. The pros and cons of each course of action are apparent. Individual research carries the risk that the individual will have insufficient time, and an insufficient grasp of the complex issues outside his area of original training, to prevent the analysis becoming superficial. Team research carries the danger of fragmentation, and lack of integration of the specialist subject components, and also poses enormous organizational and managerial problems which are well described in Chapter III.

The great surge of research interest in human ecology in Melanesia in the last two decades has centred particularly around the individual research methodology and most commonly around research conducted by individual doctoral students. This trend is well illustrated by this volume, in which six chapters report research conducted by individual students, which was later prepared for doctoral theses. This methodology brings its own special trials and joys. On the positive side it is immensely challenging to a young researcher and, particularly under the British and Australian system in which little or no training is received between first graduation and postgraduate fieldwork, it is a make-or-break experience. The researcher is thrown entirely to his own resources and must pursue his research in mental, and often physical isolation. It is a highly flexible procedure in which logistic problems are minimized and the research can change direction and respond to stimuli with little disruption or difficulty. Because the number of man-hours of productive fieldwork time is severely limited, the individual researcher is forced to define his area of interest very carefully, and there is great pressure not to collect peripheral data of doubtful importance but rather to relentlessly investigate a limited set of variables. This may well lead to tighter and more integrated research than the larger team projects, which tend to develop a "let's measure everything and decide what to do with it afterwards" mentality. Individual research projects are also attractive because they cause such little disruption to the local system under study, and this may be especially desirable when working in areas of special cultural or political sensitivity (such as the Upper Fly or Bougainville) or when working in areas where people have become sensitized towards research by previous team projects (such as Lufa or the South Fore). It is also desirable when the non-human component of the ecosystem is particularly delicate and unstable, and a good example of this is provided by Smith's research on Mt. Wilhelm reported in Chapter VII. A final advantage of individual research is that it is cheap and easy to organize and this makes it simple to abandon. This is an important consideration in times when political sensitivities necessitate the utmost flexibility and the ability to fade rapidly from the scene if necessary.

With a major team project, by contrast, flexibility becomes increasingly difficult as the juggernaut builds up its momentum and its own internal logic. Abandonment is likely to be almost impossible as, not only do the team in the field become committed to their tasks, but also a multitude of external interests, such as financial backers and academics waiting in the wings to take part in phase two during their carefully arranged sabbaticals, combine to urge the project forward without a full knowledge of the situation in the field. There is a close and pleasing analogy here with mountaineering expeditions. The small expedition with little funding and equipment can, in the face of adverse conditions, decide to go down and go home. The major expedition cannot do this and the size of the operation, combined with strong pressure from commercial and political interests, will often lead to decisions being taken for non-technical reasons which may lead to increased exposure to hazard and consequently to disaster.

The great disadvantages of the individual research approach are lack of time and inability to grasp the intricacies of other disciplines. Lack of time may in fact be an advantage if it leads to more efficient and single-minded use of time. However, the limited ability of any individual to fully master the methodologies and literature of several disciplines is a very real drawback. In every chapter in this book it is possible to identify the discipline of original training of the author and then to list several other disciplines, often with few traditional links with the author's base discipline, which the author has employed to pursue his argument. Chapter VI provides an example—the author by training is a civil engineer and yet he has employed the disciplines of geography, bacteriology, epidemiology and cultural anthropology to a substantial degree. The author of this chapter is, therefore, running the risk that he has failed to grasp the fundamentals or practice of these disciplines, so that a bacteriologist, for instance, reading Chapter VI might be highly critical. All individual researchers in human ecology run this risk and, while the more conventional scientist has to worry only about understanding his own discipline, the human ecologist has to worry about understanding several other disciplines besides. Chapter V is of particular interest here because in it a nutritionist makes some severe criticisms of the nutritional content of a major work of human ecology conducted by a social anthropologist. There is no simple answer to this problem but it is one of which those who support the individual research method, including myself, should be very aware.

Turning to team research we can identify advantages and disadvantages which follow directly from the comments already made about individual research. Team research can mobilize enormous expertise drawn from an unlimited number of disciplines and it can tackle complex research problems in a relatively short period of time. However, it has great drawbacks. The size of the operation makes it inflexible, unresponsive and often damaging to sensitive ecosystems. Team research which focuses on limited geographical regions (such as the International Biological Programme and the Harvard Biomedical Expeditions) may well antagonize the local populations and therefore promote an anti-research mood in the country which will ultimately damage all research work. Team research work will often involve short field trips by experts with no previous Melanesian experience and with little comprehension or local cultural and political sensitivities and little commitment except to their individual speciality. This can lead to unfortunate lapses as, for instance, the recent article which appeared in the *Journal of the American Medical Association* entitled "Air pollution in New Guinea: Cause of chronic pulmonary disease among stone-age natives in the Highlands" which reported research from Lufa. The word native makes one boggle at the author's lack of sensitivity, and to describe Lufa in the nineteen-seventies as stone-age reveals a certain lack of historical appreciation.

Many of the hazards of team research are well described in Chapter III and, to my mind, the greatest danger is that it often simply does not work. It is necessary to achieve integration, synthesis and co-ordination of the activities of highly specialized individuals who are concentrating on one narrow area of study. This has proved enormously difficult and it always depends on one or two people with the ability and strength of character to direct the team and then to sit down and write the synthesis of complex data. Multi-disciplinary studies can never be written by teams—this just produces multi-mono-disciplinary studies—they must be written by talented individuals who have the breadth of vision to handle the material produced by their colleagues and the capacity to coerce their colleagues into producing the right data, in the right form at the right time. I believe that the type of academic democracy, and keenness to let everyone do their own thing, that has been specially evident in the U.S.A. over the last few years, spells death for team projects. What is required is an authoritarian style of project leadership from a worker able to command the respect of the entire team or, alternatively, a team made up of a few people who know each other well and are used to working together. Without these solutions, team projects degenerate into a series of highly specialized papers published in specialized journals by people who return from the project to their many other commitments and who find it increasingly difficult to devote time to the integrated account of the project which was much talked about in the early planning stages. Sometimes, stimulated by the research funding organization, a publication such as the *Philosophical Transactions of the Royal Society*, Series B **268**, 893, is produced which does nothing more than bring together the specialized papers and provides no genuine integration of findings.

IV. POTENTIAL APPLICATIONS

Let me now return to the beginning of this chapter and to the question "what is the use of it all?" There are three possible answers here. It may be of no use, it may be of local use or it may be of global use. Clarke, in Chapter XII, argues in favour of the global use and maintains that ecological principles abstracted from the study of small societies may be applied with advantage to large industrial societies. He feels this is especially true for issues relating to the permanence of particular ecosystems. This last point is certainly true and ecologists can apply, and indeed are already applying, principles from Melanesian society to enlighten thought about other societies. However, I do not believe personally that much practical outcome will result from this export of ecological insight. Nor do I feel that those who are not steeped in the theory and practice of human ecology will take arguments based on cross-cultural transfer very seriously. Rather I suggest that the great role for human ecology, and for the findings reported in this volume, is in aiding development policy and planning in Melanesia.

The last two decades of research in the villages of Melanesia have produced a background of basic data which is second to none and which is an invaluable resource for planners in rural development. The fact that this resource is not fully appreciated or utilized by the planners is unfortunate and indicates the need for strenuous efforts to promote better communications between academics and government. However, the resource is there and it should be advertised more vigorously. For the past few years I have been engaged in research and development projects in Southern and West Africa and I am constantly amazed by the lack of background village data in these areas. In general, recent data on basic village attributes such as nutrition, health, agriculture, social change and many more are not available in much of Africa but are available in Melanesia. Development planning in Africa often seems to resemble roulette rather than rational decision making, and one sees vast sums invested in rural development projects on the slenderest of evidence and often with a total lack of sufficiently good micro-level village data. Planners are often brimming over with macro-level projections on financial returns, outputs of the product, processing capabilities, export markets and so on, but if faced with a question like "what do these people now eat and how will diet change as a result of your project" they can often provide no answers. The reason for this situation is simply that they draw up their plans in hotel rooms and offices and have to rely on the village data produced previously by academics. In Africa such information is often lacking while in Melanesia it is generally available. The basic understanding of several aspects of human ecology in rural Melanesia which we now possess provides the governments of the area with not only an invaluable planning tool but also with a protection against some of the destructive and naïve types of development policy which have been seen in Africa and elsewhere in recent years.

V. REFERENCES

Brookfield, H. C. (Ed.) (1973). "The Pacific in Transition, Geographical perspectives on adaptation and change". Edward Arnold, London.

Ward, R. G. (Ed.) (1972). "Men in the Pacific Islands". Oxford University Press, Oxford.

CHAPTER II

Human Ecology and Island Populations: The Problems of Change

TIMOTHY P. BAYLISS-SMITH

Department of Geography, University of Cambridge, England

I. ISLANDS AND HUMAN ECOLOGY

The term "human ecology", like the term "island", has tended to mean different things to different people. Human ecology first came to prominence with the Chicago School of Urban Sociology in the nineteen-twenties (Park and Burgess, 1921), and with the early attempts by geographers to redefine their discipline as the study of human ecology. More recently, the term has been revived by researchers approaching the study of man's ecology from two rather different standpoints. Moving upwards from the scale of the individual, researchers in physical anthropology, medicine, physiology and nutrition have attempted to broaden their explanations of human function and variation by considering man as an organism in relation to his environment (Sargent, 1974). At the same time workers in the social sciences have also found it increasingly useful to study the economic, social or geographical aspects of human populations in relation to the environment of those populations. Both the organism-ecology approach and the population-ecology approach are represented in this book, but in this chapter I restrict my attention to the latter. In particular, I examine the role of small islands, both real and conceptual, in advancing our understanding of man's ecology at the population level.

Insularity, whether actual or conceptual, has particular value for ecological studies. At the 1961 symposium entitled "Man's Place in the Island Ecosystem" Fosberg (1963, p. 5) identified the two essential features of real islands that made them attractive for study: their isolation, and their limited size. With limitation in size it becomes easier for the investigator to generalize, because of the greater cultural unity in small populations. It also becomes easier to analyse in depth, because the sample studied will inevitably represent a large percentage of the total population. Any isolation of a society, even if relative, also presents practical advantages: boundedness facilitates the operational definition of a population, and simplifies the measurement of material flows and migrations. If several islands are studied, then their differences in size, physical environment, culture or isolation can provide ideal, laboratory-like conditions of comparability.

In addition to these methodological considerations, insularity also provides circumstances particularly suitable for the study of human ecology, since on islands the spatial definition of man's ecosystem is relatively unambiguous. For biologists, of course, real island eco- systems have always been attractive, conceptually, for the same reasons. The land–sea interface represents a distinct boundary for most organ- isms, so that a readily defined area, the island, and the functional ecosystem of the inhabitants of that area correspond in many respects. Similarly, where the relationship between man and the ecosystem is the main focus of concern, then islands possess clear advantages over many mainland areas, where interlocking patterns of land ownership and variable spheres of influence often make it difficult to define the spatial limits of the environment that is under the control of a given population.

All these advantageous features of insularity are not necessarily confined to conventionally defined islands. In the South West Pacific several of the larger land areas, notably New Guinea, consist of a veritable chequer board of topographic and cultural diversity—many thousands of village populations that still operate essentially as islands. Whether the important decisions affecting the inhabitants of these islands are made within the community, or whether they are made in the boardrooms of companies located in Sydney or Tokyo, matters little from the methodological point of view. Any small human popula- tion that operates within well-defined boundaries and in relative isolation constitutes for human ecology an "island ecosystem".

II. THE SYSTEMS APPROACH IN HUMAN ECOLOGY

In the past 15 years two main trends within human ecology can be distinguished. The first was the adoption of an explicitly holistic viewpoint on man–environment interactions; the second was a move towards quantification. Both developments were to some extent general within the human sciences, but in studies of human ecology they resulted in part from the stimulus provided by biological concepts, and in particular from the notion of ecosystem. The influence of Fosberg's 1961 symposium was not insignificant in this respect. In pursuit of a more "scientific" and better-balanced view of man in his environment, the analysis of "systems" was seen by many as providing the necessary intellectual rigour (Ackerman, 1963; Stoddart, 1965; Watt, 1968; Clarke, 1968; Binford and Binford, 1968; Buckley, 1969; Chorley, 1971; Chapman, 1974). Stoddart, for example, wrote that

> partaking in General System Theory, the ecosystem is potentially capable of precise mathematical structuring within a theoretical framework, a very different matter from the tentative and incomplete descriptions of highly complex phenomena which too often pass for geographical 'synthesis'. (Stoddart, 1967, p. 532)

Through such advantages, systems analysis appeared to offer much to the investigator of a human society in its environment. In archaeology, for example, system models were seen by Clarke (1972) as being helpful at three levels. At the lowest level, broad problems in prehistory (e.g. the Neolithic Revolution) can be usefully "reconceptualized" by a systems approach. At a second level, and by restricting the scope of the modelling, "a more specific predictive or simulation power develops with the addition of quantitative information about the links and components of the system". And finally, with an even more tightly defined frame of reference and still more data, Clarke suggests that it becomes "possible to quantify the components and the input and output of the system and this move towards quantified, measurable and testable predictions" (Clarke, 1972, p. 30).

Ambitious claims such as these can be criticized on two grounds. The first concerns the capacity of the investigator to cope with the daunting complexity of the real world, and in particular of the interaction of man and his biotic environment. It is usually not possible to define a system, nor to identify its components, nor to specify the nature of the linkages within it, without first making subjective decisions about the critical processes in operation. When direct measurement and observation are not possible, as for example in an historical context, then the problem of system definition is even greater. Quantification of an incorrectly constructed or partially defined system merely suggests a spurious precision and a misleading degree of confidence in one's "predictions".

A second and perhaps more important problem is the difficulty of analysing change within systems in which man is included. In a natural system this problem need not arise. Ecological succession, and perhaps also evolutionary change, can be envisaged as being essentially processes of self-organization in which successively more probable states follow less probable ones through the operation of negative feedback processes (Margalef, 1968). Social systems, however, have "purposes" other than improved self-organization.

> Social systems typically progress towards greater organisation and greater levels of functional complexity. Such changes can only occur because the maintenance of a functional existence is not generally the *raison d'etre* of these systems. They occur because the systems function for a *purpose* to which the function itself is subservient. (Langton, 1972, p. 141)

Much socio-economic change, although having its ultimate origin in purposive behaviour, does not itself have "adaptive" value for any particular system (e.g. an island) within which it occurs. This contrasts with change in natural systems, which operates in many ways to achieve greater stability for the ecosystem, as through greater species diversity (Odum, 1971). Whereas ecosystems are dominated by negative feedback loops and homeostatic tendencies, all present-day systems involving social man have, in contrast, much stronger inbuilt positive feedbacks (increasing populations, rising material expectations, the impact of innovation diffusion, etc.), and in addition the factor of active control (Chorley, 1973).

The nature and effectiveness of the "control" can often be identified; even the "purpose" of a particular system can perhaps be specified in terms of the aspirations of groups and individuals, and the various constraints that make it unlikely that these goals will, in fact, be achieved. Nevertheless, there still remains the problem of continual and essentially unpredictable change in the inputs to the system. The growing interdependence of the world economy, at all scales (Brookfield, 1975), and the associated stream of innovations in information, needs and values, mean that seemingly irresistable change is the normal state. Far from being equilibrium bound, most of the real world systems that human ecologists study are increasingly dynamic, "lurching from one state of disequilibrium to another in response to changing impulses" (Chorley, 1973, p. 162). From this viewpoint, systems analysis appears far from the methodological panacea that some authors have claimed, but concomitantly the simplicity, manageable scale, and closure of island systems become even more appealing.

III. ISLAND COMMUNITIES AS ECOSYSTEMS: A NEW GUINEA EXAMPLE

The importance of change is, of course, recognized by researchers into the human ecology of island populations, but within the explicit ecosystem framework that some have adopted it is not an easy problem to tackle. Among those who have used the ecosystem model most effectively is Rappaport, whose work is discussed by several contributors to this volume (McArthur, Chapter V; Morren, Chapter X; Bayliss-Smith, Chapter XI). Rappaport's writings (1968, 1971a) about the Tsembaga Maring, a small and essentially insular community in the Bismarck Mountains of New Guinea (see Map 1), illustrate well the conceptual problem that is posed by ecosystem change.

Rappaport was concerned with two types of system: firstly, the actual montane forest ecosystem controlled and inhabited by the Maring, which he termed the "operational model" of the system; and secondly, the knowledge and beliefs concerning the environment that the people themselves possess, which he termed the "cognized model". The Maring's cognized model is dominated by the pig cycle, which is associated with religious and political rituals (see Wagner, Chapter XIII), but which also has important environmental implications through changing land use pressure. In summary, Rappaport shows that for the Maring

> The relationship of the cognized model to the operational model is similar to that of the 'memory' of an automated control device to the physical system it regulates. It is in terms of the understanding included in the cognized model that the ritual cycle is undertaken, but the ritual cycle in fact regulates material relations in the local ecological system and in the regional system. The operation of the entire cycle is cybernetic. (Rappaport, 1971a, p. 261)

Homeostatic regulation is therefore emphasized: the ritual cycle and, indeed, the whole of Maring cosmology is seen "as a functional, perhaps even adaptive, codification of reality". But two questions remain unanswered and as Vayda (1968) admits, they are probably unanswerable within a functionalist methodology that focusses largely on the mechanisms maintaining a balance between the population and its resources. The first question is how structures such as the Maring pig cycle originated; and the second is what is their future?

On the question of origins, Rappaport (1971a, p. 262) suggests that a society's cognized model will tend to be favoured by "selective forces" if it functions in an adequate way. He defines an "adequate" model as one that elicits a pattern of behaviour which contributes to the well-being of the population, and which also maintains the eco-system that is exploited in a productive state. This explanation begs a number of further questions, but for small-scale self-sufficient com-munities there must be a tendency for the process Rappaport envisages to operate.

Even for the pre-industrial world, however, it must be recognized that very similar environments are exploited in very different ways, and that many of these ways were equally "adaptive" as regards the maintenance of ecosystem stability, at least in the short term. In the longer term, severe degradation did of course take place: in the Pacific, for example, the grasslands and severely eroded *talasiga* country of many Fijian islands (Twyford and Wright, 1965), and the enlarged tropicalpine grassland zone of some New Guinea mountains that never even supported permanent settlement (Smith, Chapter VII) are evidence of long-term maladaptive land use. Different origins, tech-nologies, and degrees of interaction with neighbouring populations; and different conceptions of what constitutes an acceptable livelihood will all lead to different cultures being imposed on nature, even though nature must influence what strategies of ecosystem management have adaptive value, and so tend to persist.

Studies of Pacific island culture when they were still unchanged by European contact provide ample evidence of population controls, especially small isolated islands like Tikopia (Firth, 1936) and atolls like the Central Polynesian outliers (Bayliss-Smith, 1975). Such controls indicate clearly that isolation, acute spatial constraints on production, and a slow rate of technological innovation and social change themselves enforce negative feedback responses on to human populations (Bayliss-Smith, 1974). But the majority of the problems of island populations today concern change, and responses to innovation, rather than the dynamics of internal stability.

In studying such change, and in predicting the future of small insular populations like the Tsembaga Maring, whose cognized model of the world is now being transformed by external contacts, a steady-state ecosystem approach can offer only limited insights. Such an approach tends to view the management of the ecosystem as "the manipulation of the equilibrating operations of the ecosystem so as to achieve higher levels of production, generally within the existing structure of the system" (Chorley, 1973, p. 160). The emphasis of those who advocate this approach is therefore on maximizing existing productivity or on minimizing waste as a result of the adoption of suitable harvesting strategies, through pest control, or by scientific cropping of the native biota (e.g. Watt, 1968; Van Dyne, 1969). However desirable these aims might be, they are clearly inappropriate when studying societies at the present day, where indigenous aspirations and government planning both aim at transforming the island ecosystem, often in essentially irreversible ways.

Besides environmental alteration, this transformation involves an increase in the dependency of the community upon external inputs. In New Guinea it is being suggested that this form of economic development poses an ultimate threat to the once-isolated populations of the interior, such as the Maring. As elsewhere in the tropics, the traditional culture of these populations maintained an ecological balance through a combination of population regulation, extensive shifting cultivation, and a dominantly self-sufficient regime in energy use and nutrient cycling (see Clarke, Chapter XII). The effect of interaction with external systems tends to be a lowered subsistence diversity as cash crops replace traditional forms of livelihood, and a reduced capacity to respond to signs of degradation within the ecosystem as people's dependence upon external inputs and markets increases. In New Guinea some authors see this process as leading in the long term to social and ecological instability, and so ultimately as threatening the people's own welfare (Rappaport, 1971b; Clarke, 1973 and Chapter XII; Howlett, 1973; Waddell, 1974).

IV. QUANTIFYING THE AUTONOMY OF HUMAN SYSTEMS

If we wish to assess the degree of dependence of an island economy upon the outside world, or in other words the extent to which the island has lost its functional autonomy, then we must have some unit of measurement which will tell us how much interaction there is within the island compared to how much exists between the island and the outside world. Quantification, which is a second major trend in recent research, must therefore be considered, to determine what form of measurement might be appropriate.

In human ecology part of the value of the ecosystem concept—even at the "boxes and arrows" level—has been the way it has focussed attention on "relationships", and hence on the exact response of other components in the system that might follow from the changed state of any one component. As a result, since the nineteen-sixties there has been an increasing concern with precise measurement. The potential benefits of quantifying these relationships seem self-evident, as are the advantages of small-scale units like islands for accurate and complete measurement, census-taking and mapping. Less obvious are the disadvantages of a rigidly numerical approach, which is clearly inappropriate if it involves the exclusion of the intangible ethical and cultural values that so strongly influence behaviour.

Within the social sciences, economics has always been the most quantified discipline, but for the analysis of environmental relationships measurement in purely monetary terms is clearly not adequate. Within ecology, the dynamics of ecosystems were increasingly studied in terms of nutrient cycles and energy flows, but the direct relevance of these approaches to human ecology seemed at first to be limited. For this reason Stoddart (1967) saw the importance of the ecosystem model as lying mainly in its General System characteristics. Chorley (1973) has also pointed out that the biologist's model cannot be expanded to incorporate the complexity of modern social systems.

> The idea that flows of capital investment, population, technological information, generated energy, water and the like, together with such constraints as involved interest policies and the mechanisms of group decision-making, can be reduced to comparable units so as to be structured into energy linkages similar to those of ecosystems is clearly an illusion. (Chorley, 1973, p. 157)

On the other hand, there are certain aspects of the environmental and external relationships of communities that can usefully be analysed in energy terms, a theme which is examined for Pacific island populations in Chapter XI.

It is clear, therefore, that a balanced view of man in relation to his environment is going to require the analysis of more than one kind of measure of interaction. As Flannery (1973) remarked, human ecology must be defined as "the study of the interrelationships of man's exchanges of matter, energy and information". To ignore information and to concentrate entirely on matter and energy exchange must inevitably produce a distorted view of man–environment systems. On the other hand, the converse is also true: although information and it's diffusion remains one of the concerns of anthropologists and sociologists, is usually studied within social systems from which the environment has been excluded. In only one study has the "information" content of man–environment relations been successfully quantified within a strict information theory framework (Chapman, 1974). Meanwhile, material exchanges continue to be studied in monetary terms by economists, and in nutrient and production terms by ecologists and agronomists.

Serious attempts to integrate these approaches have not been made, since most so-called interdisciplinary research projects tend to have one dominant emphasis (often biomedical or economic), and so inevitably operate within the framework of existing theory. It may be, as Feachem (Chapter I) suggests, that this is an inevitable consequence of it being impossible for one person to be that superman of the human sciences, the human ecologist. If so, then the full implications of this purely practical constraint surely deserve to be explored.

V. REFERENCES

Ackerman, E. A. (1963). Where is a research frontier? *Ann. Ass. Am. Geogr.* **53**, 429–440.

Bayliss-Smith, T. P. (1974). Constraints on population growth: the case of the Polynesian Outlier atolls in the precontact period. *Hum. Ecol.* **2**, 259–295.

Bayliss-Smith, T. P. (1975). The Central Polynesian Outlier populations since European contact. *In* "Pacific Atoll Populations" (Ed. V. Carroll). University of Hawaii Press, Honolulu, pp. 286–343.

Binford, S. R. and Binford, C. R. (Eds) (1968). "New Perspectives in Archaeology". Aldine, Chicago.

Brookfield, H. C. (1975). "Interdependent Development". Methuen, London.

Buckley, W. (1969). "Sociology and Modern Systems Theory". Prentice-Hall, New Jersey.

Chapman, G. P. (1970). Perception and regulation: a case study of farmers in Bihar. *Trans. Inst. br. Geog.* **62**, 71–94.

Chorley, R. J. (1971). The role and relations of physical geography. *In* "Progress in Geography" Vol. 3 (Eds C. Board *et al.*). Methuen, London, pp. 89–109.

Chorley, R. J. (1973). Geography as human ecology. *In* "Directions in Geography" (Ed. R. J. Chorley). Methuen, London, pp. 153–170.

Clarke, D. L. (1968). "Analytical Archaeology". Methuen, London.

Clarke, D. L. (1972). Models and paradigms in archaeology. *In* "Models in Archaeology" (Ed. D. L. Clarke). Methuen, London, pp. 1–60.

Clarke, W. C. (1973). The dilemma of development. *In* "The Pacific in Transition" (Ed. H. C. Brookfield. Methuen, London, pp. 275–298.

Firth, R. (1936). "We, the Tikopia". Allen and Unwin, London.

Flannery, K. V. (1973). Introduction. *In* "The Use of Land and Water Resources in the Past and Present Valley of Oaxaca, Mexico" (Ed. A. V. T. Kirkby). Memoirs of the Museum of Anthropology No. 5, University of Michigan.

Fosberg, F. R. (1963). The island ecosystem. *In* "Man's Place in the Island Ecosystem" (Ed. F. R. Fosberg). Bishop Museum Press, Honolulu, pp. 1–6.

Howlett, D. R. (1973). Terminal development: from tribalism to peasantry. *In* "The Pacific in Transition" (Ed. H. C. Brookfield). Methuen, London, pp. 249–274.

Langton, J. (1972). Potentialities and problems of adopting a systems approach to the study of change in human geography. *In* "Progress in Geography", Vol. 4 (Eds C. Board *et al.*). Methuen, London, pp. 125–180.

Margalef, R. (1968). "Perspectives in Ecological Theory". University of Chicago Press, Chicago.

Odum, E. P. (1971). "Fundamentals of Ecology", 3rd edn. Saunders, Philadelphia.

Park, R. E. and Burgess, E. W. (1921). "Introduction to the Science of Sociology". University of Chicago Press, Chicago.

Rappaport, R. A. (1968). "Pigs for the Ancestors: Ritual in the Ecology of a New Guinea People". Yale University Press, New Haven.

Rappaport, R. A. (1971a). Nature, culture, and ecological anthropology. *In* "Man, Culture, and Society", 2nd edn (Ed. H. L. Shapiro). Oxford University Press, London, pp. 237–267.

Rappaport, R. A. (1971b). The flow of energy in an agricultural society. *In* "Energy and Power" (Scientific American pubn). W. H. Freeman, San Francisco, pp. 69–82.

Sargent, F. (1974). Nature and scope of human ecology. *In* "Human Ecology" (Ed. F. Sargent). North-Holland, Amsterdam, pp. 1–25.

Stoddart, D. R. (1965). Geography and the ecological approach. *Geography* **50**, 242–251.

Stoddart, D. R. (1967). Organism and ecosystem as geographical models. *In* "Models in Geography" (Eds R. J. Chorley and P. Haggett). Methuen, London, pp. 511–548.

Twyford, I. T. and Wright, A. C. S. (1965). "The Soil Resources of the Fiji Islands" Vols 1 and 2. Government Printer, Suva.

Van Dyne, G. M. (Ed.) (1969). "The Ecosystem Concept in Natural Resource Management". Academic Press, New York and London.

Vayda, A. P. (1968). Foreword. *In* "Pigs for the Ancestors" (Ed. R. A. Rappaport). Yale University Press, New Haven.

Waddell, E. W. (1974). Frost over Niugini. *New Guinea* **8**, 39–49.

Watt, K. E. F. (1968). "Ecology and Resource Management". McGraw-Hill, New York.

Part 2

Environments and the Human Organism

Human Ecology and Biomedical Research: A Critical Review of The International Biological Programme in New Guinea

RICHARD W. HORNABROOK

Wellington Hospital, New Zealand

I. INTRODUCTION

A. HUMAN ECOLOGY AND BIOLOGY

In general, the study of the biological attributes of man has been firmly in the hands of medical scientists and, to a less pronounced extent, of physical anthropologists. The latter's contributions have been primarily in taxonomic fields whilst the wide spectrum of biological disciplines have been considered to lie within the domain of the former. Advances in the field have probably been limited by the rather restricted nature of traditional training in medicine. A medical education has concentrated attention on the phenomenon arising when an individual is affected by some pathological process. The very word "medicine" has connotations of sickness and pharmacy, and the training designed to produce physicians skilled in the management of sickness does not necessarily provide a desirable foundation for the study of human ecology.

In fact, ecological and biological principles have been an integral component of the general framework of medical science since its modern development, but only in the last one or two decades has there been an awareness of a need to fully recognize their significance and to consider human biology as a discipline in its own right.

Several influences have been instrumental in the broadening of the medical horizon. For one thing, the enormous increase in human population in recent decades has underlined the importance of considering populations as opposed to individuals. There is an evident need to understand the human species as a population, and the natural forces which control it. This may be linked with the recognition of the environment as having a pervasive importance which has played a considerable role in the development of a general ecological approach to human problems. Human ecology necessarily emphasizes the relationship of man and his society with the environment.

Interest in human ecology has also derived a stimulus from the advances which have been made across the general field of biology following the application of ecological concepts. This has suggested that similar progress may follow this introduction in the study of mankind. Indeed, already this has been demonstrated by progress in a number of traditional medical fields, and one may anticipate further advance with an increasingly wide application of general biological and ecological principles.

Acceptance of the desirability of developing human ecology as a discipline falls short of a developed methodology with which the study can be handled. The development of human ecology has been hampered by a variety of philosophical and methodological problems. The fact that some of the ecological concepts have long been recognized in medicine and that they are now being considered with somewhat different emphasis, is the source of some confusion. Ecology has brought with it a framework of terminology which is either new or borrowed from other disciplines and the new terminology has been responsible for misconceptions and failures of communication. At times there have been problems in conceptualization: the terms human ecology, human adaptability and human biology are often employed as if they were synonyms. Recent monographs on human ecology and human biology contain material which is virtually identical and differs only in the nosology employed.

Many biologists and scientists, entering the field without a wide background in human studies, tend to overlook the unique nature of man. This uniqueness, which largely results from the development of the cerebral hemispheres, results in the study of human ecology offering many more challenges than are presented by the studies of other vertebrates or less complex life forms. The cerebral influence which is responsible for man's complex socio-cultural and behavioural adaptation has no parallel in other life forms. It is this aspect of human ecology which emphasizes the desirability for the planning of research projects in the subject to incorporate adequate representation of socio-cultural and environmental besides straight human biological disciplines.

B. PAPUA NEW GUINEA INSTITUTE OF MEDICAL RESEARCH

Some of the practical methodological scientific difficulties which hamper the development of human ecology are illustrated by the early development of the Institute of Human Biology of Papua New Guinea, and they will be discussed in this chapter. The awakening interest in the general study of man coincided with moves to establish a research institute in Papua New Guinea, and was instrumental in the introduction of the title "an Institute of Human Biology" rather than "an Institute of Medical Research". Attention was drawn to the fact that there was a prime need for investigation of the biology of normal as opposed to pathological phenomena. The decision to set up a research institute in Papua New Guinea was inspired to a large extent by the wide variety of human societies and the range of genetic variation which existed in that country. These were associated with the diversity of ecosystems in Papua New Guinea. The combination of circumstances suggested immense possibilities for research, a situation which was enhanced by the fact that some Papua New Guinean societies had but recently experienced their first contact with Western technology, and prior to that time the culture had been remarkably isolated from external influence (Hornabrook, 1970a to 1972).

C. THE INTERNATIONAL BIOLOGICAL PROGRAMME

The Institute's foundation coincided with the plans that the Royal Society of London and the Australian Academy of Science had in train to undertake an ambitious multi-disciplinary study of human adaptability in a tropical forest ecosystem (Hornabrook, 1970, 1971; Walsh, 1971). These plans were the basis for a joint Anglo-Australian contribution to the International Biological Programme (IBP). Human adaptability comprises one of the seven sections under which the IBP was divided. The whole objective of the programme was "to provide a world plan of research into the biological basis of productivity and human welfare", the human adaptability section of the programme being distinct from the other sections in being restricted to the study of one species—man—and of course was more concerned with human welfare than, perhaps, the biological basis of productivity, although it must be said that human productivity is certainly based on effective adaptation (Weiner, 1965; Weiner and Lourie, 1969). This research project purported to study a human population in the tropical lowlands and to contrast it with a similarly sized group of people living in the montane valleys of the interior. The general intention was to bring together a variety of disciplines to investigate man and his adaptation to the different environments. Of necessity, a large investment of both capital and time was implicit in the design. The Institute was therefore involved immediately in the design and implementation of a project which aspired to investigate, in broad terms, human ecology in Melanesia.

Now that the Institute of Human Biology has been in existence for five years and the IBP research project concluded, it is profitable to look at the Institute's development and this particular research project in a general way, and to consider the technical and philosophical difficulties which have been associated with the theme and the degree to which they have achieved their overall aims. In reviewing the IBP study, the methodological difficulties which were experienced in its undertaking are in some ways as instructive as the observations which have emerged from the research.

II. A STUDY OF HUMAN ADAPTABILITY IN PAPUA NEW GUINEA

A. GENERAL ORGANIZATION AND STUDY DESIGN

1. Preliminary Arrangements

A group of representatives of the Royal Society of London, the Australian Academy of Science and the Department of Public Health of Papua New Guinea met in Madang (Map 2) in 1967. They were

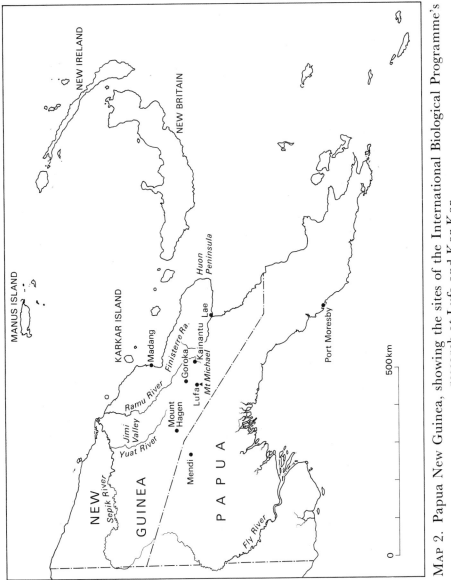

MAP 2. Papua New Guinea, showing the sites of the International Biological Programme's research at Lufa and Kar Kar.

primarily concerned with the selection of a suitable site and a population where an investigation of human adaptability in a hot, humid,
tropical climate might be undertaken. The general concept on which
the study was based required a coastal population which would be
representative of a Melanesian group living in the humid tropics,
whilst the population of the Highlands to be studied later were to be
representative of Melanesians living in the cooler altitudes of the
mountains. After viewing a number of situations on the north-east
coastal regions of the Madang district, Kar Kar Island, some 60 km to
the north and west of the town of Madang, was selected for the coastal
study (Map 2). At the time the decision concerning the site for the
investigation of the Highlands was deferred. The selection of Kar Kar
was not based on personal inspection of the island and it is, in some
ways, difficult now to appreciate why this particular site was chosen.

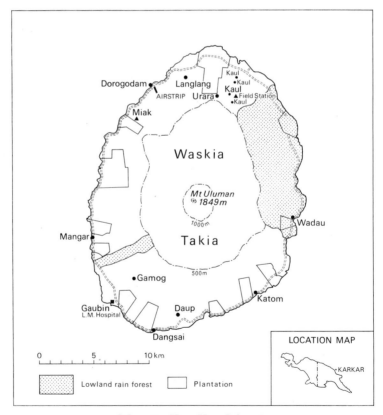

MAP 3. Kar Kar Island.

In August of 1968 a meeting of the scientists who were to participate in the various aspects of the project was convened in Madang. The disciplines represented at this meeting are noteworthy. They included a mathematician, a demographer, a physiologist with a primary interest in respiratory function, a nutritionist, a parasitologist, two environmental physiologists with interests in temperature and climatic adaptation, population geneticists and medical members of the staff of the Institute of Human Biology and the Department of Public Health of the then, Territory of Papua and New Guinea. Each scientist indicated the general objective and nature of the work which he would attempt to complete during the course of the investigation. It was agreed that the various disciplines would be responsible for the publication of their own results and that eventually all data would be transcribed on to computer tapes for subsequent integration in a comprehensive multi-disciplinary, cross-variate analysis. Following the planning meeting, the scientists journeyed to Kar Kar Island and a formal meeting of the whole party with the leaders and general population of the village of Kaul was arranged (Map 3). The general purpose of the exercise was explained and the co-operation of the villagers solicited. The villagers willingly agreed to co-operate, particularly as the medical and health implications of the project were emphasized through the discussion; and Kaul was geographically remote from the mission medical services on the island. It is perhaps only fair to say that there were communication problems as at the time few, if any, of the villagers understood English and none of the scientists understood pidgin English.

2. Logistic Requirements on Kar Kar

The Institute of Human Biology was then presented with a series of discrete specific objectives which demanded certain laboratory and housing facilities on Kar Kar Island as well as logistic support from the Madang base. The facilities included two houses of native construction for the accommodation of scientists in Kaul and a simple laboratory in the same area which was obtained by the conversion of a disused school building. In the neighbouring government station at Miak (Map 3), comparable residences were erected with a permanent, galvanized iron, concrete, steel frame, air-conditioned laboratory. Communication between the government station and the fieldworkers in the village was secured by the purchase of a four-wheel drive vehicle. Electricity for refrigeration, lighting and the laboratory was assured by the provision of suitable generators at both locations.

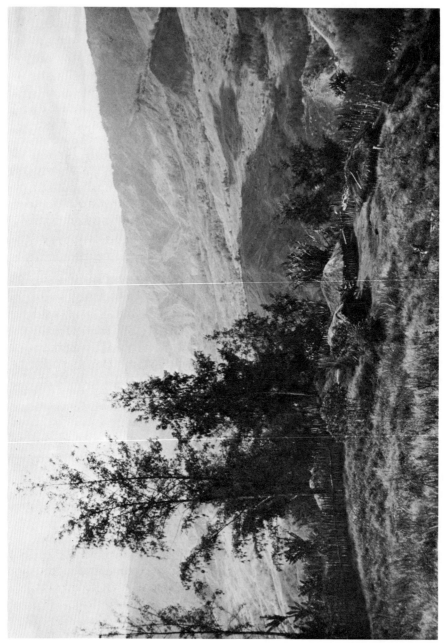

FIGURE 1. The hills and valleys of the Lufa region of the Eastern Highlands.

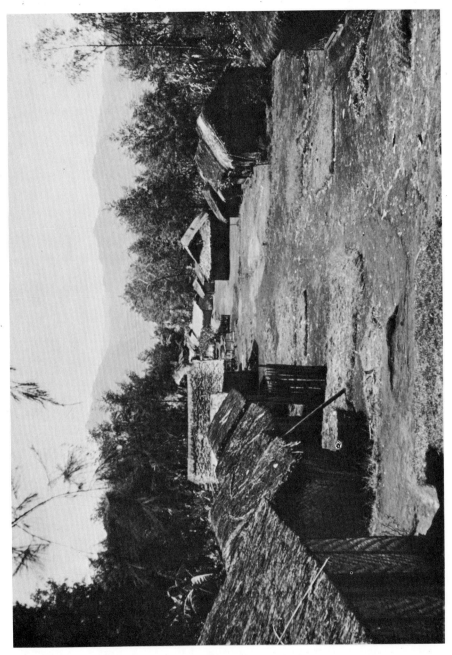

FIGURE 2. A village at Lufa.

3. Lufa—the Highlands Study Area

The general working plan was to systematically proceed with the various Kar Kar Island studies and on their completion to transport personnel and equipment to Goroka where the investigation of the Highlands was to be based. It was eventually decided that Lufa, some 60 km south and east of Goroka, would be the site for the montane population study (Map 2). As Lufa was accessible to Goroka by good road the same extensive facilities did not need to be erected, existing buildings were available for accommodation and laboratories. The setting and a village at Lufa can be seen in Figures 1 and 2.

B. RESEARCH PROCEDURES

1. Demography, Physical Anthropology and Epidemiology

Although the formal planning had envisaged the comprehensive study of a single village community in both the highland and coastal locations, this would have had but limited health and epidemiological significance as well as restricting the scope of fruitful research in population genetics and demography. To surmount these restrictions, on Kar Kar Island, epidemiological, demographic and genetic data collections were planned to be representative of the whole island.

The first research step was the compilation of a demographic inventory of the population *de jure* of the whole of Kar Kar Island. With the aid of vacationing school teachers, records of every individual, his place of residence, age, sex and family relationships, were compiled. With the completion of this documentation it was then possible to go ahead with the epidemiological investigations. For this purpose a team of two medical officers, two medical technicians, one physical anthropologist and a secretary, were involved over a period of nearly three months. There are obvious advantages in limiting the number of observers who might be involved in the acquisition of any particular set of data. The degree of error through the variable subjective interpretations of different observers is thus narrowed. Commencing in Kaul, the villagers were requested to report in family groups. It was found that approximately 50 individuals could be examined in the course of a day. The medical assessment involved a clinical examination of each individual with the completion of a questionnaire which included a note of existing or previous symptoms of ill health, and a number of parameters of socio-economic status. The Kar Kar people, in common with most contemporary Papua New Guinean societies, tend to have at best a hazy recall of previous medical incidents, and attempts to clarify symptoms according to response to interrogation proved to be so unreliable that they were eventually abandoned. Over a period of five or six years, in the course of medical surveys all over Papua New Guinea, the Institute of Medical Research has attempted to establish the significance of various symptoms. When such surveys have been based on interrogation and the recall of earlier symptoms, the responses have proved to be unreliable and misleading. People are, in the first instance, extremely suggestible and language and communication difficulties limit the accuracy of an interpretation of the responses. In many instances it has been possible to confirm quite erroneous recall. On Kar Kar, different villages replied to questions related to symptoms with such inconsistency, vagueness and lack of definition as to make the replies meaningless in any diagnostic sense. There may be a value in using recall on the few days immediately prior to interrogation, and to confining questions to symptoms such as watery diarrhoea or the existence of a productive cough which can be substantiated in the course of physical examination. Beyond these simple and limited non-specific enquiries we have not found data based on recall to be of value. This issue is discussed in Chapter VI and it is concluded that short recall periods (not more than one week) are of value if the interviewer is personally known to all the interviewees and good rapport exists. This is very seldom the case, although it was achieved in the study reported in Chapter VI.

The data obtained during the course of the medical examination was, as far as possible, recorded in a quantitative manner. This presents no difficulty when measurement is possible such as blood pressure levels, degree of anaemia and so on. Even with socio-economic status it was possible to make assessments along similar lines when the number of coconut trees and cocoa shrubs owned, the existence of a bank account and similar manifestations of affluence could be translated into a quantitative assessment. It was much more difficult to do so when attempting to gauge physical fitness in a general way, and even more specifically to quantify the presence and extent of skin or respiratory abnormalities. On the completion of the medical examination each individual was then referred to a laboratory technician for the collection of blood for genetic, biochemical and serological analysis. Finally, the villager was examined by the physical anthropologist who undertook the usual measurements along with the collection of fingerprints and standard photographs, and the assessment of colour vision. By this approach a number of objectives involving several disciplines were achieved in the course of a single attendance. The pattern of life of the village people was disrupted as little as possible and the need to attend on a number of occasions avoided. These medical and anthropological assessments were completed for the whole population (1200) of Kaul, and subsequently extended to include the inhabitants of six villages widely dispersed over the island. The sampling was considered to give an adequate representation of the whole island population.

Much of the simple laboratory work was completed in the field where the assessment of anaemia, and the examination of urine and for alimentary parasites was performed. More complex serological and biochemical investigations were analysed elsewhere, often overseas, the specimens being deep frozen and subsequently shipped on ice to the appropriate laboratory.

Demographic, genetic, medical and anthropometric data served as a foundation to three interrelated investigations which, because of their sophistication and the demands they made on resources, form the central pivotal point to the whole IBP project. They involved an assessment of energy and nutrient intake; the heat stress, and temperature control mechanisms involved in adaptation to it; and respiratory function both in relation to physical fitness and disease states. Each study was demanding in time and resources.

2. Nutrition

In the course of the energy balance investigation two nutritionists resided in Kaul for nine months and subsequently at Lufa for ten months. Their investigations necessitated the continuous presence in the field of professional workers along with a number of trained village assistants who set out to monitor the energy balance of a series of randomly selected individuals. Each subject was observed continuously over periods of five consecutive days, whilst activity records were maintained for every minute of each day. At the same time the food consumed over the five day period was weighed and suitable samples collected for later chemical analysis. The gross energy costs for the diverse activities which the subject undertook were measured by indirect calorimetry, and the total daily expenditure was derived from the amount of time spent on each activity multiplied by the respective energy costs. The use of the Douglas bag method for lying and sitting, and the Max Plank respirometer for other activities, involved the maintenance of this equipment in working order under difficult field conditions. The energy output in sleeping was derived from the basal metabolic rate with a reduction of 10% for individuals living in the coastal climate. After nine months on Kar Kar food intake measurements of 120 individuals and energy expenditure measurements for 82 had been accumulated: whilst at Lufa, in a somewhat longer period, 84 and 78 individuals were observed. The selected individuals received the concentrated attention of the researchers over the study period, but a general surveillance was maintained of the total family unit. This step was regarded as necessary in order to check that the individuals receiving concentrated study did not diverge from the ordinary pattern of family living during the period of observation.

3. Thermal Stress

Concurrently another group of observers assessed thermal stress. In Kaul some 56 men and women, and at Lufa 58 subjects, were studied intensively. Each subject was accompanied by two observers. The task of one observer was to record every 20 minutes the air temperature, humidity and rate of wind speed. The other observer made minute by minute records of activity, noting the existence of shade and evidence of discomfort from heat, such as rearranging clothing and so on. The various activities of each subject over 20 minute intervals could then be multiplied by their energy equivalents to arrive at an estimate of the subject's metabolic rate, whilst the mean radiant temperature of the subject's surroundings was calculated from the meteorological data; ultimately a measure of the overall heat stress was derived. Repeated weighings of subjects and measurement of the amount of urine passed, allowed an estimation of the balance of fluid output in sweat. Complementary laboratory studies of the same subjects explored the physiological mechanisms involved in the temperature regulations which had been observed in the field. For this purpose a specially designed air-conditioned bed was used. The apparatus employed a recording system which permitted simultaneous records of a number of different physiological processes. Thus deep body-temperature and the mean skin-temperature in several sites were monitored, in addition to the peripheral blood flow in the hands as measured by a venous occlusion plethysmograph, and the heart rate as recorded by a photo-electric pulsimeter. The thin plastic suits in which the subjects were dressed allowed the collection of sweat and its withdrawal under negative pressure. As the bed was designed to permit the raising of the environmental temperature of the subject in a controlled way the physiological response to this temperature rise could be observed.

4. *Respiratory Function*

The respiratory physiological studies involved the use of quite sophisticated equipment and measurements of vital capacity and forced
expiratory volume were obtained with a McDermot dry spirometer.
Lung volume, transfer factor and its various subdivisions, the diffusing
capacity of the alveolic capillary membrane and the volume of blood
in the lung capillaries were obtained with the use of closed circuit
helium dilution, and the single project carbon monoxide method
based on the respirometer. The physiological response to exercise was
observed with the subject exercising on a bicycle machine, whilst
ventilatory minute volume, respiratory frequency and tidal volume,
cardiac frequency and oxygen consumption during each minute of a
progressive submaximal exercise test could be recorded. The response
of the respiratory centre to carbon dioxide re-breathing was also studied
under the same general circumstances.

Both the respiratory and thermal studies were confined to young,
healthy, in the case of females, non-pregnant, subjects who manifested
a willingness to co-operate and an interest in the investigation.

All these investigations were completed within two years. Follow-up
studies on various aspects relating to genetic, demographic and
epidemiological studies have been conducted over the succeeding
three to four years.

III. RESULTS

A. DEMOGRAPHY

The outcome of the IBP project is the accumulation of a great deal of
data ranging over the description and definition of human variability,
the nutrient and energy intake and the responses of selected samples to
a number of environmental stresses. One cannot in the space available
describe in detail the results of all the investigations but it will suffice
to make a brief résumé of the most significant observations.

The structure and size of the population of Kar Kar have been
defined and a limited amount of demographic information on the
population living at Lufa was also obtained. The population *de jure* of
Kar Kar, 16 800, is a rapidly expanding one with 18·6% of the population under five years of age and 48% less than 15 years of age. This
rapid increase in population on Kar Kar is associated with a long
period of active reproduction among the coastal women who have

more children than their montane counterparts. In spite of the fact that Kar Kar men are now monogamists they fathered more children than the Lufa males, even though the latter often had more than one wife. Lufa women had fewer children, fewer pregnancies but this was somewhat counterbalanced by fewer childhood deaths. Increased childhood mortality on Kar Kar was probably attributable to the presence of holoendemic malaria. The Lufa population was demonstrably more static and probably more closely reflected the pre-contact demographic situation. The Kar Kar population was also displaying some of the results of improved education, economic development and health care (Hornabrook, 1974; Stanhope and Hornabrook, 1974).

B. PHYSICAL ANTHROPOLOGY

Significantly, the physical anthropometric study confirmed the slow rate of growth in childhood and adolescence which was associated with a delay in physiological maturity and which has been revealed by previous investigations of growth in Papua New Guinea (Malcolm, 1970; Malcolm and Wark, 1969; Malcolm, 1966, 1967, 1969, 1970). Equally striking was the rapid and uniform reduction in body musculature and physical dimensions which occurred with ageing, changes which had begun to make their appearance by the middle and late nineteen-thirties, and were quite prominent in both populations (Harvey, 1974; Sinnett, 1972 and Chapter IV).

Physical anthropometric assessments confirmed the difference in the physical structure and proportions of individuals in the two populations. The study of genetic markers also confirmed the distinctive difference in the genetic constitution (Beaven et al., 1974; Booth, 1974; Booth et al., 1972). Studies of red cell enzymes, haemoglobin and red cell antigens confirmed the presence of distinctive traits indicative of the marked heterogeneity of New Guinea populations (Serjeantson, 1975). Whether or not any or some of these genetic polymorphisms have selective advantage in the respective environments remains to be determined, but there is clearly scope for a cross-variate analysis of the genetic markers with parameters of health and fertility.

C. EPIDEMIOLOGY

Epidemiological studies confirmed the presence of malaria involving infestation with *Plasmodium falciparum*, *vivax* and *malariae* in most of the

Kar Kar population. At Lufa, it was present only in the few Highlanders who had travelled to the lowlands. Other parameters of health
revealed that the inhabitants of the warm coastal region were more
subject to a treponematosis (yaws), (Garner *et al.*, 1972, 1971), had a
higher incidence of skin disease, children were prone to trachoma and
the adults subject to tuberculosis (Hornabrook *et al.*, 1974). In the
more recently contacted Lufa people tuberculosis was unknown, skin
disease, other than scabies, was uncommon, trachoma rare. There was
neither serological nor clinical evidence of active yaws. Both populations showed a remarkable absence of any signs of the degenerative
diseases of urban and technologically sophisticated societies. Thus the
blood pressures were not elevated and tended to diminish with age
rather than to increase, diabetes was not found, there were no cases of
gout and no evidence of coronary artery disease, stroke or other
consequences of arteriosclerosis. Both populations had a high incidence
of chronic non-specific respiratory failure, first apparent in the 30–40
year age group, this problem involved larger percentages of succeeding
age cohorts and became clearly a most significant cause of chronic
disability in those over middle age (Anderson, 1974). Apart from
chronic respiratory disease, the Lufa people exhibited little sign of ill
health. A striking finding in the Kar Kar medical surveys was the
variation in morbidity within the relatively small ecosystem (Hornabrook *et al.*, 1974). Thus, alimentary parasitic infestation varied
statistically significantly between the Waskia and Takia halves of the
island (as shown on Map 3) (Hornabrook *et al.*, 1974; Hornabrook *et
al.*, 1975). There was also a marked difference in the prevalence of
filaria and malaria parasitaemia. Yaws was rather commoner on the
north and west of the island than the south and east. Each village
tended to have its own distinctive epidemiological pattern and a group
of villages might vary significantly from other groups of villages in the
absence of any apparent variation in the general ecology. The most
obvious influence which could be correlated with such variations lay
in the general field of economic development, exposure to education,
existence of health services and physical relationship to mission or
plantation. Anaemia, known to be of almost universal occurrence in
Papua New Guinea, as suspected was of major importance on Kar Kar
and less prevalent at Lufa (Crane *et al.*, 1972). Subsequent investigations have shown this to be multi-factorial in origin. Iron deficiency,
malaria, alimentary parasites and other obscure factors all playing a
part (Crane *et al.*, 1974; Hornabrook and Serjeantson, in press). It is
interesting that there were similar conspicuous variations in demographic statistics and in the presence of genetic markers, underlining
the difficulty of correlating any of these variables with each other, and

the need to give some weight to social and economic status of the communities.

D. NUTRITION

The medical investigation found little significant evidence of overt malnutrition or specific dietary deficiencies (see Figure 3). In the light of the observations on nutrient and energy intake this must be taken as a manifestation of the singularly efficient adaptation on the part of the community to the nutrients available. The mean daily energy intake in both Kar Kar and Lufa was remarkably small although at Lufa the intake was comparable with what might be expected in a Western community (Norgan et al., 1974). For Kaul men and women, energy intake of 8·12 MeJ (1940 kcal) and 5·94 MeJ (1420 kcal) was extremely low, particularly taking into account the activities of the subjects. At Lufa the corresponding figures were 10·55 MeJ (2520 kcal) and 8·81 MeJ (2105 kcal). The protein intake was correspondingly poor, being 6·7%, 6·0%, 6·5% and 7·2% of the energy value of the diet in Kaul men and women, and Lufa men and women, respectively. Fat comprised only 10% of the energy intake in the Highlands and 17% of the intake in the coastal diet. The energy intake must be taken into perspective of the daily activities of the villagers. Whilst sitting, lying and standing comprise 70% of the daily activity and 60% of the daily energy expenditure, walking comprised only 10% of the 24 hour day and only 20–27% of the energy output. Even allowing for this behavioural adaptation, the energy balance of the coastal Melanesians shows a lower intake than one might have anticipated and more strikingly there was found to be no increase in pregnancy, lactation or other physiological circumstances for which the conventionally accepted standards require an increased intake. Another interesting observation relates to the type of food which was preferred. It has usually been assumed that human beings will naturally eat the diet which is physiologically optimal; the Kaul people, although living in fairly close proximity to the sea, use the abundant fish and marine resources of the ocean to a very sparing extent. Indeed, these marine products contributed little of significance to their diet.

E. PHYSIOLOGY

The physiological reports have revealed that the Papua New Guineans sweat less than Europeans who are acclimatized to life in the tropics. The normal level for Melanesians on both the coast and in the High-

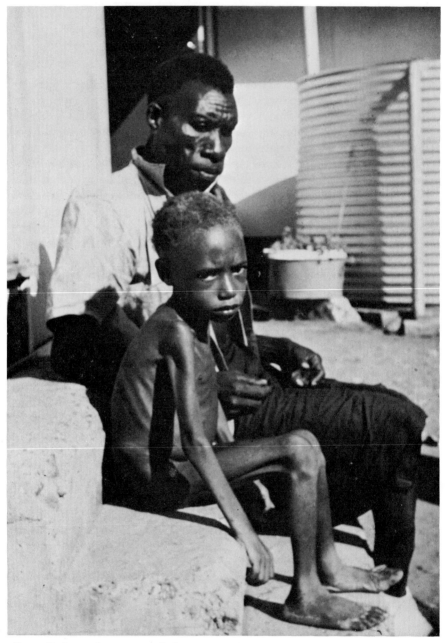

FIGURE 3. A case of marasmus at Lufa.

lands is comparable to that of unacclimatized Europeans. Heat stress in the mountains was comparable to that on the coast, the lower air temperature being counterbalanced by a higher radiant heat gain. Other physiological responses to temperature were very comparable among the Melanesians, both between the coastal people and the Highlanders and between both groups and Europeans working and living under the same environmental circumstances (Budd et al., 1974; Fox et al., 1974).

The respiratory function of Highlanders was characterized by a ventilatory capacity similar to Europeans and appreciably greater than that of people living on the coast. The Highlanders showed a significantly lower cardiac frequency in response to physical exercise than the coastal inhabitants. This probably reflects the increased amount of physical activity involved in life in the rugged mountain zone and with the respiratory ventilatory complex renders the Highlanders physically fitter than their coastal counterparts. The investigations did not clearly define whether such physiological differences could be attributed to genetic or purely environmental factors (Anderson et al., 1974; Cotes et al., 1974).

During the IBP a detailed assessment of the environment was not defined. In general, the Kar Kar people were swidden agriculturalists dwelling primarily in a secondary tropical rain forest, much of which had been transformed into plantation mono-cultures. The Kar Kar people lived in proximity to the sea with its rich resources of marine foods and in the hinterland had access to the central forested peak of the island where wild pig and small mammals were occasionally hunted. In contrast, the Lufa people might best be regarded as rotational horticulturalists living in an *Imperata*, wild cane (*Miscanthus*) grassland in proximity to the forested peak of Mt. Michael (Figure 1). Whilst sweet potato (*Ipomoea batatas*) and other vegetable crops were the staple food, these people also used the neighbouring forest as a source of game and for various forest resources for fencing, housing and other domestic uses. They were much more concerned with the maintenance of pig herds and had less contact with the outer world and less access to imported bought produce.

IV. GENERAL DISCUSSION OF THE IBP HUMAN ADAPTABILITY PROJECT IN PAPUA NEW GUINEA

Five years have elapsed since the planning meetings of the New Guinea Human Adaptability project. A large expenditure of money and human endeavour have been expended in the course of the study. Now it is timely to consider whether the original objectives have been attained. It is also proper that one should subject the project to an overall critical scrutiny. Were the endeavours worthwhile? Could the project have been improved upon?

In actual fact, it is not possible to ascertain whether the project attained its original objectives. A failure to adequately define aims was an unfortunate hallmark of the study from its inception, and an ambiguity in the definition of prime objectives of the IBP New Guinea investigation, and a vagueness in concept, limited the thrust of the total study.

1. General Limitations of Multi-disciplinary Studies

A multi-disciplinary study—human ecology in the tropical ecosystem, human biology and human adaptability—in reality suggest a comprehensive investigation of man in relation to his environment. This was not attained. A clear definition of what is implied by these phrases is required so that the data collection may be organized in a systematic manner to permit its directed analysis. Failure to clearly delineate aims permits an erratic, disorganized and rather random collection of facts. The multi-disciplinary study readily became transformed in practice into multi-mono-disciplinary studies. A study in human ecology may degenerate into a series of discrete studies of comparative physiology. It is easy to lose sight of the general ecosystem whilst being preoccupied with a local research project in a restricted discipline. These developments all arose in the course of the New Guinea work, and are an inevitable consequence of the failure to define in clear and unambiguous terms the aims of the exercise and the managerial steps required for their implementation. Perhaps the IBP project was hampered from its inception by an undue respect of the terminology employed—"multi-disciplinary, multi-variate, ecological investigation of human adaptability". Idealistic as these concepts may be they fail to materialize in the absence of a basis for integration, which must be carefully planned in advance of the investigation.

2. Difficulties in Project Design and Concept

Some specific examples may clarify the manner in which the hopes of the organizers were thwarted. The project purported to study a "typical Melanesian community of the lowlands of Papua New Guinea" but the initial decision to concentrate attention on Kar Kar was not based on any sound background information of the island or its inhabitants. If the study had intended to obtain baseline data on a typical Melanesian community of the lowlands of Papua New Guinea, Kar Kar Island would never have been selected. At the time of the study Kar Kar had already had 100 years of Western contact. The island had established a significant degree of economic development which was far ahead of that of most of the rest of the region. Its rich volcanic soil, the long period of Western contact and its island situation, rendered it in the first instance an atypical location with an atypical population. Of less importance, the logistic problems associated with undertaking research on an island as opposed to a mainland location, compounded the difficulties and expenses involved in the completion of the study. The Lufa people were at least representative of the populations of the valleys of the central cordillera, and in 1968 had experienced relatively little economic advancement.

3. Failure of Organization and Integration of Disciplines

The general planning sessions in the formative stages of the project tended to resolve into a gathering of individual scientists who had individual specific interests in certain restricted phenomena. There was, therefore, a natural tendency for the researchers to utilize the IBP venue as a medium for the advancement of their particular interest. There was, as a result, a tendency for the study to develop into a series of unrelated exercises in comparative physiology or geographic pathology which often did not lend themselves to integration with other disciplines and often did not justify themselves in their relevance to the local population. In some fields this idiosyncratic approach to a multi-disciplinary project reached excessive proportions and even at best any attempt at integration of the disciplines into a meaningful whole was seriously handicapped. No computer can integrate the various disciplines without definition in advance of the data that might be suitably correlated.

4. Absence of Social and Environmental Science

Perhaps the most glaring failings in the general organization of the IBP were the omissions in the overall range of studies undertaken. There was little or no attempt to gather a detailed description of the environment. Some climatic variables—temperature, humidity and wind speed—were measured for a short period during the project, but the nature of the vegetation, the use and influence of man on the fauna and flora and the physical resources, both water and soil, were not catalogued. An even more serious oversight was the failure to consider socio-cultural adaptive processes. Both at Lufa and on Kar Kar the continuing involvement of a trained social anthropologist would have greatly enhanced the value of almost all aspects of the project, and almost all specialized biological investigations may have been complemented and extended. Thus, even such accurately identifiable and measurable quantitative variables as genetic markers can often only be sensibly interpreted in terms of a knowledge of the prevailing customs in marriage and the kinship structure of the society. Social anthropological techniques would have provided also essential background information on the dietary practices of the population and would qualify and facilitate the measures of energy expenditure. Anthropology would also have given a greater balance to the whole enterprise as there seems little doubt that a prime factor in adaptation to any environment is the cultural and social behaviour of the human population in that environment.

5. *Limitations of Quantification of Biological Data*

Another range of problems mitigated against the success of work in the individual disciplines. These were not always satisfactorily surmounted. In the epidemiological studies there is no doubt that the single medical survey, as undertaken during the course of this investigation, leaves much to be desired. Whilst they are relatively easy to undertake, it is frequently forgotten that such surveys can only elucidate pathological processes which are either chronic or leave some persistent hallmark of their prior occurrence. The chronic infectious diseases such as tuberculosis, yaws or leprosy, or the chronic degenerative diseases such as raised blood pressure, diabetes mellitus, chronic renal disease, renal failure or joint disease, may be detected. The persistence of serological antibodies may confirm that the population at some stage in the past was exposed to measles or a particular arbovirus infection. Such surveys cannot, from their brief and transitory duration, assess the significance of acute infectious illnesses which leave neither longstanding disability nor the stigmata of infection in the form of altered biological or serological parameters in the blood or tissue fluids. For this reason, pneumonia, meningococcal meningitis, and many other bacterial processes are completely overlooked, whilst at the same time sub-acute but lethal degenerative diseases such as neoplasms, many vascular events and other sub-acute illnesses, are underestimated.

6. *Limitations of Cross-sectional Data*

To obtain good reliable medical information on the prevalence of pathological processes, particularly those which are relevant to the survival of the individual and the community, one must consider the feasibility of prospective and continuous monitoring of the population. Even here there are great handicaps—difficulties in diagnosis, particularly difficulties in uniform standard of diagnosis when a number of different observers are involved in the long-term study. Furthermore, the very presence of medical and other staff over a long period of time introduces another factor into the ecosystem and materially alters the nature of the community. Perhaps the greatest handicaps to the prospective studies are the problems arising from human failings. There are few research workers who can be induced to remain in the field for a prolonged period. At the same time the village subjects become either bored or irritated, or even antagonistic, especially if there is no immediate and obvious tangible benefit.

Much that is relevant and significant from an epidemiological viewpoint cannot readily be quantitated and attempts to do so may render a spurious accuracy to what is, in fact, a subjective assessment. In regard to the physiological and nutritional observations, they were unfortunately limited to subjects who could co-operate both intellectually and physically. The physiologists were indeed investigating the response of the villagers to certain environmental stressors, but it is clear that the environmental stresses so studied and the human response to them has been restricted to both in the sampling of the subjects studied, and in the type of stresses examined. Thus, attention is directed to the healthy, young, better educated adults. This section of the community is the least subject to environmental stresses. Perhaps the greatest value of determining the impaired physiological response in such circumstances might be to detect their appearance and the manner of their development in the aged or in the very young, and for a variety of reasons this was impracticable.

It is not surprising that those aspects of a study of this sort which were most readily analysed and had the fewest limitations from sampling error are those where a clear quantitative measure of some biological variable may be obtained, for example, anthropometric measurements and blood group and serological genetic markers. These can be gathered in a quantitative sense from the total population and they are unlikely to fluctuate capriciously from season to season or week to week.

V. ETHICAL PROBLEMS

Social and economic developments and their attendant political changes are sweeping across the island populations of the Pacific with accelerating momentum. The IBP project did not precede these events but was underway before they had deeply permeated through the villages of Kar Kar and Lufa. It would not now be possible to contemplate a similar project either in these locations or anywhere else in Papua New Guinea. To some extent the IBP itself has played a part in creating a situation where a critical and perhaps even suspicious appraisal of such enterprises prevails in many, if not all, of the developing countries. In the first place, the whole concept of an "expedition", for whatever purpose and no matter how prestigious its sponsors may be, is unacceptable to educated Papua New Guinea nationals. Intellectual tourism tends to display the unacceptable face of science, and like many forms of tourism may be degrading both to the visitors and the visited. There are also more explicit objections which arise when Europeans are involved in the study of indigenes, particularly when the barely avoided phrases of "primitive man" enter into the project's conception. The expedition mentality also evokes visions of colonialism in an age when colonialism is synonymous with all that is wrong with the past. Inadvertently at times, projects such as the IBP New Guinea adaptability investigation, easily and thoughtlessly arouse national antagonism and upset local sensitivities. It is of little significance to local people to tell them that they should be proud to be the most studied population in the world. The practice of distributing plastic badges with "IBP" inscribed on their faces to volunteers during some of the IBP studies may have appeared a harmless exercise to the scientists involved, but could have been and was construed as an act of patronizing condescension by some citizens of the country.

The practical issue of obtaining informed consent is also fraught with problems under circumstances in which sophisticated, educated researchers are required to communicate with less sophisticated and often uneducated villagers. At Kaul, the arrival of a fleet of cars with a large body of Europeans in some ceremony, with the attendance of senior officers in the Administration, was likely to arouse a wealth of expectations which might not have been within the scope of the visitors to fulfil. These impressions tended to be exaggerated by the preliminary orations in English which explained the nature of the work and solicited co-operation of the villagers. Such presentation from English speaking expatriates to pidgin-English speaking villagers required at least one interpreter and lent themselves to exaggeration and distortion. Furthermore, there was a tendency to naturally exaggerate and enhance the possible beneficial aspects of the project. The ultimate consequences to the village people proved to be less than the expectations which had been aroused. The outcome of such projects may well be to induce a state of apathy, disappointment, frustration and disillusionment. Benefits which may not have been promised, but which were assumed from the villagers to devolve from the project, never materialized.

On Kar Kar the villagers of Kaul were presented with a water supply pumping system as a gesture of appreciation for their co-operation. This was installed at the completion of the project. It worked most effectively for 12–18 months but after a period of two or three years the whole supply system now lies derelict. The villagers are unwilling to provide the necessary funds to maintain it in serviceable condition. They now feel that they have been left with nothing, whilst at the inception of the project there was a prevailing view that at least a general hospital would materialize in the community. At Lufa, although an elaborate meeting did not precede the research, the people did conceive that material benefits would eventually flow. There remains today a similar feeling of disillusionment to that which exists on Kar Kar. They are aware that co-operation was offered, blood was collected, people attended regularly for examination and review, but their daily lives are in no way altered. It is difficult for the average villager to appreciate that benefits which might arise may be long term, and the concept of contributions to knowledge as such as worthy of their inconvenience and discomfort during tests, is singularly unlikely to appeal.

There will always exist a problem in regard to the obtaining of informed consent whilst uneducated people are the subject of research projects. How this may be circumvented remains to be defined, but there seems no doubt that it is incumbent on researchers to understate the benefits which may arise from their sojourn in a community rather than to overstate them. The possible benefits should be voiced in low key, and the inconveniences and temporary disadvantages of the project placed in the forefront before one can reasonably claim to have obtained the co-operation of the community on a sound basis.

VI. SUMMARY OF HUMAN ADAPTABILITY STUDY

We have commented at some length on the methodology of the human adaptability studies in Papua New Guinea and have also stressed the shortcomings of the project both in its orientation and in its relation with the subjects who were investigated. It is suggested that much may be gained from this analysis in order that future projects involving studies of human ecology in developing countries may achieve a greater scientific yield at the cost of less disruption and frustration in the village and community in which the study has been pursued.

It seems essential that investigations relating to human ecology should clearly indicate the objectives and at the same time define methodology prior to the collection of data. The procedures enumerated by Brooke Thomas (1973) in relationship to the investigations of human adaptation in high Peru, appear to present an ideal basis for such planning, namely the identification of environmental stressors, the strategy employed by the community in adaptation, the resources which are essential for the maintenance of this adaptation and the factors involved in making these resources available; the immediate object of such a project being the establishment of a model which might provide administrators with a basis for prospective planning when new modifications and changes might influence its structure. Such a definition of objectives would have ensured that in the human adaptability study in New Guinea an adequate description of the physical and biotic environment should have been obtained. It would also have guaranteed that the physical environmental stressors, not only temperature and radiation, were involved in the data collection, and would have provided more adequate consideration of the abiotic and biotic environment of man. One cannot avoid also the need to emphasize the vital necessity for the representation of social, cultural and economic factors in any investigation relating to human ecology. If anything, the IBP data suggests that man's health and biological status is influenced to a far greater degree by his socio-cultural adaptive processes than it is by the environment as such. One might put this alternatively by suggesting that the environment influences man's biological characters indirectly through varying his socio-cultural adaptation. The IBP investigation on Kar Kar suggests that the populations of Papua New Guinea are enormously variable, that each village has its own peculiar and unique demographic pattern, its distinctive genetic traits and an epidemiological history which is in many respects peculiar to itself. These variations may well reflect changes and differences in history of cultural contacts, in the proximity to hospitals or schools, the presence of returning migrant labourers and so on. The impact of environmental and ecological variables on the human community would appear to be much less effective in modifying the character of the community.

In conclusion one must question if the type of study undertaken in the course of the IBP, which presumed to undertake an overall assessment of human ecology on a community, can or could ever succeed. Such a project, with its aspirations to ascertain the overall nature of the human community in all its many facets in relation to a complex environment, may well set its sights at an unscaleable peak. The number of disciplines involved, the range of personnel and the duration of the work may be neither practicable in execution nor acceptable to the subjects under study. This point is further discussed in Chapter I.

There remains also the question concerning so-called quantitative studies in human ecology. Are these likely to provide a tangible benefit to human health? Whilst it seems clear that ecological studies of this nature may provide essential background data to projects involving engineering, industrial exploitation and perhaps even nutrition, there is less evidence that they may be rewarding in the immediate sense in the fields of health or medicine. There are, however, abundant examples of more limited ecological investigations which have, on the other hand, proved eminently rewarding in their practical results and have made very significant contributions leading to advancement of medical science. If one regards human ecology as the study of man in relation to the environment and considers that this includes man's biological and socio-cultural characteristics and the influence which the environment has on these, this may serve as a basis to an ecological perspective which when analysed critically may provide the key to the understanding of disorders which arise from disturbances in the equilibrium established at the man–environment interface. One may refer to medical ecology as a study of those disorders which are more or less directly related to a breakdown in the man–environment interaction. In rather different terms it is possible to consider the ecological circumstances which permit the existence of the development of any disease as an entity. For example, an epidemic can be regarded as a biological entity which is composed of a smaller or greater number of individual cases which comprise its component parts, its growth depending on the size and extent of these components which are influenced by environmental factors favourable or unfavourable. Minor changes in the environment may result in conditions unfavourable for the growth of the disease and lead eventually to its extinction, whilst of course the reverse may occur.

At this point it is helpful to discuss two instances of disease arising from a breakdown in a delicately established ecological balance.

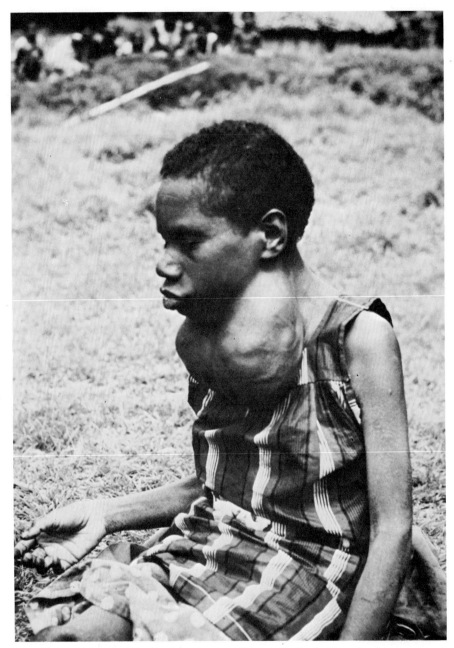

FIGURE 4. A lady with goitre from the upper Wario valley in the Owen Stanley range.

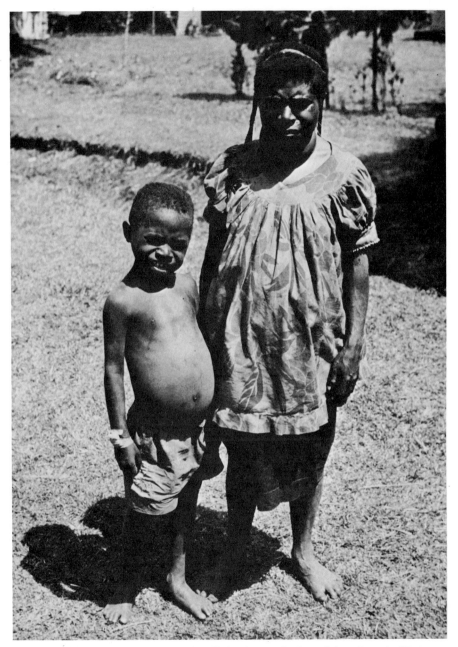

FIGURE 5. Mother with goitre, and son suffering from endemic cretinism; from the Wantoat valley, Huon Peninsula.

VII. SPECIFIC EXAMPLES OF ECOLOGICALLY DETERMINED DISEASE

A. ENDEMIC CRETINISM

Endemic cretinism occurs in scattered foci throughout Papua New Guinea. The regions of high prevalence are characterized by a geological formation of mesozoic rocks or of recent volcanic deposition. The areas share in common a deficiency of iodine in the soil and water and in the staple foodstuffs. Enlargement of the thyroid gland is a physiological adaptation which compensates for the iodine deficiency by permitting a greater utilization of available iodine and a supply of sufficient hormonal substances for physiological demands (Figure 4). Only in very rare instances is the goitre sufficiently large that it may compress neighbouring organs and interfere with function (McCullagh, 1963). In Papua New Guinea, and in other developing countries, endemic goitre occurs in association with a rural population which is exposed to a high degree of infection and subsists on a diet which is known to be poor in protein and often also in calories. In such regions women are prone to bear children with damage to the brain and central nervous system (Figure 5), a syndrome which is described as endemic cretinism (Hornabrook, 1971a, 1971b, 1975; Buttfield and Hetzel, 1969, 1971; Buttfield et al., 1965). The actual cause of the neurological damage has not been firmly established (Hetzel, 1972; Hornabrook, 1972, 1974). Iodine deficiency is certainly central and basic, but whether this is due to deficiency of the element itself or to the thyroid hormones is not clear. Women treated with iodine by injection continuing to live in the region do not bear defective children. On the other hand, both dietary deficiency and repeated infection may be necessary in the background to aggravate the iodine deficiency and produce disease. Women with goitres in relatively affluent societies do not appear to produce endemic cretinous children. The condition of endemic cretinism is a serious public health problem in those regions where it occurs, and in ancient times would have certainly threatened the survival of the community. It is interesting that in many regions of Papua New Guinea, where goitre has been long familiar to the inhabitants, it is maintained that children born with mental defect have been a more recent phenomenon. In the Jimi valley in the Western Highlands (Map 1) there is evidence that the first cases of endemic cretinism began to appear shortly after the initial contact with government patrols. It seems that the incidence of the disease increased rapidly with increasing contact until large numbers of children born in the late nineteen-fifties and early nineteen-sixties had evidence of damage to the nervous system. In what way has Western contact precipitated the incidence of this serious consequence of iodine deficiency? It appears that early patrols rewarded services by trade in rock salt, deficient in elemental iodine. Carriers would be paid in this commodity and food and other services rendered by the population rewarded in a similar manner (Pharoah and Hornabrook, 1974). It is known that the inhabitants of the valley had a craving for salt and valued the commodity. It is also known that in the pre-contact era salt was traded into the Jimi valley from the neighbouring Simbai valley, where a simple industry involving the distillation of water from certain mineral pools was the source of a crude material which passed as salt in the area. Analysis of the distillate from these pools has revealed that it is extremely rich in iodine. The salt prepared from the pools contains sufficient iodine to provide a reasonable supplement to a diet known to be iodine deficient. The appearance of Western contact and the introduction of iodine deficient rock salt obviated the need for the arduous time-consuming practice of distillation and manufacture of native salt which ceased to be used. Thus the Jimi people, through the use of native salt, had provided themselves with sufficient iodine to achieve an adequate and efficient adaptation to an environment in which the obvious stress of iodine deficiency might otherwise have hampered population growth and development. The result of contact with a new socio-economic system was to disrupt the delicate ecological balance which had been achieved. Primitive trade and migration had unconsciously allowed the development of a system in which a deficient diet was enriched. The disruption of the practice suddenly deprived the population of a significant iodine supplement and created a situation where, within a short time, the decompensation was manifested by the appearance of cases of endemic cretinism. The incidence of such cases rapidly increased as the magnitude of the deficiency increased. An understanding of this phenomenon has permitted the mass treatment of the region with supplementary iodine and an early and significant reduction in defective children has resulted in the generations born after the initiation of treatment (Pharoah, 1971).

B. KURU

In contrast to the case history of endemic cretinism kuru (Gajdusek, 1958, 1963; Hornabrook, 1966, 1968), offers an equally illustrative example of the ecological principles which may underly the existence of a particular health hazard. In the case of epidemic kuru in the Eastern Highlands, the presence of a fatal and sub-acute degenerative disease of the nervous system has resulted from the existence of socio-cultural practices which provided an environment which was condu-cive to the proliferation and spread of a pathogenic virus through an otherwise healthy population (Hornabrook and Moir, 1970).

Kuru has been shown to result from infection with a virus-like particle which invades the central nervous system, and after a lengthy incubation period, causes the death and destruction of neurones, first in the cerebellum, later spreading through the cerebral cortex and nuclear masses of the brain stem (Gajdusek, 1965, 1967; Gajdusek and Gibbs, 1964; Gajdusek *et al.*, 1966). The pathological appearances of kuru and the nature of the clinical disease have some similarities with a widespread but very rare disease of universal occurrence—Creutzfeldt-Jakob disease (Gajdusek and Gibbs, 1968, 1971). Creutzfeldt-Jakob disease is known to appear in all populations of the world in the form of isolated sporadic cases. It is a rare and chance event. In contrast, kuru was extremely common in the late nineteen-fifties and early nineteen-sixties in the Fore population of the Okapa subdistrict. Of approximately 30 000 people, 130–150 were dying each year of the disease. It was obviously so common that if its prevalence continued the population might well have fallen into serious decline and become extinct. Much speculation arose as to how this state of affairs had come about. It was generally thought that some inherent genetic character of the Fore people had rendered them extremely susceptible to a newly introduced infection, or that even a new pathogen may have arisen by mutation. The other viewpoint was that there was in the general ecology of the region a reason which created a local situation which favoured the spread and development of a lethal disease. Intensive investigations were directed to elucidating whether either of these alternative theories may have been responsible for the disease but it was the social anthropologists, R. Glasse and S. Lindenbaum, who drew attention to the fact that the Fore people organized elaborate mortuary feasts at the time of a death. On these occasions gifts were distributed among the relatives and kin of the deceased whilst the body was dismembered and distributed among close relatives in an organized way. Females and young children participated in the practice, whilst the males refrained from doing so. It was females and young children who were the principal victims of kuru. With the appearance of the Australian Administration and the attendant missions who entered the region, the practice of cannibalism was frowned upon and soon ceased. By 1964 it was apparent that kuru was no longer affecting young children, and in the succeeding years the incidence of the disease has shown an overall decline, whilst the mean age of the patients each year tends to increase (Alpers, 1965;

Alpers and Gajdusek, 1965). Even more informative is the fact that the disease has shown its greatest reduction in incidence in those regions which first came under administrative control, and that the change in incidence was less marked in the more remote and inaccessible areas (Mathews, 1965). The epidemiological evidence therefore suggested that epidemic kuru retreated in parallel with the advance of mission and governmental influences. About this time, Gajdusek and his colleagues showed that kuru was indeed the result of the invasion of the nervous system by an infectious particle. They were able to induce the disease in chimpanzees who were injected with suspensions of material obtained at post-mortem examinations of the brains from kuru patients. It seems that the infective material was transmitted from the deceased to the family group and kin at the time of the mortuary feasts. This event favoured an exposure of people in a family group in a most intimate way to the remains of the kuru victims (Hornabrook and Moir, 1970; Mathews; Glasse and Lindenbaum).

There seems little doubt that an infective agent which might, under ordinary circumstances, rarely have the opportunity for invasion of a host, was able to proliferate and invade the population through the adoption by the population of a particular and specific social practice. It even seems possible that an individual suffering from Creutzfeldt-Jakob disease may have succumbed of that disease in the region, and formed the initial nidus on which the growth and proliferation of kuru developed. It is interesting to contemplate that the socio-cultural practice which favoured the appearance and development of kuru may in turn have stemmed from the general protein deficiency which pervades the whole Highlands region of Papua New Guinea.

Both endemic cretinism and kuru may well be regarded as diseases which owe their existence to a derangement of the normal ecological equilibrium which is essential for good health and well-being. Both case histories provide illustrations of the application of ecological principles to the solution of specific health problems. The two specific instances quoted reveal the benefits which may arise when investigation of a medical problem is oriented in an ecological direction. The example of the IBP suggests that great improvements in methodology are required before a formal ecological approach is likely to produce the rewards which are commensurate with the efforts and the resources deployed. On the other hand, the examples we have quoted indicate the importance of doing specific case studies in an ecological perspective. It is doubtful, however, whether any attempt to analyse these diseases through formal complex quantitative multi-disciplinary investigation would have been fruitful.

It is worth remembering also that Papua New Guinea is remarkable

for the absence of many disorders which are prevalent in the technologically sophisticated and urban societies of the world. Virtually all
the serious degenerative diseases ranging from arteriosclerosis with its
consequences of stroke, myocardial infarction and renal failure,
through high blood pressure, diabetes mellitus and gout, do not occur
in Melanesia or are exceedingly rare (Maddocks, 1967; Maddocks and
Rovin, 1965; Sinnett, 1970; MacGregor *et al.*, 1969). Their abundance
and universal penetration of the "Western and urban" communities
suggest that the ecology of such communities favours their appearance
in some peculiar and ill-defined manner. It could be that an enquiry
concerning the characters of the Melanesians which protect and shield
them from the impact of these diseases may be completed before
societies have been so modified that the problem becomes obscured by
the complex changes. An answer to the problem would be of the
greatest significance, not only to the future health of Melanesians, but
to the world at large. Perhaps careful consideration and comparative
studies of the ecology of communities in different socio-cultural settings
may provide the fundamental information towards unravelling the
problems of degenerative diseases.

A final word should be said concerning the Institute of Human
Biology of Papua New Guinea. In 1972, four years after its formation,
the governing Council agreed that the name of the Institute should be
changed to the Papua New Guinea Institute of Medical Research.
Essentially the factors influencing this change in nomenclature
stemmed to some degree from the issues to which we have alluded in
this essay. If human ecology and biology are to be accepted as worthy
of support by government they must be able to clearly demonstrate
their utility and immediate relevance to the community at large. The
alteration in the name of the Institute, whilst not implying any material
change in the nature of its work, indicates to a degree, that most
societies are not yet ready to accept investigations which are regarded
as primarily being of academic significance. It also underlines the
significance of considering the general social and political appeal of
research and perhaps an exercise in human relations which is involved
in the acceptance of studies of this sort presents the various disciplines
involved with their greatest challenge.

VIII. REFERENCES

Alpers, M. P. (1965). Epidemiological changes in kuru 1957–1963. *In* "Slow, Latent and Temperate Virus Infections", NINDB. Mono. 2. U.S. Government Printing Office, Washington, D.C.

Alpers, M. P. and Gajdusek, D. C. (1965). Changing patterns of kuru: epidemiological changes in the period of increasing contact of the Fore people with Western civilization. *Am. J. trop. Med. Hyg.* **14**, 852.

Anderson, H. R. (1974a). The epidemiology and allergic features of asthma in the New Guinea Highlands. *Clin. Allergy* **4**, 171.

Anderson, H. R. (1974b). Smoking habits and their relationship to chronic lung disease in a tropical environment in Papua New Guinea. *Bull. physiopath. Resp.* **10**, 619.

Anderson, H. R. (1975). A clinical and lung function study of chronic lung disease and asthma in coastal Papua New Guinea. *Aust. N.Z. J. Med.* **5** (4), 329–336.

Anderson, H. R. and Cunnington, A. M. (1974). House dust mites in the Papua New Guinea Highlands. *Papua New Guin. med. J.* **17**, 304.

Anderson, H. R., Anderson, J. A. and Cotes, J. E. (1974). Lung function values in healthy children and adults from highland and coastal areas of Papua New Guinea: prediction nomograms for forced expiratory volume and forced vital capacity. *Papua New Guin. med. J.* **17**, 165.

Beaven, G. H., Fox, R. H. and Hornabrook, R. W. (1974). The occurrence of haemoglobin-J (Tongariki) and of thalassaemia on Kar Kar Island and the Papua New Guinea mainland. *Phil. Trans. R. Soc.* Ser. B **268**, 269.

Blake, N. M., Saha, N., McDermid, E. M., Kirk, R. L. and Crane, G. G. (1974). Additional electrophoretic variants of 6-phosphogluconate dehydrogenase. *Humangenetik* **21**, 347.

Booth, P. B. (1974). Genetic distances between certain New Guinea populations studied under the International Biological Programme. *Phil. Trans. R. Soc.* Ser. B **268**, 257.

Booth, P. B., McLoughlin, K., Hornabrook, R. W. and MacGregor, A. (1972). The Gerbich Blood Group System in New Guinea. III. The Madang District, the Highlands, the New Guinea Islands and the South Papuan Coast. *Hum. Biol. Oceania* **1**, 267.

Brooke Thomas, R. (1973). Human adaptation to a High Andean energy flow system. Pennsylvania State University occasional papers, University Park, Pennsylvania.

Budd, G. M., Fox, R. H., Hendrie, A. L. and Hicks, K. E. (1974). A field survey of thermal stress in New Guinea villagers. *Phil. Trans. R. Soc.* Ser. B, **268**, 393.

Buttfield, I. H. and Hetzel, B. S. (1966). The aetiology and control of endemic goitre in Eastern New Guinea. *Papua New Guin. med. J.* **9**, 114.

Buttfield, I. H. and Hetzel, B. S. (1967). Endemic goitre in Eastern New Guinea. *Bull. Wld Hlth Org.* **36**, 243.

Buttfield, I. H. and Hetzel, B. S. (1969a). Endemic goitre in New Guinea and the prophylactic program with iodinated poppy-seed oil. Report of a meeting of PAHO Science Group on Research on Endemic Goitre, PAHO No. 193. Washington.

Buttfield, I. H. and Hetzel, B. S. (1969b). Endemic cretinism in Eastern New Guinea. *Australas. Ann. Med.* **18**, 217.

Buttfield, I. H. and Hetzel, B. S. (1971). Endemic cretinism in Eastern New Guinea. Its relation to goitre and iodine deficiency", Institute of Human Biology, Papua New Guinea, Mono. 2. Goroka.

Buttfield, I. H., Black, M. L., Hoffman, M. J., Mason, E. K. and Hetzel, B. S. (1965). Correction of iodine deficiency in New Guinea natives by iodized oil injection. *Lancet* **2**, 767.

Cotes, J. E., Anderson, H. R. and Patrick, J. M. (1974). Lung function and the response to exercise in native New Guineans: role of genetic and environmental factors. *Phil. Trans. R. Soc.* Ser. B **268**, 349.

Crane, G. G., Hornabrook, R. W. and Kelly, A. (1972). Anaemia on the coast and highlands of New Guinea. *Hum. Biol. Oceania* **1**, 234.

Crane, G. G., Jones, P., Delaney, A., Kelly, A., MacGregor, A. and Leche, J. (1974). The pathogenesis of anaemia in coastal New Guineans. *Am. J. clin. Nutr.* **27**, 1079.

Fox, R. H., Budd, G. M., Woodward, Patricia M., Hackett, A. J. and Hendrie, A. L. (1974). A study of temperature regulation in New Guinea people. *Phil. Trans. R. Soc.* Ser. B **268**, 375.

Gajdusek, D. C. (1958). Kuru: an acute degenerate neurological disorder in Melanesian natives. *Trans. Am. neurol. Ass.* 156–158.

Gajdusek, D. C. (1963). Kuru. *Trans. R. Soc. trop. Med. Hyg.* **57**, 151.

Gajdusek, D. C. (1965). Kuru in New Guinea and the origin of the NINDB study of slow, latent and temperate virus infections of the nervous system of man. *In* NINDB Mono. 2 (Eds D. Gajdusek, C. Gibbs and M. Alpers). Public Health Publ. 1378, pp. 3–12.

Gajdusek, D. C. (1967). Slow virus infections of the nervous system. *New Engl. J. Med.* **276**, 392.

Gajdusek, D. C. and Gibbs, C. J. (1964). Attempts to demonstrate a transmissible agent in kuru, amyotrophic laterial sclerosis and other subacute and chronic system degenerations in man. *Nature* **204**, 257–259.

Gajdusek, D. C. and Gibbs, C. J. (1968). Degenerative neurological diseases of viral etiology: scrapie, kuru and Creutzfeldt-Jacob disease. Proc. Conf. on atypical virus infections: possible relevance to animal models and rheumatic disease. Atlanta, December.

Gajdusek, D. C. and Gibbs, C. J. (1971). Transmission of two subacute spongiform encephalopathies of man (kuru and Creutzfeldt-Jacob disease) to new world monkeys. *Nature* **230**, 588–591.

Gajdusek, D. C., Gibbs, C. J. and Alpers, M. (1966). Experimental transmission of a kuru-like syndrome to chimpanzees. *Nature* **209**, 794–796.

Garner, M. F., Hornabrook, R. W. and Backhouse, J. L. (1972a). Yaws in an island and in a coastal population in New Guinea. *Papua New Guin. med. J.* **15**, 136.

Garner, M. F., Hornabrook, R. W. and Backhouse, J. L. (1972b). The prevalence of yaws on Kar Kar Island, New Guinea. *Br. J. vener. Dis.* **48**, 350.

Glasse, R. M. and Lindenbaum, Shirley (1976). Kuru at Wanitabe. *In* "Essays on Kuru" Mono. 3 (Ed. R. W. Hornabrook) Papua New Guinea Institute of Medical Research. E. W. Glassey, Faringdon, p. 38.

Harrison, G. A., Hiorns, R. W. and Boyce, A. J. (1974). Movement, relatedness and the genetic structure of the population of Karkar Island. *Phil. Trans. R. Soc.* Ser. B **268**, 241–249.

Harrison, G. A., Boyce, A. J., Hornabrook, R. W. and Craig, W. J. (1976). Associations between polymorphic variety and anthropometric and biochemical variation in two New Guinea populations. *Ann. hum. Biol.* **3** (6) 557–568.

Harrison, G. A., Boyce, A. J., Platt, C. M. and Serjeanston, S. (1975). Body composition changes during lactation in a New Guinea population. *Ann. hum. Biol.* **2** (4), 395–398.

Harvey, R. G. (1974). An anthropometric survey of growth and physique of the populations of Karkar Island and Lufa Subdistrict, New Guinea. *Phil. Trans. R. Soc. Ser.* B **268**, 279–292.

Hetzel, B. S. (1970). The control of iodine deficiency. *Med. J. Aust.* **2**, 615–622.

Hetzel, B. S. (1971). The history of endemic cretinism. *In* "Endemic Cretinism" (Eds B. S. Hetzel and P. O. D. Pharoah), Institute of Human Biology, Papua New Guinea Mono. 2. Goroka, p. 5.

Hornabrook, R. W. (1966). Kuru. Some misconceptions and their explanation. *Papua New Guin. med. J.* **9**, 11–15.

Hornabrook, R. W. (1968). Kuru—subacute cerebellar degeneration. Natural history and clinical features. *Brain* **91**, 53–74.

Hornabrook, R. W. (1970a). The Institute of Human Biology—new development. *Papua New Guin. med. J.* **13**, 2–3.

Hornabrook, R. W. (1970b). International Biological Programme Investigation on Kar Kar Island. *Sop. Coq. Bull.* **20**, 15–17.

Hornabrook, R. W. (1970c). The Institute of Human Biology, of Papua New Guinea. *Science* **167**, 146–147.

Hornabrook, R. W. (1971a). Neurological aspects of endemic cretinism in Eastern New Guinea. *In* "Endemic Cretinism" (Eds B. S. Hetzel and P. O. D. Pharoah). Institute of Human Biology, Papua New Guinea Mono. 2. Goroka, p. 105.

Hornabrook, R. W. (1971b). Neurological damage which is associated with a high prevalence of endemic goiter. Proceedings of the Third Asian and Oceanian Congress of Neurology, Bombay, 1971. Reprinted from Neurology India, Suppl. IV, June 1973, p. 670.

Hornabrook, R. W. (1971c). "Essential tremor syndromes in New Guinea". Proceedings of the Third Asian and Oceanian Congress of Neurology, Bombay, 1971. Reprinted from Neurology India, Suppl. IV, June 1973, p. 581.

Hornabrook, R. W. (1972). Institute of Human Biology. *In* "Encyclopaedia of Papua and New Guinea" **1**, 573–574.

Hornabrook, R. W. Kuru. International Congress Series No. 319. (ISBN 90 219 0227 3). Proceedings of Tenth International Congress of Neurology, Barcelona, 1973. Excerpta Medica, Amsterdam.

Hornabrook, R. W. (1974). The demography of the population of Kar Kar Island. *Phil. Trans. R. Soc. Ser.* B **268**, 229–239.

Hornabrook, R. W. (1975a). Kuru. *In* "Topics on Tropical Neurology" (Ed. R. W. Hornabrook). Contemporary Neurology Series. F. A. Davis Company, Philadelphia, p. 71.

Hornabrook, R. W. (1975b). Endemic cretinism. *In* "Topics on Tropical Neurology" (Ed. R. W. Hornabrook). Contemporary Neurology Series. F. A. Davis Company, Philadelphia, p. 91.

Hornabrook, R. W. (1976). Kuru: the disease. *In* "Essays on Kuru" Mono. 3 (Ed. R. W. Hornabrook) Papua New Guinea Institute of Medical Research. E. W. Glassey, Faringdon, p. 53.

Hornabrook, R. W. and Moir, D. J. (1970). Kuru: epidemiological trends. *Lancet* **2**, 1175–1179.

Hornabrook, R. W., Fox, R. H. and Deaven, G. H. (1972). The occurrence of haemoglobin-J (Tongariki) and the p-thalassaemia trait on Kar Kar Island and the mainland of Papua and New Guinea. *Papua New Guin. med. J.* **15**, 189.

Hornabrook, R. W., Crane, G. G. and Stanhope, J. M. (1974). Kar Kar and Lufa: an epidemiological and health background to the human adaptability studies of the International Biological Programme. *Phil. Trans. R. Soc. Ser.* B **268**, 293–308.

Hornabrook, R. W., Kelly, A. and McMillan, B. (1975). Parasitic infection of man on Kar Kar Island, New Guinea. *Am. J. trop. Med. Hyg.* **24**, 250.

Lindenbaum, Shirley (1976). Kuru Sorcery. *In* "Essays on Kuru" Mono. 3 (Ed. R. W. Hornabrook) Papua New Guinea Institute of Medical Research. E. W. Glassey, Faringdon, p. 28.

McCullagh, S. F. (1963a). The Huon Peninsula endemic. I. Effectiveness of an intramuscular depot of iodized oil in the control of endemic goitre. *Med. J. Aust.* **1**, 769–777.

McCullagh, S. F. (1963b). The Huon Peninsula endemic. II. The effect in the female of endemic goitre on reproductive function. *Med. J. Aust.* **1**, 806–808.

McCullagh, S. F. (1963c). The Huon Peninsula endemic. III. The effect in the female of endemic goitre on reproductive function. *Med. J. Aust.* **1**, 844–849.

McCullagh, S. F. (1963d). The Huon Peninsula endemic. IV. Endemic goitre and congenital defect. *Med. J. Aust.* **1**, 884–890.

Maddocks, I. (1963). Dietary factors in the genesis of hypertension. Nutrition Proceedings Fifth International Congress on Nutrition, Edinburgh 1963. Livingstone, Edinburgh.

Maddocks, I. (1964). Blood pressure and race. *Papua New Guin. Sci. Ann. Rep. Proc.* **16**, 10–18.

Maddocks, I. (1967). Blood pressure in Melanesians. *Med. J. Aust.* **1**, 1123–1126.

Maddocks, I. and Rovin, L. (1965). A New Guinea population in which blood pressure appears to fall as age advances (Chimbu). *Papua New Guin. med. J.* **8**, 17–21.

Malcolm, L. A. (1967). Age estimation of New Guinean children. *Papua New Guin. med. J.* **10**, 122.

Malcolm, L. A. (1969a). Determination of the growth curve of the Kukukuku people of New Guinea from dental eruption in children and adult height. *Arch. Phys. Anthropol. Oceania* **4**, 72–78.

Malcolm, L. A. (1969b). Growth, malnutrition and mortality in the infant and toddler of the Asai Valley of the New Guinea Highlands. *Am. J. clin. Nutr.* **23**, 1090–1095.

Malcolm, L. A. (1969c). Growth and development of the Kaiapit children of the Markham Valley, New Guinea. *Am. J. phys. Anthrop.* **31**, 39–52.

Malcolm, L. A. (1969d). Growth and development of the New Guinea child. *Papua New Guin. med. J.* **12**, 23–32.

Malcolm, L. A. (1970a). Growth retardation in a New Guinea boarding school and its response to supplementary feeding. *Br. J. Nutr.* **24**, 297–305.

Malcolm, L. A. (1970b). The growth and development of the Bundi child of the New Guinea Highlands. *Hum. Biol.* **42**, 293–328.

Malcolm, L. A. (1970c). "Growth and development in New Guinea. A study of the Bundi people of the Madang District of New Guinea", Institute of Human Biology, Papua New Guinea Mono. 1.

Malcolm, L. A. and Wark, L. (1969). Growth and development of the Lumi child in the Sepik District of New Guinea. *Med. J. Aust.* **2**, 129–136.

Mathews, J. D. (1965). The changing face of kuru. *Lancet* **1**, 1138–1141.

Mathews, J. D. (1967a). A transmission model for Kuru. *Lancet* **1**, 821–825.

Mathews, J. D. (1967b). The epidemiology of kuru. *Papua New Guin. med. J.* **10**, 76–82.

Mathews, J. D. (1976). Kuru as an epidemic disease. *In* "Essays in Kuru" Mono. 3 (Ed. R. W. Hornabrook) Papua New Guinea Institute of Medical Research. E. W. Glassey, Faringdon, p. 83.

Morris, P. J., Bashir, Helen, MacGregor, A., Batchelor, J. R., Case, J., Kirk, R., Ting, A., Hornabrook, R. W., Boyle, A., Dumble, L., Law, W., Lightfoot, A., Johnston, J., Guinan, J. and Brotherton, J. (1973). Genetic studies of HL-A in New

Guinea. In "Histocompatibility Testing 1972" (Eds J. Dausset and J. Colombani). Munksgaard, Copenhagen, pp. 267–274.

Norgan, N. G., Ferro-Luzzi, A. and Durnin, J. V. G. A. (1974). The energy and nutrient intake and the energy expenditure of 204 New Guinean adults. *Phil. Trans. R. Soc.* Ser. B **268**, 309.

Patrick, J. M. and Cotes, J. E. (1974). Anthropometric and other factors affecting respiratory responses to carbon dioxide in New Guineans. *Phil. Trans. R. Soc.* Ser. B **268**, 363.

Pharoah, P. O. D. (1971). Epidemiological studies of endemic cretinism in the Jimi River Valley in New Guinea. *In* "Endemic Cretinism" (Eds B. S. Hetzel and P. O. D. Pharoah), Institute of Human Biology, Papua New Guinea Mono 2. Goroka, p. 109.

Pharoah, P. O. D. and Hornabrook, R. W. (1974). Endemic cretinism of recent onset in New Guinea. *Lancet* **2**, 1038.

Schamschula, R. G., Barmes, D., Keyes, P. J. and Gulbinat, W. (1974). Prevalence and inter-relationships of root surface caries in Lufa, Papua New Guinea. *Community Dent. Oral Epidem.* **2**, 295.

Serjeantson, S. The population genetic structure of Kar Kar Island, New Guinea (in preparation).

Sinnett, P. (1972). Nutrition in a New Guinea Highland community. *Hum. Biol. Oceania* **1**, 299–305.

Sinnett, P. "The ecology of a Highland community". Papua New Guinea Institute of Medical Research, Mono. 4 (in press).

Sinnett, P. and Solomon, A. (1968). Physical fitness in a New Guinea Highland population. *Papua New Guin. med. J.* **2**, 56.

Sinnett, P., Maddocks, I. and Hornabrook, R. W. (1970). Studies in New Guinea. 1. Coronary artery disease in a New Guinea Highland population. 2. Studies of Melanesians (Cardiovascular Epidemiology). WHO Report 1970.

Stanhope, J. M. and Hornabrook, R. W. (1974). Fertility patterns of two New Guinea populations: Kar Kar and Lufa. *J. biosoc. Sci.* **6**, 439.

Walsh, R. J. (1971). The International Biological Programme in New Guinea. *Med. J. Aust.* **1**, 1235.

Walsh, R. J. (1974). Geographical, historical, and social background of the people studied in the I.B.P. *Phil. Trans R. Soc.* Ser. B **268**, 223.

Weiner, J. S. (1965). "A guide to the human adaptability proposals".

Weiner, J. S. and Lourie, J. A. (1969). "Human Biology: a guide to field methods", IBP Handbook 9. Blackwell Scientific Publications, Oxford.

CHAPTER IV

Nutritional Adaptation Among the Enga

PETER F. SINNETT

University of Papua New Guinea

I. INTRODUCTION

Two questions recur in all population-based nutritional studies. What are the factors that limit nutrition in a particular community, and to what extent can any characteristic be taken as an objective indicator of malnutrition?

The nutritional status of a community is determined by the inter-action of many factors, including physical environment, socio-economic organization, levels of technology, standards of hygiene, disease prevalence and levels of health care. Ultimately, all such factors can be grouped into those that control the quantity and quality of food intake on the one hand and those that influence nutritional require-ments on the other.

A suggested model of the major determinants of nutritional status and their interactions in a self-contained subsistence community is presented in Figure 1. In this model economic structure, political orientation and educational standards are seen as related social variables which by establishing both the community's priorities and its technological capabilities, interact with such factors in the physical environment as soil composition, rainfall, altitude, temperature and humidity

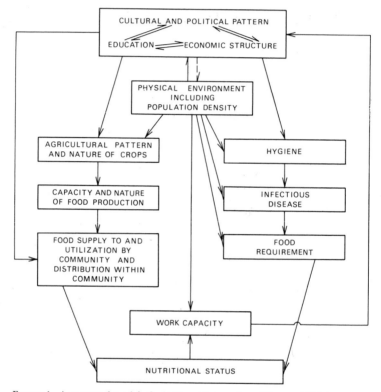

FIGURE 1. A suggested model of nutritional interactions (Sinnett, 1972a).

to determine the nature and level of agriculture and in turn the capacity for food production and hence, in a subsistence economy, the level of nutritional supply. Similarly, socio-economic factors interact with environmental characteristics, including population density, to determine the level of hygiene, the prevalence of infectious disease, and thus the nutritional requirements. The balance between nutritional supply and demand in turn determines the physical and psychological potential of the group and influences the community's socio-economic organization and its capacity to modify its environment.

The assessment of nutritional status is an essentially subjective matter. In the absence of absolute criteria, the various individual and population characteristics used in evaluation purely reflect the nature and extent of the cultural and biological adaptation imposed by nutritional stress.

In the majority of tropical subsistence communities, a low protein intake and exposure to repeated immunological challenge are central factors which determine the morphological, biochemical and demographic characteristics of the people. The growth pattern of children, the body build and physical fitness of young adults, and age-related changes in body composition, the levels of haemoglobin, serum proteins, blood urea nitrogen and serum lipids, as well as the population's demographic patterns, are all parameters which reflect the extent of adaptation to nutritional stress. It is realized that as these characteristics differ in their relationship to the body's homeostatic mechanisms, they are not all equally serviceable as indicators of nutritional status. Indeed, the more basic a characteristic is for the maintenance of homeostasis the less variance the characteristic will show and the less sensitive it will be as an indicator of environmental stress. Thus biochemical signs of overt clinical disease, such as serum protein levels, are usually insensitive and are of only limited use in the assessment of nutrition in population studies.

The importance of culture as an adaptive mechanism cannot be underrated, for cultural mechanisms generally represent the initial adaptive response to an environmental stress. It is only when the cultural response is not completely adequate to cope with the environmental challenge that biological adaptation becomes the central survival strategy. Man has progressively used social adjustment to limit the need for direct biological adaptation, for as pointed out by Dubos (1965), Darwinian fitness achieved through genetic mechanisms accounts for only a small part of the adaptive responses made by man and his societies.

II. THE PEOPLE OF MURAPIN

The major determinants of nutritional status and the problems of nutritional assessment are here considered in relation to a single self-contained Papua New Guinea population of 1500 people. This population is the subject of a longitudinal epidemiological survey commenced in 1966 under the auspices of the National Heart Foundation of Australia. The objective of this study is to investigate the influence of social, nutritional and other environmental factors on the anthropometric, biochemical and other physiological characteristics as well as on the disease pattern of the people under study (Sinnett, 1972a, 1972b, 1972c; Sinnett and Solomon, 1968; Sinnett and Whyte, 1973a,

1973b; Sinnet *et al.*, 1970). These people form the entire membership of Murapin, a complete Yandapu-Enga* phratry, or tribal community. Their clan territory is centred on the hamlet of Tukisenta within the Lagaip subdistrict of the Western Highlands of Papua New Guinea, 160 km north-west of Mt. Hagen and 25 km from Laiagam, the headquarters of the subdistrict (see Map 1).

They are hamlet dwellers; their homesteads of timber and grass extend along the valleys of the Lagaip, Puriok and Tibirit rivers at an altitude of 1800 to 2600 m and are scattered among sweet potato gardens and beech trees which grow in the narrow river valleys and on the foothills of the mountain forests. They are pre-literate farmers and pig herders whose subsistence economy depends almost entirely on the cultivation of a single staple food, the sweet potato. Theirs is a singularly self-contained society; their tribal land fully supplies their needs for food, energy and building materials, while their farming methods and limited technology assure that there is a minimum disruption to the ecosystem of which they are so completely a part. In adaptive terms, they can be viewed as a mountain people who live at altitudes close to the upper limits of cultivation of the staple on which they depend for their subsistence. Many of their cultural and biological characteristics are seen as adaptations to altitude, the factor in their physical environment which poses the greatest threat to their survival. The significance of any environmental challenge is increased by the fact that the Highlands of Papua New Guinea are occupied by a series of small, and for practical purposes, culturally identical societies, each of which is virtually a closed ecosystem. As a result of their isolation, their limited technology and their lack of cultural diversity, the impact and the response to a given environmental stress will be identical for adjacent communities and, therefore, the development of survival strategies based on mutual support is largely pre-empted.

III. HISTORICAL BACKGROUND

It is claimed that the first human migrations into Papua New Guinea occurred from South East Asia between 20 000 and 50 000 years ago (Golson, 1970). Humans have occupied the Highlands of Papua New Guinea for at least 10 000 years (Bulmer, 1964). On the basis of ethnobotanical evidence, Robbins (1963) suggests that human migration

---

* Yandapu-Enga is one of 13 dialects of the Enga language and is spoken by 14 000 people living mainly in the Lagaip subdistrict of the Western Highlands of Papua New Guinea (Capell, 1962).

into the Highlands occurred from coastal regions in an east to west direction via the Markham valley.

Bulmer and Bulmer (1964) postulate that following initial settlement of the Highlands there has been continuous occupation of the region by the original population. The changing pattern of their existence has been the result of progressive adaptation to their environment, together with the introduction of crops and technology from outside the area rather than the result of large scale intrusions into the Highlands by other migrant groups.

Gradually the initial hunting and gathering economy was replaced by a semi-nomadic agriculture based on a stone-age technology and associated with the cultivation of taro, bananas, yams and sugar cane which, according to Brookfield (1964), restricted the population to altitudes below 2100 m.

The final stage in the agricultural development of the Highlands was associated with the introduction of the sweet potato (*Ipomoea batatas*) some 350 years ago (Conklin, 1963). This crop made possible development of relatively large settled communities and the colonization of altitudes up to 2700 m. The occupation of altitudes above 2100 m, presumably as the result of population pressure, leads to a heavy dependence on the sweet potato and to a restricted range of food intake; an important factor in view of the low protein content of the sweet potato and its susceptibility to frosts. It is also postulated that the greater productivity of the sweet potato increased the number of pigs that could be maintained and thus assisted in the development of the large ceremonial exchange systems typical of the societies of the Papua New Guinea Highlands (Westerman, 1968).

IV. PHYSICAL ENVIRONMENT

Situated 650 km to the south of the equator, the clan's territory lies at the boundary of two land systems (CSIRO, 1965). To the north lies the Ambum system, characterized by mountainous terrain, humic brown clay soils on a substratum of soft non-calcareous sedimentary rock and vegetation consisting of sword grass and low montane forest in which beech and casuarina trees predominate. To the south lies the Womgum system, the main characteristics of which are low rounded hills and ridges, humic brown and reddish clay soils based on soft sedimentary rocks, and sword grass as the dominant vegetation.

As would be anticipated from the area's proximity to the equator, seasonal variations in temperature and humidity were not marked, however as a consequence of altitude, diurnal variations were relatively large. During the periods of fieldwork thermohygrographs standardized against a wet and dry bulb thermometer were used to continuously monitor temperature and relative humidity. The daily temperature ranged through 11 to 16°C, often falling to 4°C between 4.0 and 6.0 a.m. and rising to 21°C between 2.0 and 4.0 p.m. Relative humidity readings reached values of 95% between 10.0 p.m. and 8.0 a.m. and fell to 30% at midday. The use of two thermohygrographs permitted continuous seven-day records of temperature and relative humidity to be obtained simultaneously in the open and inside local houses. The average diurnal variation in temperature was 11°C in the open and 5°C inside the houses tested. Similarly, the mean daily range of relative humidity was 40% in the open but only 10% inside the local houses. The design of the traditional grass house thus represents a cultural adaptation which effectively limits the impact of climatic extremes (Sinnett and Whyte, 1973a).

Although the rainfall is distributed throughout the whole year, there is nevertheless a definite wet season that extends from November to April. Rainfall records kept at Laiagam, report a mean annual rainfall of 2160 mm and show that rain falls on an average of 239 days per year (CSIRO, 1965). Winter droughts do occur, but they rarely present a serious threat to food production unless they are associated with frosts. From June until September 1972 severe frosts did occur during a dry winter season and destroyed the majority of the sweet potato gardens, not only within the clan's territory but throughout much of the Enga territory and beyond. It would be an over-simplification to blame the 1972 disaster solely on the occurrence of frosts during a winter drought, for many factors combine to render this community's food supply tenuous. The high altitude of the terrain and the clan's consequent heavy dependence on a single staple, the sweet potato which is frost susceptible, poor communications, the cultural and technological similarity of adjacent communities, the absence of a technology for food storage and the dependence on a subsistence economy which precludes the purchase of alternate food supplies, are all factors which in association with the frosts contributed to the 1972 food shortage. In order to compensate for this environmental threat it would be necessary to implement a policy which combined crop diversification, development of a food storage technology, improved communications and economic expansion.

V. AGRICULTURE

Traditional agriculture is based on the intensive cultivation of a single staple food, the sweet potato (*Ipomoea batatas*). Some 24 varieties of this plant are grown within the clan territory. Sweet potato is planted in raised mounds 0·6–1 m high and measuring up to 11 m in circumference at the base. A single mound contains 6–20 sweet potato plants. A medium sized garden measuring 30 m by 23 m contains some 50 potato mounds. As these gardens are generally constructed on mountain slopes, the building of mounds conserves the topsoil and minimizes erosion during the heavy rains that fall between November and April. Furthermore, it is claimed by Waddell (1968) that the construction of mounds alters the plants' microclimate, the minimum temperature in the mounds being higher than those in the intervening troughs by as much as 3°C, it also facilitates cold air drainage. Waddell (1973) has drawn attention to the relationship which exists between increasing altitude and mound dimensions throughout the Enga territory of the Western Highlands. At higher altitudes the mounds are significantly higher and wider and the sweet potato plants are increasingly concentrated towards the top of the mounds. He further stresses the importance of mound building as an adaptive strategy which minimizes the impact of altitude and environmental temperature, claiming that "generalized mound topography serves as a critical mechanism by means of which an ecologically vulnerable crop is cultivated in a marginal environment" (Waddell, 1973).

The clearing of the garden site and much of the work of garden preparation, including the digging of irrigation ditches and the building of fences to keep out pigs, is undertaken by the men, while the women in the family, although assisting in garden preparation, are mainly responsible for the maintenance of the garden and the harvesting of the crops. Once planted, the sweet potato takes about ten months to mature. The gardens are planted in rotation to ensure a continuous supply of sweet potato. After harvesting, a garden plot is left fallow while another plot, usually adjacent to the first and within the same garden site, is cleared and planted. The period of fallow is highly variable, but at Tukisenta the pattern appears to be one of "continuous cultivation" where "cultivation is repeated at frequent intervals, with or without short intervening rest periods, for as long as a generation or more, without any intervening spell of years under idle fallow" (Brookfield and Hart, 1971). Although the garden sites of a family are often widely scattered throughout the clan territory, there is no evidence that this is due to shortage of land. In view of the amount of land that has subsequently been converted to cash cropping, the capacity for food production would seem to be well in excess of the present land requirements of the community.

Other crops cultivated include taro (*Colocasia esculenta*), which is now grown only to a limited extent although informants claim that one to two generations ago this crop was extensively cultivated throughout the area; pit-pit (*Saccharum sponataneum*); sugar cane (*Saccharum officinarum*) and pandanus palms (*Pandanus* sp.). Further, European contact has resulted in the planting of potatoes, corn, peas, beans, lettuce, cabbage and celery, but with the exception of potatoes, these other items make only a minimal contribution to the dietary intake of these people. Extensive herds of pigs are maintained and, during exchange ceremonies, large amounts of pork are consumed. However, in terms of the overall dietary intake, pork is a minor food source.

VI. NUTRITIONAL INTAKE

A diet survey was undertaken involving 90 subjects, in which all food consumed by each individual was weighed over a period of seven consecutive days. Sweet potato supplied over 90% of their total food intake, while non-tuberous vegetables accounted for less than 5% of the food consumed and the intake of meat was negligible. A similar heavy dependence on a single vegetable staple has been reported for other Papua New Guinea Highlands communities (Hipsley and Clements, 1947; Oomen *et al.*, 1961; Venkatachalam, 1962; Bailey and Whiteman, 1963; Hipsley and Kirk, 1965; Malcolm, 1970; Norgan *et al.*, 1974).

Chemical analysis was carried out on the 14 separate varieties of the sweet potato consumed by subjects during the dietary survey. This analysis was considered necessary as significant differences have been reported in the chemical composition of the sweet potato (Oomen *et al.*, 1961; Bailey, 1968; Malcolm, 1970). As predicted, chemical composition varied widely between the different varieties of sweet potato analysed; for example, protein content ranged from 1·01 to 1·97% of wet weight and energy values varied from 111·8 to 154·9 calories per 100 g edible portion. The low protein content of the staple is the major factor imposing a serious limitation on the nutritional status of this population.

The daily energy intake was 2300 calories in the case of males and 1770 calories for females. Of these, 94·6% were derived from carbohydrate, 3% from protein and only 2·4% from fat. Male subjects consumed 25 g and female subjects 20 g of protein per day. By contrast, Australians derive 40% of their calories from fat and consume approximately 100 g of protein per day (Woodhill et al., 1969). These results are in keeping with the majority of dietary surveys carried out in the Highlands of Papua New Guinea (Hipsley and Clements, 1947; Oomen and Malcom, 1958; Venkatachalam, 1962; Bailey and Whiteman, 1963; Hipsley and Kirk, 1965) which in general show levels of calorie and protein intake far below the recommended allowance for both Australians (National Health and Medical Research Council, 1965) and New Guineans (Langley, 1947). Indeed the dietary studies of Reid and Gajdusek (1969) in the Fore district and of Norgen et al. (1974) at Lufa in the Eastern Highlands are the only two works to report a calorie intake above the New Guinea allowance recommended by Langley. The dietary intake of pregnant and lactating females appeared barely sufficient to meet their increased nutritional demands as reported by the World Health Organization (WHO, 1973). Thus in the present study lactating women had an average daily intake of 1997 calories and 23·6 g of protein, only a slight increase on the intake of non-lactating women. On the other hand, however, the dietary intake appeared to be reduced during pregnancy, as intakes of 1683 calories and 18 g of protein were recorded for pregnant women in this study. In spite of the low levels of calorie and protein intake there was no evidence of nutritional impairment among these women.

The energy intake for young adult subjects in this study was 41·5 calories per kilogram body weight per day for males and 37·5 for females. These are corrected values based on the recommendations of the Food and Agriculture Organization of the United Nations (FAO, 1957). In general these results are marginally below the most recent FAO/WHO recommendations of 46 calories per kilogram for moderately active men and 40 calories per kilogram for women in the same group (WHO, 1973). However in the absence of information on the basal metabolic rate and energy expenditure of these people, it is impossible to conclude that their calorie intake is not optimal (Sinnett, 1972a). Indeed it would be surprising if the food intake of adults was not adequate to cover energy requirements as there was no evidence of any restriction of food availability.

In spite of uncertainties as to the true protein requirements of man (Clements, 1971), it would be hard to deny that the protein intake of this group is marginal. The central problem in this case is the low percentage contribution made by dietary protein to the total calorie intake. As pointed out by an expert committee on protein requirement (WHO, 1965), if the protein content of the diet contributes less than 5% of the total calorie intake, an optimum intake of protein cannot be achieved as appetite is satisfied before protein requirements are met. In the present study protein accounts for less than 4% of total calorie intake. In consequence, it would not be possible to improve significantly the protein intake of these people by simply increasing the amount of sweet potato consumed, due to the low protein-to-calorie ratio of this crop. This claim implies that the achievement of an optimum nutritional status by the people living in the Highlands of Papua New Guinea must await the introduction of foods of higher protein content than their present staple.

Attempts have been made to explain the adjustment of these populations to their low protein diet in terms of biological adaptation. The fixation of atmospheric nitrogen by intestinal bacteria and the re-utilization of urea nitrogen are two mechanisms commonly proposed.

The finding of a negative nitrogen balance among sweet potato eaters living in the Baiyer river area of Papua New Guinea led Oomen and Cordon (1970) to postulate that nitrogen fixation by intestinal bacteria may augment the limited protein intake of these people, this undisclosed source of nitrogen being claimed to account for the observed negative nitrogen balance. In view of the immense technical difficulties involved in carrying out balance studies under field conditions, the findings of this study must be interpreted with caution and final judgement must await the demonstration that labelled atmospheric nitrogen so fixed can be transported across the mucosa of the intestine and incorporated into body protein.

The concept of urea re-utilization may be significant. Although it would not explain the negative nitrogen balances observed by Oomen and Cordon, it would nevertheless be one physiological mechanism capable of conserving nitrogen in a population whose nitrogen intake is marginal.

Widdowson (1956) drew attention to the high values found for the total body water of protein-deficient persons when urea was used as the test substance, and suggested that the reason for these spuriously high readings might be in the fact that urea nitrogen was being used to alleviate the protein deficiency in these subjects. She further raised the possibility that utilization of urea nitrogen might account for the low levels of urea found in the serum of children with kwashiorkor. This suggestion is supported by the work of Snyderman et al. (1962) who found that the administration of unessential nitrogen in the form of either glycine or urea was capable of establishing both normal nitrogen retention and weight gain when fed to protein restricted infants. By the use of N^{15}-urea and N^{15}-ammonium chloride, they demonstrated the incorporation of unessential nitrogen into the haemoglobin and plasma proteins of infants on low protein intake. Similarly,

Giordano (1963), in a study of uraemic and normal patients, demonstrated that positive nitrogen balance could be achieved in protein-restricted individuals fed either ammonium salts, glucine, glutamic acid or urea. Likewise, Tripathy *et al.* (1970a) demonstrated the utilization of exogenous urea as a nitrogen source in studies carried out on malnourished males. Urea was effective whether given intravenously or orally. In this study dietary protein abolished the utilization urea.

There is thus strong evidence that urea provides a nitrogen source in protein-restricted individuals and further urea utilization may serve as a useful biological adaptation to marginal protein intakes. The mechanism of this action is obscure. Orally administered urea could be split by the action of bacterial urease in the gut and the liberated ammonia subsequently incorporated in glutamine. Alternately, it has been claimed (Giordano, 1963) that reversal of the citrulline cycle in the liver is thermodynamically feasible. This latter mechanism would be energetically expensive.

VII. SERUM PROTEINS AND HAEMOGLOBIN

Among the people of Murapin, young males in their twenties had a mean serum protein level of 8·4 g/100 ml, a serum albumin level of 4·5 g/100 ml, and a serum globulin level of 3·9 g/100 ml. Females in the same age group had a total protein level of 8·1 g/100 ml, an albumin level of 4·2 g/100 ml and a globulin level of 3·9 g/100 ml.

Serum protein patterns characterized by a low serum albumin and a high gamma globulin level are typical of many tropical communities and are usually taken to imply a significant exposure to infectious disease in the presence of nutritional deficiency (Curtain *et al.*, 1965; Curtain, 1966).

The serum albumin levels in the present study are higher than those previously reported for populations living in the Highlands of Papua New Guinea (Venkatachalam, 1962; Curtain *et al.*, 1965; Malcolm, 1970; Vines, 1970). These findings however do not necessarily imply a satisfactory state of nutrition as levels of serum protein are maintained in states of protein-calorie deficiency at the expense of tissue proteins. That this is in fact occurring in the present population is suggested by the marked decrease in body weight and more especially in muscle which accompanies ageing.

The lack of sensitivity of serum albumin as an index of nutritional status has been stressed by Arroyave (1961), who pointed out that adaption to chronically sub-optimal intakes of protein is not accompanied by changes in fundamental protein components like albumin until the deficiency is very severe. Indeed Whitehead *et al.* (1971) pointed out that the serum albumin levels can be normal in marasmus in spite of the presence of gross muscle wasting.

The finding of high globulin levels in this population is taken to indicate exposure to a significant immunological challenge. In spite of the apparent priority given to the maintenance of γ-globulin levels and overall immunological competence, there is little doubt that protein deficiency interferes with the function of the immune system in man and renders him more susceptible to infectious disease (Scrimshaw *et al.*, 1968; Smythe *et al.*, 1971; Geefhuysen *et al.*, 1971). On the other hand, as pointed out by Jose and Good (1972), malnourished children may be capable of producing an adequate antibody response in the face of an acute immunological challenge but at the expense of developing overt symptoms of protein-calorie deficiency.

Nalder *et al.* (1972) have shown that progressive reduction in the protein content of the diet of weanling rats leads to a proportionate decrease in antibody production. Further, Jose and Good (1971) have demonstrated a reduction in the humoral immune response as measured by depression of haemagglutinating, cytotoxic and blocking antibody titres in mice fed diets in which less than 10% of the calories were derived from protein. By contrast, cell-mediated immunity was not impaired until the protein intake was reduced to 3% of calories. Thus it is claimed that the humoral immune mechanism is more sensitive to protein deficiency than the cell-mediated component. However, studies on children with kwashiorkor (Geefhuysen *et al.*, 1971) indicate that severe protein malnutrition is capable of deranging cell-mediated immunity.

These effects of protein deficiency on the immune response may be significant in explaining disease prevalence in populations with low protein intakes. Certainly high prevalence rates of infectious disease would be expected, while Jose and Good (1971) further claim that the continued efficiency of the cell-mediated response functioning without the impairment of serum blocking antibodies would be expected to result in a decreased prevalence of malignant conditions.

As in the case of albumin, haemoglobin levels are maintained at the expense of tissue proteins and are thus poor predictors of nutritional status. In the present study the mean haemoglobin value was 17·5 g/100 ml for males and 15·6 g/100 ml for females. These results reflect a successful adaptation to altitude and indeed agree closely with values predicted by Walsh *et al.* (1959) for subjects living at altitudes between 2100 and 2400 m (7000 and 8000 ft).

VIII. BLOOD UREA NITROGEN

Extremely low levels of blood urea nitrogen were recorded in the present study. These results, in the order of 4·8 mg/100 ml for males and 5·7 mg/100 ml for females, reflect the subjects' low protein intake of 25 g/day. Although liver enlargement is common in the Highlands of Papua New Guinea (Blackburn et al., 1966), there is little evidence that the low levels of blood urea nitrogen found in this population were significantly influenced by liver pathology (Sinnett, 1972a; Sinnett and Whyte, 1973a).

In spite of the obvious influences of hepatic and renal function, it appears that the measurement of blood urea nitrogen provides a simple and useful index for assessing the level of protein intake in population studies. Indeed as early as 1942, Longley and Miller (1942) demonstrated that in normal subjects an increase in dietary protein is associated with an increase in fasting blood urea nitrogen levels over a range of 0·3–2·8 g protein/kg. This relationship has been repeatedly confirmed in studies involving groups with contrasting protein intakes (Phillips and Kenney, 1952; Barnicot and Sai, 1954; McFarlane et al., 1970).

It has been suggested (Sinnett, 1972a) that a measurement of the body's urea nitrogen pool provides valuable insight into the level of nitrogen metabolism and thus of protein intake in comparative population studies.

San Pietro and Tittenberg (1953a, 1953b) pointed out that the size of the body's urea nitrogen pool is related to the rate of oxidative metabolism of proteins. They noted that the urea nitrogen space is coextensive with total body water and thus the total urea nitrogen content of the body can be calculated from a knowledge of the blood urea nitrogen level and the total body water according to the formula:

Total body urea nitrogen (mg) = 10 × blood urea nitrogen
$$(mg/100 ml) \times total body water (l).$$

By way of example, if it is assumed that the total body water is 54% of total body weight in the case of males (Alper, 1968), then from a knowledge that young male subjects in the present survey had a mean body weight of 59·8 kg and a blood urea nitrogen level of 4·8 mg/100 ml, it can be calculated that the total urea nitrogen pool of young males was 1550 mg. By contrast, a hypothetical Australian male weighing 70 kg with a blood urea nitrogen level of 13 mg/100 ml would have a total urea nitrogen pool of 4914 mg. This calculation provides insight into the relative difference in the level of protein metabolism in the two groups. The use of the urea nitrogen pool is preferable to the use of blood urea nitrogen levels as it compensates for differences in body mass.

IX. SERUM LIPIDS

Extensive epidemiological studies reviewed by Lowenstein (1964) and Stamler (1967) have shown that in affluent communities such as those of the United States of America, the levels of serum cholesterol, triglycerides and β-lipoproteins are all elevated. In such populations, a dietary pattern characterized by a high intake of total calories, saturated fat, cholesterol and refined carbohydrate is associated with low levels of habitual physical activity and obesity. By contrast, people from economically less developed areas of Africa and the Asian-Pacific region, who subsist largely on vegetable staples and have a low consumption of total calories, saturated fats, cholesterol and sugar, but whose diet contains a relatively high content of complex carbohydrates and fibre, are usually found to have low serum cholesterol and triglyceride levels.

The lipid pattern of the people of Murapin differs from those reported for both affluent communities and for most developing areas in that here a low level of serum cholesterol is associated with elevated triglyceride values. Thus cholesterol values of 158 mg/100 ml for males and 168 mg/100 ml for females were recorded in the present study, while the triglyceride levels were 140 mg/100 ml in the case of males and 150 mg/100 ml in the case of females.

There are at least four dietary factors which contribute to the low cholesterol values in this study: energy intake, the quantity and quality of dietary fat, the level of protein intake and the fibre content of the diet.

In the first place, the total calorie intake is low. Keys et al. (1950) have shown that low calorie diets are associated with a reduction in serum cholesterol levels even when the intake of dietary lipids is constant, further Mann et al. (1955) demonstrated that a calorie induced increase in cholesterol could be prevented by a programme of exercise sufficient to dissipate the excess calories. Thus the high level of physical activity of these people is a significant factor contributing to their low cholesterol levels.

The low level of dietary fat intake is a second factor determining low cholesterol levels. The mean daily consumption of fat was 6·4 g for males (2·4% of calories) and 9·8 g for females (4·8% of calories). The fact that this fat was derived from vegetable sources is also significant, for as pointed out by Hegsted *et al.* (1965), serum lipid levels are influenced by the quality in addition to the quantity of dietary fat. Dietary cholesterol and saturated fats increase serum cholesterol levels while polyunsaturated fats have the reverse effect. In spite of the foregoing, there is no general agreement as to the relationship between fat ingestion and resulting lipid levels, either in individual subjects or in international epidemiological studies (McGandy *et al.*, 1967). Notable among population studies in which low levels of serum cholesterol have been reported in spite of high dietary intakes of animal fat, are those of the Masai and Samburu tribesmen of Kenya (Shaper *et al.*, 1961; Mann *et al.*, 1964). Valuable insight has been provided by indepth metabolic studies of the Masai tribesmen reported by Biss *et al.* (1971) and Taylor and Ho (1971). These workers confirmed previous observations that the Masai were, in fact, consuming 3000 calories per day, 66% of which was derived from animal fat. In spite of this the serum cholesterol level was a modest 135 mg/100 ml. These studies demonstrated that the Masai had a much greater capacity to suppress endogenous cholesterol synthesis than the North Americans. Further, these workers claim that a similar mechanism is operative in the Eskimo population of Point Hope in Alaska (Ho *et al.*, 1971).

In addition to the influence of their low calorie, low fat intake, the low protein content of the diet is another factor affecting serum lipid levels. Olson *et al.* (1958) demonstrated that a reduction in protein intake to 25 g/day resulted in a significant decrease in serum cholesterol and β-lipid proteins, even when the total calories and the fat intake were maintained constant. Moreover Tripathy *et al.* (1970b) have demonstrated that protein supplements increase cholesterol levels in malnourished subjects. Thus below a critical level in protein intake there is a reduction in cholesterol levels which can be wholly corrected by protein replacement. It is interesting that this critical level (25 g/day) corresponds to the observed level of protein intake for the subjects in this study. Hodges *et al.* (1967) reported that replacement of animal protein by equal quantities of vegetable protein resulted in a decrease in serum cholesterol. Methionine is generally the limiting amino acid in vegetable proteins and it has been postulated that low levels of this amino acid result in a decrease in available methyl groups and a subsequent reduction in choline systhesis, which is partly responsible for the low cholesterol values reported for subjects on vegetable diets (Ahrens, 1957).

The fourth factor which has a possible influence on the serum cholesterol levels in this study is the fibre content of the sweet potato. The diet consumed is high in fibre content and this is predicted to decrease serum cholesterol levels by binding of bile acids (Trowell, 1972).

The high triglyceride readings recorded in this study are, in all probability, the consequence of a high carbohydrate diet. A carbohydrate induced hypertriglyceridaemia has been reported in clinical studies (Ahrens et al., 1961; Albrink, 1962; Yudkin and Rooday, 1964; Yudkin, 1967). Some caution is, however, needed in interpreting these relatively short-term clinical studies, as the work of Antonis and Bersohn (1961) indicated that the hypertriglyceridaemia resulting from high carbohydrate diets was a transitory phenomenon. In the present study, people derived 90% of their calories from complex carbohydrates, ingestion of simple sugars was negligible and less than 5% of total calories were derived from fat. It appears inevitable under these conditions that the plasma triglycerides must arise as the result of endogenous formation from complex carbohydrates.

X. GROWTH AND AGE-RELATED CHANGES IN BODY BUILD

The adaptation to a low calorie, low protein diet is reflected not only in the biochemical parameters but is manifest in the growth patterns and age-dependent changes in the body build of these subjects. Thus the values for height and weight of Murapin children are lower at all ages than those of Australians (Patrick, 1951; Meyers, 1956; Australian Institute of Anatomy, 1957). Growth in both these parameters is not completed until the age of 18 years in females and 24 years in the case of males. Such findings are common in Papua New Guinea communities (Malcolm, 1970). By contrast, British children reach adult stature by the age of 15 years in females and 17 years in the case of males (Tanner et al., 1966).

In spite of the delayed growth curves of children, young adults in this population, although of short stature, are extremely well built (Figure 2). Young men are 98% standard weight and women in their twenties are 102% standard weight when compared with American subjects aged 20–24 years who are of the same sex and height (Society of Actuaries, 1959). In addition young adults were found to have a high level of physical fitness as assessed by both the Harvard Pack Test and by bicycle ergometry. Indeed the mean result for the people of Murapin was significantly superior to the results quoted for Royal Australian Air Force personnel serving in the Pacific during World War II (MacPherson, 1949). Further, high levels of physical fitness were

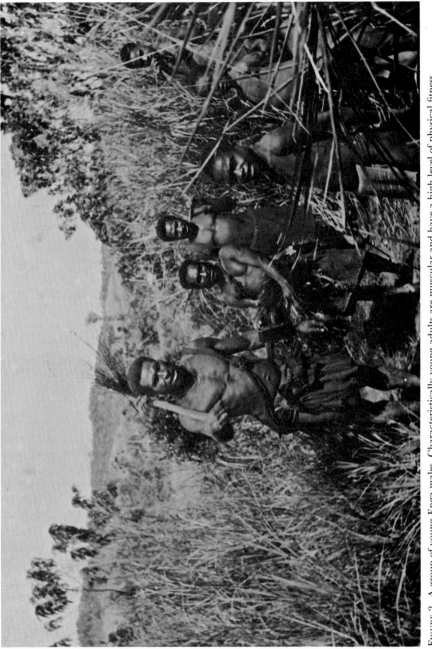

FIGURE 2. A group of young Enga males. Characteristically young adults are muscular and have a high level of physical fitness.

maintained well into the fifth decade (Sinnett and Solomon, 1968). Thus in spite of the low protein diet and consequent growth retardation, young adults are well built, physically fit and apparently well adapted to their environment.

Many Caucasian populations show a progressive increase in body weight from maturity through middle age and even into the seventh and eighth decades. By contrast, a decrease in body weight associated with advancing age has been reported for a number of groups in Papua New Guinea (Hipsley and Clements, 1947; Whyte, 1958; Venkatachalam, 1962; Jansen, 1963; Bailey, 1963; Hipsley and Kirk, 1965; Vines, 1970). The subjects of the present study are typical of other Papua New Guinea populations in that their body weight reaches a maximum between the ages of 20 and 29 years. In this age group the mean body weight is 59·8 kg for male subjects and 50·9 for females; thereafter both sexes show a progressive decrease in body weight with advancing age. By the seventh decade the average body weight has decreased by 13·3 kg or 23·3% in the case of men (Figure 3) and 13·5 kg or 25% in the case of women.

There is evidence that the lean body mass of adults falls progressively with advancing age even in those populations in which a cumulative caloric excess leads to an increase in body weight during adult life (Allen *et al.*, 1960). Based on longitudinal studies of total body potassium content, Forbes and Reina (1970) have pointed out that after maturity is reached anabolic processes are "superseded by catabolic events which slowly erode the lean body mass. The adult should be looked upon as being in a continuous state of negative potassium (and hence nitrogen) balance". These authors have developed an interesting concept of "desirable" body weight—"if one assumes that the goal is of no increase in body fat, then the male should strive to weigh 12 kg less at age 65–70 years than at age 25 years and the female 5 kg". This implies that between the third and seventh decades there should be a reduction in body weight of 16·4% in male subjects and 8·5% in the case of females. By contrast, male subjects in the present study lose 23·3% of their body weight between the third and seventh decades while females in the study experienced a weight reduction of 25% over the same age span. The marked decrease in body weight that accompanies ageing in this population implies a rate of catabolism and a degree of negative nitrogen balance far greater than that reported for the Caucasian subjects reviewed by Forbes and Reina (1970). This is taken to reflect the low protein intake of the people of Murapin. It has been shown that muscle loss is a major factor in accounting for this age-dependent decrease in body weight. Further, the finding that both blood pressure and electrocardiographic voltage fall progressively with advancing age

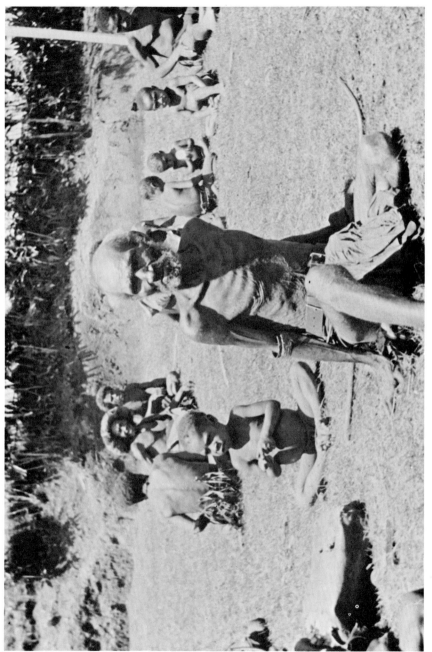

FIGURE 3. An elderly Enga man showing evidence of marked weight loss. Ageing is associated with a marked loss of muscle mass in this population.

suggests that the nutritionally based muscle loss in this population may be associated with deterioration in myocardial function (Sinnett, 1972a; Sinnett and Whyte, 1973b).

XI. POPULATION STATISTICS

The population of Murapin is predominantly a young one; 43·6% of the subjects are less than 15 years of age. This suggests a satisfactory level of population growth; by contrast, 29·4% of Australians are under the age of 15 years (Commonwealth Bureau of Census and Statistics, 1968).

In the absence of accurate birth registration, the number of children under the age of five years per 1000 women of child-bearing age (15–45 years) provides some indication of fertility (Barclay, 1958). For Murapin, the ratio was 772 per 1000. By way of comparison, the ratio for Australians, excluding Aboriginals, was 427 per 1000 (Commonwealth Bureau of Census and Statistics, 1968).

The population of Murapin was found to have a crude birth-rate of 42 per 1000, a death-rate of 15 per 1000, and thus a rate of natural increase of approximately 2·7% per annum. In contrast, the Australian population had a crude birth-rate of 19·3 per 1000, a death-rate of 9·0 per 1000, and a rate of natural increase of 1·03% per annum (Commonwealth Bureau of Census and Statistics, 1969). The high rate of natural increase for the population of Murapin testifies to its successful biological adaptation. However, the death-rate, and more specifically the infant mortality rate, are high in comparison to Australian figures. Of the 140 children born during the survey, 12 died before reaching the age of one year; hence the infant mortality rate is 85 per 1000 live births compared to 18 per 1000 in the case of Australia (Commonwealth Bureau of Census and Statistics, 1969). The infant mortality for Murapin is similar to the figure of 67 per 1000 reported by Malcolm (1970) for the Bundi people of Madang district and the rate of 74 per 1000 recorded by Becroft et al. (1969) for the people of the Baiyer river. The infant mortality rates for these three populations of the Highlands are considerably lower than the rate of 123·7 deaths per 1000 live births reported for the highlands by Vines (1970). In keeping with the high infant mortality rate there was a high death-rate in childhood; 42·8% of children in the present study died before they reached the age at which they were eligible for marriage.

XII. PATTERNS OF DISEASE

Infectious diseases appear to predominate in those communities which depend on a subsistence economy, while degenerative diseases dominate in those populations whose economy is based on high levels of technology. Fenner (1970) in his review of the effects of changing social organization on the prevalence of infectious disease, suggested that human infections date from the development of an agricultural economy which provided the population density and other conditions necessary for the transmission of respiratory and enteric microbes. Most traditional communities in Papua New Guinea, including the people of Murapin, are subsistence farmers and among these people infectious diseases are the major cause of morbidity and mortality. Gastrointestinal and respiratory infections, leprosy and parasitic infestations, together with trauma, constitute the major public health problems while degenerative disease, including degenerative cardiovascular disease, is of relatively little significance. Of the cardiovascular diseases diagnosed, those associated with primary pulmonary disease or secondary rheumatic fever were the most commonly encountered in the present study. Indeed no case of coronary artery disease, peripheral vascular disease, previous cerebrovascular accident or diabetes was detected in this population. Malaria and tuberculosis, although common in most tropical areas, were virtually absent from this population. The low prevalence of malaria is to be expected in view of the high altitude at which these people live. Peters *et al.* (1958) have pointed out that malarial transmission is extremely rare above 2400 m. It is more difficult to explain the virtual absence of tuberculosis. Wigley (1967) has pointed out that tuberculosis is by and large a predominantly coastal disease. He claims prevalence rates of the condition are proportional to the duration of European contact and the degree of urbanization.

As previously pointed out

> Many factors currently operating in Papua New Guinea can be expected to change the disease patterns of the country. Economic development; improved standards of education, nutrition, and hygiene; increased technology as well as developments within the health services; are likely to decrease the infant and toddler mortality rate and increase life expectancy. As a result there will be a net increase in population size and also a change in the age structure of the population, with more people living into the coronary-prone age groups. In addition, improvements in diagnostic services will increase case detection and place a further burden on health services.

As economic development cannot be expected to be uniform, but will in all probability be greatest in relatively few industrial centres, a shift in population along an economic gradient to such developing urban centres, with attendant social disruption, appears inevitable. Such migrations will add a further burden to the health services, especially in the area of control of communicable disease.

Thus, social and economic development is likely to result not simply in a replacement of infectious disease by chronic degenerative disease, but rather in an increase in the total spectrum of disease in which vascular disease, diabetes, hypertension, and cancer will be added to the existing problems of infectious disease. Further, it is likely that marked regional differences in disease patterns will develop, reflecting differences in social and economic development. (Sinnett and Buck, 1974)

XIII. ADAPTIVE PROCESSES AND NUTRITIONAL ASSESSMENT

The assessment of the nutritional status of the community is a subjective matter and depends to a large extent on the standpoint from which the assessment is made. Thus, if the traditional concept of Darwinian fitness is applied then the people of Murapin must be considered to have an adequate nutritional status. The high birth-rate and the high level of fertility, as judged by the child–woman ratio, together with the large proportion of the population under the age of 15 years, testify to a satisfactory level of population growth. Further, young adults are well built, have normal levels of haemoglobin and serum albumin and high levels of physical fitness which are maintained well into middle age. Using this frame of reference, these people are well adapted to their low protein intake and to the other rigours imposed by their environment. However from the standpoint of the individual, the situation is less clear. The levels of the crude death-rate and the infant mortality rate, although not unduly high by New Guinea standards, do support the contention that nutritional factors and disease levels pose significant health problems to this group.

Generally little attention has been given to the role of adaptive processes in assessing morphological and biochemical differences observed in comparative population studies. Such findings as slow growth rates, delayed attainment of maturity and the marked decrease in body weight which accompanies ageing, as well as the low levels of blood urea nitrogen and serum cholesterol, all support the contention that the nutritional status of this community is sub-optimal. However, they do so only in the light of our knowledge of the morbidity and mortality patterns of the community and our evaluation of their acceptability. Seen in isolation, they purely reflect a low level of nutritional intake, but give no indication as to the adequacy or otherwise of the people's adaptation to their nutritional intake. The assessment of delayed growth curves is an example of this problem. It is customary to regard those populations showing the fastest growth curves as being the best nourished. Leaving genetic factors aside, they may well have the highest levels of nutritional intake—however this does not imply that their state of nutrition is optimal. Indeed, mortality figures from coronary artery disease suggest that such levels of nutritional intake are positively harmful (Stamler, 1967).

For the people of Murapin, altitude is the dominant environmental stress, and adaptation to this stress is of prime importance in determining the cultural and biological characteristics of the people. Migration into this area has led to a decrease in the range of crops cultivated and a consequent increased dependence, by the people, on a single staple which is frost sensitive and has a low protein content. The agricultural practice of mound building represents one significant cultural adaptation which minimizes the influence of altitude and environmental temperature on the staple crop. Cultural adaptation has been only partly successful as under favourable conditions the dietary intake of protein is a marginal 25 g/day, while periodic frosts and winter droughts threaten the viability of the community. The resulting adaptation to the low protein intake is reflected in the demographic, morphological and biochemical characteristics of these people as well as in their disease patterns.

The assessment of the nutritional status of a community and the analysis of the interactions that govern human nutrition included clearly both require a multi-disciplinary approach. It is only by establishing an appropriate conceptual model to serve as a basis for research and welfare programmes that specialist expertise can be co-ordinated into a unified plan of action. Failure to set up such a model can result in a failure to correctly identify those factors limiting the nutritional status in a particular community and, in consequence, result in the development of expensive programmes which may be singularly inappropriate in the light of the social and economic factors operating in the community. Thus any significant improvement in the nutritional status of the people of Murapin cannot be achieved by increasing the production of the existing staple alone, but must ultimately depend on the implementation of policies which combine crop diversification, development of food storage technology, improved communication and economic expansion.

XIV. REFERENCES

Ahrens, E. H. (1957). Nutritional factors and serum lipid levels. *Am. J. Med.* **23**, 928–952.

Ahrens, E. H., Hirsch, J., Oette, K., Farquhar, J. W. and Stein, Y. (1961). Carbohydrate-induced and fat-induced lipaemia. *Trans. Ass. Am. Physns* **74**, 134–146.

Albrink, M. J. (1962). Triglycerides, lipoproteins and coronary artery disease. *Archs. intern. Med.* **109**, 345–359.

Allen, T. H., Anderson, E. C. and Langham, W. H. (1960). Total body potassium and gross body composition in relation to age. *J. Geront.* **15** (Sect. A), 348–357.

Alper, C. (1968). Fluid and electrolyte balance. *In* "Modern nutrition in health and disease" (Eds M. G. Wohl and R. S. Goodhart) Lea and Febiger, Philadelphia, pp. 404–409.

Antonis, S. and Bersohn, I. (1961). The influence of diet on serum-triglycerides in South African white and Bantu prisoners. *Lancet* **1**, 3–9.

Arroyave, G. (1961). Biochemical evaluation of nutritional status in man. *Fedn. Proc. Fedn. Am. Soc. exp. Biol.* **20** (Suppl. 2), 39–47.

Australian Institute of Anatomy (1957). "Standard height–weight tables for Australians". Commonwealth Department of Health, Canberra.

Bailey, K. V. (1963). Nutritional status of East New Guinean populations. *Trop. geog. Med.* **15**, 389–402.

Bailey, K. V. (1968). Composition of New Guinea Highland foods. *Trop. geog. Med.* **20**, 141–146.

Bailey, K. V. and Whiteman, J. (1963). Dietary studies in the Chimbu (New Guinea Highlands). *Trop. geogr. Med.* **15**, 377–388.

Barclay, G. W. (1958). "Techniques of population analysis." John Wiley and Sons, New York and London.

Barnicot, N. A. and Sai, F. T. (1954). Blood urea levels of West Africans in London. *Lancet* **1**, 778–779.

Becroft, T. C., Stanhope, J. and Burchett, F. M. (1969). Mortality and population trends among the Kyaka-Enga, Baiyer Valley. *Papua New Guin. med. J.* **12**, 48–55.

Biss, K., Ho, K. J., Mikkelson, B., Lewis, L. and Taylor, C. B. (1971). Some unique biological characteristics of the Masai of East Africa. *New Engl. J. of Med.* **284**, 694–699.

Blackburn, C. R. B., Arter, W. J., Burchett, P., Murrell, T., Radford, A., Meehan, E., Ma, M. and McGovern, V. J. (1966). Hepatomegaly: an epidemiological study in the Eastern and Western Highlands districts of New Guinea. *Papua New Guin. med. J.* **9**, 21–26.

Brookfield, H. C. (1964). The ecology of highland settlement: some suggestions. *Am. Anthrop.* **66**(4), 20–38.

Brookfield, H. C. and Hart, D. (1971). "Melanesia. A geographical interpretation of an island world." Methuen, London.

Bulmer, S. (1964). Radiocarbon dates from New Guinea. *J. Polynes. Soc.* **73**, 327–328.

Bulmer, S. and Bulmer, R. (1964). The prehistory of the Australian New Guinea Highlands. *Am. Anthrop.* **66**(4), 39–76.

Capell, A. (1962). "A linguistic survey of the South-Western Pacific," South Pacific Commission Technical Paper No. 136. Noumea.

Clements, F. W. (1971). The present status of our knowledge of protein needs of man. Presented at Twelfth Pacific Science Congress, August 1971, Canberra.

Commonwealth Bureau of Census and Statistics. (1968). "Age structure of the population excluding aborigines at the census of 30th June, 1966, adjusted for misstatement of age." Canberra.

Commonwealth Bureau of Census and Statistics. (1969). "Summary of vital and population statistics: June quarter, 1969." Canberra.

Conklin, H. C. (1963). The Oceanian-African hypothesis and the sweet potato. In "Plants and the migration of Pacific peoples" (Ed. J. Barrau) Symposium, Tenth Pacific Science Congress, Honolulu.

CSIRO (1965). "Lands of the Wabag-Tari area, Papua-New Guinea," Land Research Series No. 15. Commonwealth Scientific and Industrial Research Organization, Melbourne.

Curtain, C. C. (1966). Hypergammaglobulinaemia in New Guinea. *Papua New Guin. med. J.* **9**, 145–151.

Curtain, C. C., Gajdusek, D. C., Kidson, C., Gorman, J., Champness, L. and Rodrigue, R. (1965). A study of the serum proteins of the peoples of Papua and New Guinea. *Am. J. Trop. Med. Hyg.* **14**, 678–690.

Dubos, R. (1965). "Man adapting." Yale University Press, London.

FAO (1957). "Calorie requirements," Food and Agriculture Organization of the United Nations Nutritional Studies No. 15. Rome.

Fenner, F. (1970). The effects of changing social organization on the infectious diseases of man. In "The impact of civilization on the biology of man" (Ed. S. V. Boyden). Australian National University Press, Canberra, pp. 48–76.

Forbes, G. B. and Reina, J. C. (1970). Adult lean body mass declines with age:- some longitudinal observations. *Metabolism* **19**, 653–663.

Geefhuysen, J., Rosen, E. V., Katz, J., Ipp, T. and Metz, J. (1971). Impaired cellular immunity in kwashiorkor with improvement after therapy. *Br. med. J.* **4**, 527–529.

Giordano, C. (1963). Use of exogenous and endogenous urea for protein synthesis in normal and uremic patients. *J. Lab. clin. Med.* **62**, 231–246.

Golson, J. (1970). Foundations for New Guinea nationhood. Presidential Address, ANZAAS, August 1970. Port Moresby, Papua.

Hegsted, D. M., McGandy, R. B., Myers, M. L. and Stare, F. J. (1965). Quantitative effects of dietary fat on serum cholesterol in man. *Am. J. clin. Nut.* **17**, 281–295.

Hipsley, E. H. and Clements, F. W. (1947). "Report of the New Guinea nutrition survey expedition, 1947." Department of External Territories, Canberra.

Hipsley, E. H. and Kirk, N. E. (1965). "Studies of dietary intake and the expenditure of energy by New Guineans," South Pacific Commission Technical Paper No. 147. Noumea.

Ho, K. J., Feldman, S. and Taylor, C. B. (1971). Cholesterol dynamics of Arctic Eskimos. *Circulation* **34** (Suppl. 11), 4.

Hodges, R. E., Krehl, W. A., Stone, D. B. and Lopez, A. (1967). Dietary carbohydrates and low cholesterol diets: effects on serum lipids of man. *Am. J. clin. Nutr.* **20**, 198–208.

Jansen, A. A. J. (1963). Skinfold measurements from early childhood to adulthood in Papuans from Western New Guinea. *Ann. N. Y. Acad. Sci.* **110**, 515–531.

Jose, D. G. and Good, R. A. (1971). Absence of enhancing antibody in cell-mediated immunity to tumour homografts in protein-deficient rats. *Nature* **231**, 323–325.

Jose, D. G. and Good, R. A. (1972). Immune resistance and malnutrition. *Lancet* **1**, 314.

Keys, A. Brozek, J., Henschel, A., Mickelsen, O. and Taylor, H. L. (1950). "The biology of human starvation," Vol. I. University of Minnesota Press, Minneapolis.

Langley, D. M. (1947). Food consumption and dietary levels. In "Report of the New Guinea nutrition survey expedition, 1947." Department of External Territories, Canberra.

Longley, L. P. and Miller, M. (1942). The effect of diet and meals on the maximum urea clearance. *Am. J. med. Sci.* **203**, 253–263.

Lowenstein, F. W. (1964). Epidemiological investigations in relation to diet in groups who show little atherosclerosis and are almost free of coronary ischaemic heart disease. *Am. J. clin. Nutr.* **15**, 175–186.

Malcolm, L. A. (1970). "Growth and development in New Guinea—a study of the Bundi people of the Madang Subdistrict," Institute of Human Biology Mono. 1. Madang.

Mann, G. V., Shaffer, R. D., Anderson, R. S. and Sandstead, H. H. (1964). Cardiovascular disease in the Masai. *J. Arterioscler. Res.* **4**, 289–312.

Mann, G. V., Teel, K., Hayes, O., McNally, A. and Bruno, D. (1955). Exercise in the disposition of dietary calories. Regulation of serum lipoprotein and cholesterol levels in human subjects. *New Engl. J. Med.* **253**, 349–355.

McFarlane, H., Akinkugbe, O. O., Adejuwon, A. C., Oforofuo, I. A. O., Onayemi, O. A., Longe, O., Ojo, O. A. and Reddy, S. (1970). Biochemical normals in Nigerians with particular reference to electrolytes and urea. *Clinica chim. Acta* **29**, 273–281.

McGandy, R. B., Hegsted, D. M. and Stare, F. J. (1967). Dietary fats, carbohydrates and atherosclerotic vascular disease. *New Eng. J. Med.* **277**, 186–192.

MacPherson, R. K. (1949). "Tropical fatigue," University of Queensland Papers Vol. I, No. 10.

Meyers, E. S. A. (1956). Height–weight survey of New South Wales school children. *Med. J. Aust.* **1**, 435–453.

Nalder, B. N., Mahoney, A. Q., Ramakrishnan, R. and Hendricks, D. G. (1972). Sensitivity of the immunological response to the nutritional status of rats. *J. Nutr.* **102**, 535–542.

National Health and Medical Research Council, Nutritional Committee. (1965). "Dietary allowances for Australians." Canberra.

Norgan, N. G., Ferro-Luzzi, A. and Durnin, J. V. G. A. (1974). The energy and nutrient intake and the energy expenditure of 204 New Guinean adults. *Philosophical Trans. R. Soc.* Ser. B **268**, 309–348.

Olson, R. E., Vester, J. W., Gursey, D., Davis, N. and Longman, D. (1958). The effect of low protein diets on the serum cholesterol of man. *Am. J. Clin. Nutr.* **6**, 310.

Oomen, H. A. P. C. and Corden, M. W. (1970). "Metabolic studies in New Guinea. Nitrogen metabolism in sweet potato eaters," South Pacific Commission Technical Paper No. 163. Noumea.

Oomen, H. A. P. C. and Malcolm, S. H. (1958). "Nutrition and the Papuan child," South Pacific Commission Technical Paper No. 118. Noumea.

Oomen, H. A. P. C., Spoon, W., Heesterman, J. E., Ruinard, J., Luyken, R. and Slump, P. (1961). The sweet potato as the staff of life of the Highland Papuan. *Trop. geograph. Med.* **13**, 55–56.

Patrick, P. R. (1951). Heights and weights of Queensland school children, with particular reference to the tropics: a report of an anthropometric survey by Queensland school health services. *Med. J. Aust.* **1**, 324–331.

Peters, W., Christian, S. H. and Jameson, J. L. (1958). Malaria in the Highlands of Papua and New Guinea. *Med. J. Aust.* **1**, 409–416.

Phillips, P. G. and Kenney, R. A. (1952). Plasma urea levels in West Africa. *Lancet* **2**, 1230.

Reid, L. H. and Gajdusek, D. C. (1969). Nutrition in the kuru region. II. A nutritional evaluation of traditional Fore diet in Moke village in 1957. *Acta Tropica* (Basel) **26**, 331–345.

Robbins, R. G. (1963). Correlations of plant patterns and population migrations into the Australian New Guinea Highlands. *In* "Plants and the migration of Pacific peoples" (Ed. J. Barrau), Symposium Tenth Pacific Science Congress, Honolulu.

San Pietro, A. and Rittenberg, D. (1953a). A study of protein synthesis in humans. I. Measurement of the urea pool and urea space. *J. biol. Chem.* **210**, 445–455.

San Pietro, A. and Rittenberg, D. (1953b). A study of protein synthesis in humans. II. Measurement of the metabolic pool and the rate of protein synthesis. *J. biol. Chem.* **201**, 457–473.

Scrimshaw, N. S., Taylor, C. E. and Gordon, J. E. (1968). "Interactions of nutrition and infection." World Health Organization, Geneva.

Shaper, A. G., Jones, M. and Kyobe, J. (1961). Plasma-lipids in an African tribe living on a diet of milk and meat. *Lancet* **2**, 1324–1327.

Sinnett, P. F. (1972a). "The people of Murapin. A study in human biology." Thesis accepted for the degree of Doctor of Medicine, University of Sydney.

Sinnett, P. F. (1972b). "A society in transition," World Health, February–March 1972. World Health Organization, Geneva.

Sinnett, P. F. (1972c). Nutrition in a New Guinea Highland community. *Hum. Biol. Oceania* **1**, 299–305.

Sinnett, P. F. and Buck, L. (1974). Coronary heart disease in Papua New Guinea: present and future. *Papua New Guin. med. J.* **17**, 242–247.

Sinnett, P. F. and Solomon, A. (1968). Physical fitness in a New Guinea Highland population. *Papua New Guin. med. J.* **11**, 56–60.

Sinnett, P. F. and Whyte, H. M. (1973a). Epidemiological studies in a Highland population of New Guinea: environment, culture, and health status. *Hum. Ecol.* **1**, 245–277.

Sinnett, P. F. and Whyte, H. M. (1973b). Epidemiological studies in a total Highland population, Tukisenta, New Guinea. Cardiovascular disease and relevant clinical, electrocardiographic, radiological and biochemical findings. *J. Chronic Diseases* **26**, 265–290.

Sinnett, P. F., Blake, N. M., Kirk, R. L., Lai, L. Y. C. and Walsh, R. J. (1970). Blood, serum proteins and enzyme groups among Enga-speaking people of the Western Highlands, New Guinea. *Arch. Phys. Anthropol. Oceania* V, 236–252.

Smythe, P. M., Schonland, M. Brereton-Stiles, G. G., Coovadia, H. M., Grace, H. J., Loening, W. E. K., Mafoyane, A., Parent, M. A. and Vos, G. H. (1971). Thymolymphatic deficiency and depression of cell-mediated immunity in protein-calorie malnutrition. *Lancet* **2**, 939–944.

Snyderman, S. E., Holt, L. E., Dancis, J., Roitman, E., Boyer, A. and Balis, M. E. (1962). "Unessential" nitrogen: a limiting factor for human growth. *J. Nutr.* **78**, 57–72.

Society of Actuaries. (1959). Build and blood pressure study. *Chicago* **1**, 16.

Stamler, J. (1967). "Lectures on preventive cardiology." Grune and Stratton, New York.

Tanner, J. M., Whitehouse, R. H. and Takaishi, M. (1966). Standards from birth to maturity for height, weight, height velocity and weight velocity for British children, 1965. *Archs. Dis. Child.* **41**, 454–613.

Taylor, C. B. and Ho, K. J. (1971). Studies on the Masai. *Am. J. clin. Nutr.* **24**, 1291–1293.

Tripathy, K., Klahr, S. and Lotero, H. (1970a). Utilization of exogenous urea nitrogen in malnourished adults. *Metabolism* **19**, 253–261.

Tripathy, K., Lotero, H. and Bolanos, O. (1970b). Role of dietary protein upon serum cholesterol level in malnourished subjects. *Am. J. clin. Nutr.* **23**, 1160–1168.

Trowell, H. (1972). Fiber: a natural hypocholesteremic agent. *Am. J. clin. Nutr.* **25**, 464–465.

Venkatachalam, P. S. (1962). "A study of the diet, nutrition and health of the people of the Chimbu area (New Guinea Highlands)." Department of Public Health Mono. 4, Territory of Papua and New Guinea.

Vines, A. P. (1970). "An epidemiological sample survey of the highlands, mainland and island regions of the Territory of Papua and New Guinea." Department of Public Health, Territory of Papua and New Guinea, Port Moresby.

Waddell, E. W. (1968). The dynamics of a New Guinea Highlands agricultural system. Ph.D. dissertation, Australian National University, Canberra.

Waddell, E. (1973). Raiapu Enga adaptive strategies: structure and general implications. *In* "The Pacific in transition" (Ed. H. Brookfield). Australian National University Press, Canberra.

Walsh, R. J., Cotter, H. and MacIntosh, N. W. G. (1959). Haemoglobin values of natives in the Western Highlands, New Guinea. *Med. J. Aust.* **1**, 834–836.

Westerman, T. (1968). "The mountain people. Social institutions of the Laiapu-Enga." Thesis prepared for the Committee for Scholarly Research and the Board for Missions of the Lutheran Church, Missouri Synod.

Whitehead, R. G., Frood, J. D. L. and Poskitt, E. M. E. (1971). The value of serum albumin measurements in nutritional surveys: a reappraisal. *Lancet* **2**, 287–289.

WHO (1965). "Protein requirements." World Health Organization Technical Report Series No. 301, Geneva.

WHO (1973). "Energy and protein requirements." World Health Organization Technical Report Series No. 522, Geneva.

Whyte, H. M. (1958). Body fat and blood pressure of natives of New Guinea: reflections on essential hypertension. *Australas. Ann. of Med.* **7**, 36–46.

Widdowson, E. M. (1956). Urea metabolism in protein deficiency. *Lancet* **2**, 629.

Wigley, S. (1967). Personal communication *cited* by Vines, A. P. (1970). *In* "An epidemiological sample survey of the highlands, mainland and island regions of the Territory of Papua and New Guinea." Department of Public Health, Territory of Papua and New Guinea, Port Moresby.

Woodhill, J., Palmer, J. and Blackett, R. (1969). Dietary habits and their modification in a coronary prevention programme for Australians. *Fd. Technol. Aust.* **21**, 264–271.

Yudkin, J. (1967). Evolutionary and historical changes in dietary carbohydrates. *Am. J. clin. Nutr.* **20**, 108–115.

Yudkin, J. and Roody, J. (1964). Levels of dietary sucrose in patients with occlusive atherosclerotic disease. *Lancet* **2**, 6–8.

CHAPTER V

Nutritional Research in Melanesia:
A Second Look at the Tsembaga*

MARGARET McARTHUR

University of Sydney, Australia

I. INTRODUCTION

In recent years anthropologists, geographers and others with little or no formal training in nutrition have collected and analysed data on the production, consumption and exchange of food as part of their studies in human ecology. One of the most widely acclaimed is Rappaport's "Pigs for the Ancestors" (1968), a study of ritual in the ecology of the Maring people of New Guinea. Nutrition is likely to be an important part of such enquiries, because feeding exchanges are perhaps the most important and typical of the relations between living organisms and non-living substances that ecologists study. But much of the literature on nutrition is oriented to the concerns and problems of developed Western countries, and before it can be used to interpret the quite different diets of subsistence societies there is a need to assess

* This chapter is a slightly abridged version of a paper published in *Oceania*, Vol. XLV, no. 2 (December, 1974) and is reproduced by kind permission of the editor and publisher.

its underlying foundations and their relevance to other conditions. Failure to appreciate this accounts for many of the weaknesses of Rappaport's study, but to place my criticisms of his material in perspective it is only fair to add that no such assessment is readily available. This is what I shall attempt to provide, using his data to make points of more general relevance.

For the most part I limit myself to data that were available to the author, indicating more recent information in footnotes for those who may wish to pursue the subject further. Occasionally I make exceptions if I consider later material makes the same point as earlier reports, and will be more relevant for the student.

To help readers follow and assess my criticisms, I begin with a brief outline of the author's aims and a thumbnail sketch of the book's contents. Following this I deal with the nutritional aspects of his study. After outlining and commenting on his methods for collecting data on Tsembaga food consumption, I look at how he assesses the nutritional adequacy of the diet. He first compares it with the results of earlier surveys, and subsequently with recommended "requirements".* Next I return to his suggestion that ritual regulates the slaughter of pigs and the distribution and consumption of the meat, so as to enhance its value in the diet by assuring people high quality protein when they most need it. It sounds very plausible, and he acknowledges that its confirmation would require physiological tests, but I propose that in the meantime, anthropologists who wish to pursue this line should collect details about the exact stage in situations of misfortune or emergency when pigs are sacrificed, and follow not only the distribution of meat but also its consumption.

The only other nutrient he discusses is salt, and in the course of reviewing his opinions I cite evidence, in Section V, that some New Guineans seem to have adapted satisfactorily to very low sodium intakes. Hence their physiological responses cannot be predicted from studies on subjects who habitually take large amounts. In Section VI I examine his assertion that "sanctity is a functional alternative to political power among the Maring". I suggest he reaches this conclusion by limiting politics to hierarchical authority relations. If we take the broader view that politics concerns an aspect of behaviour, namely that dealing with competition for the power to determine matters of policy, and is not a particular kind of activity, there is a whole dimension to Maring society he mentions only briefly. Many influences, of which ritual conventions are only one, regulate relations between subgroups within a local population, but there is also a competitive political

---

* I enclose requirements in inverted commas whenever I refer to a scale of recommendations, to distinguish them clearly from biological needs.

aspect to relations between these larger groups, too. As he notes, the ritual system contains no requirement specifying the size of pork gifts at a *kaiko*, though larger prestations confer prestige. Unfortunately, he does not explore the consequences of this for pork production or the timing of the festival.

II. AN OUTLINE OF RAPPAPORT'S WORK

Rappaport applies concepts developed by animal ecologists to communities living in the Simbai valley of New Guinea (Map 1). He distinguishes two systems—the ecosystem and the regional system—in both of which a "local population" participates. He considers the Tsembaga, who number approximately 200, and whom he also refers to as a "territorial group" or a "local group", a local population in the animal ecologist's sense

> a unit composed of an aggregate of organisms having in common certain distinctive means whereby they maintain a set of shared trophic relations with other living and non-living components of the biotic community in which they exist together. (Rappaport, 1968, p. 224)

The ecosystem consists of the trophic exchanges that take place within the group's territory; of these I shall concentrate on food production for humans and their domestic animals by hunting, gathering and cultivation. He introduces the regional system to accommodate other, usually non-trophic, exchanges such as the interaction or transfer of persons and the movement of goods between populations occupying separate localities. It is a vaguely bounded entity that seems to have no place in animal ecology but which

> may in some instances be more or less coterminous with other aggregates distinguished by anthropologists, ethologists, and geneticists by application of other criteria. These are 'societies', aggregates of organisms that interact according to common sets of conventions; and 'breeding populations', aggregates of interbreeding organisms capable of persisting through an indefinite number of generations in isolation from similar aggregates of the same species. (Rappaport, 1968, p. 226)

For his purpose the regional system includes those groups with which the Tsembaga marry, trade, fight and conduct their ceremonies. It extends beyond the Maring to neighbouring linguistic groups.

Many studies of religion have analysed the events, processes or relations that occur within a social group of some sort. Rappaport's interests in ecology lead him to examine how ritual affects a different set of relations, namely those between the local population and entities external to it, of which there are two types. The first comprises the non-human components of the immediate environment—the plants, animals and supernatural beings—with which the members constitute an ecosystem, and the second, other local populations similar to themselves that live outside their territory. He contends that

through ritual the following are effected:

1. Relationships between people, pigs and gardens are regulated. This regulation operates directly to protect people from the possible parasitism and competition of their pigs and indirectly to protect the environment by helping to maintain extensive areas in virgin forest and assuring adequate cultivation–fallow ratios in secondary forest.
2. The slaughter, distribution, and consumption of pig is regulated and enhances the value of pork in the diet.
3. The consumption of nondomesticated animals is regulated in a way that tends to enhance their value to the population as a whole.
4. The marsupial fauna may be conserved.
5. The redispersal of people over land and the redistribution of land among territorial groups is accomplished.
6. The frequency of warfare is regulated.
7. The severity of intergroup fighting is mitigated.
8. The exchange of goods and personnel between local groups is facilitated. (Rappaport, 1968, pp. 3–4)

The first half of the list are effects of ritual within the ecosystem, the second half effects between groups within the regional system. In addition he argues that ritual is very important in relating the two systems (Rappaport, 1968, p. 229).

The Tsembaga, like most New Guinea rural people, are subsistence agriculturalists who rely on their gardens for much of their food. They keep pigs, whose numbers fluctuate over the years, and a few chickens and cassowaries. Rappaport describes their diet, and concludes that while it probably contains enough protein to meet their everyday needs, persons undergoing stress may suffer. Consequently, how the scarce supplies from game and domestic pigs are distributed may be significant. Enquiries revealed that a set of taboos ensures that most game goes to women and children, whose needs for protein are greatest, and he was told that in the years between festivals owners kill their pigs in situations of misfortune—such as sickness, injury or death—or in rituals associated with warfare; he suggests that in all cases those under stress receive pork. The Tsembaga told him they pay most of their debts to affines at festivals, but Mrs Lowman-Vayda informed him that the Kauwasi, a comparable Maring group in the Jimi valley, kill more pigs in non-festival years to make affinal prestations than to deal with misfortunes and warfare.

Calculations, based on data he collected (some of which he admits leave much to be desired), suggest that the Tsembaga and their pigs in 1962–63, the year he observed their *kaiko* festival, were far below "carrying capacity", or in other words the maximum numbers that the territory could support for an indefinite period at existing levels of food intake without depleting the environment.

Maring have two kinds of relations with other local groups. With some, usually neighbours sharing a boundary on the same side of the valley, they fight; with others they marry, trade and are friends.

Between warring groups armed confrontation alternates with long periods of ritually sanctioned mutual avoidance. Suspicions of sorcery, and offences against women and property of the type common in Melanesia are proximate causes of conflict, but Rappaport suggests, though he can produce only the scantiest evidence, that these wrongs would increase in number with increasing population density. The Maring deny they fought over land. Again, as in other Melanesian societies, the outcome of quarrels does not rest solely on the precipitating event; the state of relations between the parties is an equally important consideration. Pressures to settle are strongest between members of the same local population, and weakest between long-standing enemies who are accustomed to fighting each other. Erstwhile friendly groups presumably occupy an intermediate position.

Most fights have two stages, distinguished by the weapons used and the rituals performed; he suggests the first or "small fight" that lasts several days, provides an opportunity to suppress rather than encourage hostilities. If those in favour of peace prevail the fight is dropped. More often, it seems, the conflict escalates into the second phase, the "true" or "axe fight", after both parties conduct rituals in which they seek the help of several types of spirits. They sacrifice two pigs; the principal combatants and their allies eat the salted pork fat from one before they go to the battle ground, and the remainder of the meat when they return at the end of the day. All residents of the local group that initiated the battle assume taboos, including a ban on trapping marsupials, eating eels, or eating marsupials and pandanus fruit together. Men are forbidden to eat pork from the festivals of other groups, many kinds of marsupials, some yams and greens, or to share certain foods with women.

No doubt the duration of this phase depends on the speed and success with which the warriors achieve their respective objectives. Sometimes it ends in a rout, and families scatter to take refuge with relatives living elsewhere. The victors could not occupy the vacated lands immediately for fear of supernatural punishment. The only mention of any doing so was a plan about which details are uncertain, conflicting and never put into effect, because, he says, the arrival of Administration officials thwarted the takeover. With the passage of years, refugees become more and more absorbed into the life of their host group, and those far from their natal territory might never return. Others living close by might gradually reoccupy their lands, at first under the protection of their hosts; in time they can invite immigrants to swell their numbers and accept others who come of their own initiative.

Rappaport was given the impression that if the combatants are more evenly matched they might engage each other at intervals for several months before agreeing to stop fighting. Each party formally plants *rumbim* (*Cordyline* sp.) in its own territory to initiate the truce. Each group thanks their ancestors and allies for help in the recent conflict, and offers them a small quantity of pork as a token of what they can expect when sufficient pigs are available. Henceforth each promises to avoid all contact with the other, and that, of course, includes fighting, and to devote themselves to raising the pigs and food for the *kaiko* ceremony at which they will make the presentations. This might take up to 20 years, though the average is perhaps 10 or 12 years.

The cycle culminates in the *kaiko*, a year-long festival, that begins with the men of a local group such as the Tsembaga, assisted by their allies, planting stakes at the boundaries of their territory. If the enemy remains on his land or has since returned and planted *rumbim*, the boundary between their two territories does not change. If not, the victors presume it has been abandoned by both its former occupants and their ancestors, and they can annex it. In practice, they are likely to blame ancestors of their former enemies for misfortunes that befall them on land they have taken over, and they may then move to safer ground.

About the time men plant the stakes, they move their families from homesteads and hamlets to the local group's traditional dance ground, where they also build accommodation for visitors. They live there for the following year while they plant large gardens. During this time they perform rituals at which they renounce food taboos assumed earlier, uproot the *rumbim* planted at the cessation of hostilities, and entertain other local groups singly or in small groups for a night of dancing. Just before the climax, young men are ritually dedicated to the red spirits, and when all is in readiness the host group invites its former allies to assemble together. They kill most of their mature pigs, make prestations they have postponed months or years before, and present salted pork to their guests from behind a ceremonial fence that they then break down. After a night of dancing and a morning of trade exchanges, the crowd departs and the *kaiko* is over. Traditionally, fighting can then begin again, though a means exists for re-establishing permanent peace.

III. FOOD CONSUMPTION AND NUTRITIONAL ADEQUACY

A. THE METHODOLOGY OF NUTRITIONAL SURVEY

To assess the significance of pork for the Tsembaga, Rappaport first had to determine the quality of their normal diet, which like that of most New Guinea rural communities is almost entirely vegetarian. He gathered the required food consumption data on approximately 240 days between March and November 1963. Each day all vegetable foods brought home to the four hearths of Tomegai clan were weighed, but he does not say by whom. They included some that were fed to the pigs, and it is not absolutely clear what he did about those. On p. 278 he says "the harvester was asked to set aside the ration for pigs", but on p. 59 "records were kept of rations set aside for pigs at the four households of Tomegai clan for a period of a little over three months. . . . The pig consumption figures were then extended to cover an additional five months for which harvesting and consumption figures were compiled for the Tomegai, and during which the pig and human populations were fairly constant". It seems likely, then, that for five months the amount fed to the pigs was not weighed.

To estimate the edible portion of the food for human consumption, he next subtracted a factor for waste that he derived from test weighings. Finally, he guessed how much vegetable food people ate away from home (p. 279), but he does not say if he simply added a constant weight or if somebody checked each day with all or most people in the sample.

He kept no records of wild animal foods because most of them are not brought back to the houses. Women and children eat rats, frogs, birds and insects frequently, but in small quantities. He thinks larger animals like eels, snakes, marsupials and cassowaries, though caught less often, probably contribute more, but in 1963 six wild pigs supplied most from this category. All 200 Tsembaga received meat from the two largest. A series of taboos and avoidances ensures that women and immature children benefit most from this wild game.

Like other New Guineans, the Maring rarely kill domestic pigs except to fulfil ritual or ceremonial obligations. The ritual cycle culminates in a year-long festival, the *kaiko*, which the Tsembaga celebrated while he was there. They subordinated all other needs for pigs to this major undertaking, and Rappaport has therefore to rely on their accounts of why they kill pigs in non-festival years, how they distribute the pork and so on. As I noted earlier, he and Lowman-Vayda received different impressions about this.

In short, he has weights of vegetable foods only, though he says these make up approximately 99% of the usual Tsembaga diet. Taro accounts for 26% of the total, sweet potato 21%, yams 9%, bananas 8%, fruits and stems 17%, leaves 10% and pandanus, manioc and miscellaneous vegetables the remainder.

Obviously, the aim of a nutrition survey is to determine the weight of food eaten by a person or a group during a specified period. The results have little meaning unless they accurately reflect normal consumption. To this end, it is important to devise a method compatible with the usual procedures housewives follow in preparing, cooking and allocating food. That is why a nutritionist aims to be present whenever food is being prepared, and weighs it before or after it is cooked, watches how it is distributed and, if possible, waits to see it eaten.

Unfortunately, Rappaport does not tell us whether Tsembaga women are accustomed to separating the raw food intended for humans and pigs, as they did for three months at his request. If they are, we are left to wonder why he did not weigh the pig feed separately for eight months. If they are not, the division they made to please him may not be very reliable. It is impossible to know, too, how accurately people predict a day's food needs for their household when this does not form part of their normal routine. Any such method of estimating consumption should be tested at intervals to see how the amounts selected agree with what is actually eaten. Without such a check, the reliability of the results remains in doubt.

An important decision in any nutrition survey is how long it should continue. Food supplies may fluctuate from day to day or at different periods of the year. The weather and the health of family members may cause variations. So, too, may work schedules, depending on whether a couple is preparing a new garden, harvesting an old one, bringing in an annual crop, searching for missing pigs, building a house, preparing for a ceremony and so on. Ideally, the results should reflect the relative significance of all these influences. But it is tedious for any housewife to have an outsider weighing food as she prepares it, and the risk of losing her co-operation effectively limits this type of survey to a week or ten days at most, and sometimes to as little as a day at a time. The same households can be revisited at a later date, or a sample selected to include a series of families. Either way, those chosen should comprise a cross section of the population, because food requirements are presumed to follow a normal distribution. Differences between household figures then indicate the likely range any family might experience, and the results apply to the whole population, not to segments within it.

Rappaport chose to deal with fluctuations in supply by weighing the food of a single group of 16 people, 6 men, 4 women and 6 children, for a period of 8 months. The duration is excellent, but not the choice of sample. Presumably 15 of the 16 are members and wives of Tomegai clan, and though the members could not demonstrate a common ancestry they believed they were related (Rappaport, 1968, p. 18). Not only that, the Tsembaga population has a higher proportion of children than his sample, approximately 9 under the age of 20 years for every 10 adults, compared to his 6. On both points his sample is not representative of the local group.

All fieldworkers are familiar with the problem of deciding how best to spend their limited time, and we can sympathize with Rappaport's dilemma. Accurate and reliable information about food consumption is tedious to collect and takes a great deal of time when women and children cook at irregular hours, in houses that may be scattered over a considerable area. Even if an observer is present, it is often hard to keep track of food once it is cooked, and while many gifts cancel out over time, this is not always so; for example, contributions to elderly relatives or others in need.

The trouble with approximations like Rappaport's is that we do not know how big an error they embody. This uncertainty limits their usefulness for some purposes, such as, for instance, his questioning of the accuracy of results from other surveys.

TABLE I

Comparative values of six New Guinea diets

Place	Per-capita daily intakes		
	Calories	Protein (g)	Total daily intake (g)
Busama	1225	19	790
Kaiapit	1610	25	1010
Patep	1900	24	1390
Kavataria	1600	41	1260
Chimbu	1930	21+	1630
Tsembaga	2015	35+–47+	2290

In Table I, I reproduce some of the data Rappaport presents on p. 283 of his book, comparing the Tsembaga with five other local groups. The second and third columns list the mean calorie and protein contents of their respective diets, and the fourth column the weight of food; all values have been calculated on a daily per-capita basis, and thus ignore sex and age differences. Food was weighed in the first four villages in 1947 by the New Guinea Nutrition Survey team (Hipsley and Clements, 1953). Lucy Hamilton collected the data on Chimbu diet for Venkatachalam's nutrition study (1962).

Readers will note that on these figures the Tsembaga diet provides more calories, more protein with the possible exception of the Kavataria diet, and considerably more bulk than any of the other tribal diets considered. The uncertainty about protein derives from two sources. As I have already noted, Rappaport did not weigh any animal foods; hence the plus signs after the Tsembaga protein figures in Table I. His two estimates of protein, 35 g and 47 g, are derived from the vegetable component only. The composition of natural foodstuffs differs according to botanical variety, soil composition, methods of cultivation, time of harvesting etc., but in addition compilers of food composition tables do not all use the same figures to convert the results of chemical analyses into the quantities of nutrients that become available to consumers. These differences are largely irrelevant for Western type diets in which highly refined foods are relatively uniform in composition, and none is eaten in an amount that gives it a predominant place, but the variations may be very significant in New Guinea diets that depend heavily for calories and protein on many varieties of one or two root crops. Rappaport used the upper and lower limits of the range of values for taro, sweet potatoes, yams and manioc from the tables of Massal and Barrau (1956) to arrive at a maximum estimate of 47 g of protein and a minimum of 35 g. He accepted a single figure for the protein content of all other foods.

Commenting on the implications of Table I, he notes that the comparison

> suggests the marked superiority of the Tsembaga diet over those of the other groups. The differences between the Tsembaga and several of the other groups are so large, however, they are suspect. The size of the disparities becomes increasingly apparent when gross intake is compared. Langley reports Busama intake to be 794 grams per day. Tsembaga intake was almost three times as great. Langley states that there was a food shortage at Busama at the time of the survey, but no mention is made of a food shortage at Kaiapit, where the reported daily intake was only 1,013 grams, less than half that of the Tsembaga.

The methods employed by the New Guinea Food Survey expedition in

1947 are not made fully explicit, so it is impossible to judge whether different procedures led to different results. My belief is, nevertheless, that figures for Busama, Kaiapit, Patep and Kavataria, which were derived from a limited number of visits to houses at mealtimes, do not adequately represent per capita consumption in those communities. With the exception of Patep, they seem much too low. (Rappaport, 1968, pp. 283–284)

I consider Langley explains clearly how she worked (Hipsley and Clements, 1953, pp. 94–105), and it is certainly true that her method differed from his. Perhaps part of the discrepancy is due to a higher proportion of children in her samples.

But rather than pursue this line of argument, it might be more enlightening to examine other published figures. Table II contains some that were collected by nutritionists in four different areas but from adults only, and therefore they should be higher than the per-capita figures in Table I. The results for coastal Kaporaka and for Sepik valley and lakeside Ajamoroe villages are comparable to coastal Busama and Kavataria, and to the Markham valley village of Kaiapit cited in Table I. All of these lowland diets have energy values below those for the mountain villages of Patep (1100 m) and the Chimbu district (1500–2100 m); the Tsembaga live around 1500 m and would thus fall into this category. The difference between highland and lowland areas is of the order of 20%, and Hipsley and Kirk (1965, pp. 109–115) suggest why this should be so. Hence Rappaport's doubts about the accuracy of Langley's data seem unwarranted. From all of this evidence it seems difficult to escape the conclusion that if his figures are correct the Tsembaga enjoy a diet that is superior to many in New Guinea, especially in protein content.

Average per-capita figures are adequate for such overall comparison of diets, but food requirements vary throughout the life cycle. An apparently satisfactory overall mean can mask deficiencies in specific sections of a population, if the food available is not divided in accordance with physiological need. Some may get more, some less than they need. Rappaport wanted to know what the members of different age and sex groups ate, so that he could assess the dietary significance of the unequal distribution the Tsembaga make of scarce food, especially meat. As he correctly points out, he would have had to take up more or less permanent residence next to the larder of a single household to get this information (Rappaport, 1968, p. 282). That is how the data for adults in Table II were obtained. It is even more tedious and time consuming to weigh the food eaten by individuals than by groups. Unfortunately, there is no short cut, especially for people whose eating pattern differs in important respects from Western diets that have been more thoroughly studied.

TABLE II

Comparative values of five New Guinea diets

Place	Daily intakes, adults only		
	Calories	Protein (g)	Total daily intake (g)
Kaporaka[b]			
Men	1640	31	1230
Women	1365	22	1140
Sepik[a]	1395	19	1050
Ajamoroe[a]	1380	37	910
Chimbu[a] (Jobakogl)	1830	25	1705
Chimbu[b] (Pari)			
Men	2360	20	1770
Women	1620	17	1380

[a] From Oomen and Malcolm (1958, p. 33).
[b] From Hipsley and Kirk (1965, pp. 77 and 110).

TABLE III

The protein value of the vegetable portion of the Tsembaga diet compared with recommended FAO/WHO and Langley's New Guinea standards

Category	Trophic units per capita	Protein (g)			
		Rec. daily intake (Langley corrected)	Rec. daily intake (FAO/WHO) corrected[a]	Estimated daily intake of vegetable protein	
				Min.	Max.
Adult males	25·0	32	37	43·2	58·2
Adult females	21·0	32	33	36·3	48·9
Adolescent females	20·5	56	27	35·4	47·3
Children (5–10 yr)	13·0	44–53	21	22·5	30·3
Children (3–5 yr)	12·0	42	15	20·7	28·0
Children (0–3 yr)	8·5	33	10	14·7	19·8

[a] Corrected for protein with a biological value of 70.

Being unable to weigh individual portions, he managed with some calculations from a set of calorie allowances suggested by Langley in 1947. Briefly, he divided her figures for specified age and sex categories by 100 to produce the "trophic units" that I have listed in the second column of Table III. Next he calculated the product of trophic units and consumer days for each category, added them all together, and divided this figure into the total amount of each nutrient contained in the food eaten by the whole group. He derived the daily intake of each nutrient for each category of persons from this "trophic unit day value for each nutrient". In the last two columns of Table III, I reproduce his estimates of the minimum and maximum values for protein, calculated in this way, but I omit his figures for calories and calcium because they do not bear on this argument. The third and fourth columns list the daily intakes of protein recommended by Langley and the 1965 Food and Agriculture Organization/World Health Organization (FAO/WHO) committee respectively, both corrected for body size, and the United Nations figures also adjusted for protein quality.

Rappaport's estimates of Tsembaga minimum protein consumption equal or exceed the FAO/WHO recommendations for all age groups, but even his maximum estimates for children fall short of Langley's. He concludes that her suggestions, which include a wide margin of safety, may be unrealistically high,* but he is cautious about accepting the FAO/WHO series which has no such margin. His main basis for doubt seems to be that he saw some symptoms that are often considered to indicate protein deficiency, namely, the condition of children's hair, enlargement of their parotid glands and their slow rate of growth, symptoms that suggest to him that the Tsembaga achieve nitrogen balance at a low level. He admits that "a clinical assessment of the nutritional status of the children would have indicated more clearly than the comparison of estimated intakes to standard recommendations whether or not there was sufficient protein in their diets" (Rappaport, 1968, p. 77), but he could not arrange it.

Unfortunately, the type of data he provides are quite useless for the purpose he has in mind. In the first place, we have no way of assessing the validity of his estimates of protein in the diets of the different age and sex groups. Secondly, even if they were reliable figures, obtained by painstakingly weighing the food eaten by a cross section of the population, the next step of comparing them with the amounts

* To anyone familiar with nutritional investigations in New Guinea, selection in the nineteen-sixties of Langley's suggested allowances is a strange choice. She compiled them following the first attempt to study village food consumption patterns systematically, 15 years before Rappaport went into the field. Hipsley's charts (1961), based on work completed in the intervening period and incorporating the results of more recent enquiries throughout the world, would have provided a more up to date scale.

recommended for persons in the various categories would not tell us how well individuals were nourished. His use of standards as a yardstick for measuring nutritional status suggests a misunderstanding about them that seems to be widespread, so I shall digress to explain briefly why they should not be used in this way.

B. RECOMMENDED CALORIE AND PROTEIN REQUIREMENTS

There are many scales of so-called "requirements" or "recommended", "suggested" or "optimal" allowances, drawn up by national or international bodies with a variety of purposes in mind. To assist people who lack a detailed knowledge of nutrition, I examined in an earlier paper (McArthur, 1964) the evidence, assumptions and guesses on which the FAO committee of experts based their 1957 scale of calorie "requirements", and their proposals for adjusting them to suit populations with different body weights, age structure, environmental conditions and so on. I showed by some examples why it is not inevitable that a group or population that fails to reach these so-called "requirements" is undernourished. Sukhatme (1961), an FAO statistician, had proposed a method for deriving the proportion of a population that is hungry by comparing household intakes with the FAO calorie "requirements". I applied it to the 1962 Japanese National Nutrition Survey, to produce the startling result that between one-quarter and one-third of the Japanese people were not getting enough to eat in 1962, a conclusion that was meaningless in the light of all the other evidence available.

There was nothing new in all this (Keys, 1949), for there are many reasons why a comparison of intakes and "requirements" does not measure the adequacy of a diet. First, all scales of "requirements" are based on certain assumptions and guesses. For example, the FAO calorie scale specifies the age, weight and level of activity of its reference adults, and suggests, using data of varying degrees of reliability, how these may be modified to suit populations with other characteristics. It makes no such adjustments for children up to the age of puberty, because many in developing countries are thought to be underweight as a result of previous malnutrition. In other words, all children regardless of actual body size, are assumed to "require" the same as their North American and European counterparts of the same age. Yet it is well known that the bulky nature of many vegetable diets prevents small children, especially, from eating the quantities that would supply the calories specified for their age group. If the "requirement" is even 25% above the amount of their traditional diets that children who are considered well fed actually eat—and there is evidence the figure may be higher than that—I estimate that this factor alone would account for a deficit of about 10% in per-capita daily consumption, relative to the mean "requirement", for populations in many developing countries. Similarly, other assumptions and guesses on which the scale is based but which do not apply to a specific population might contribute to a discrepancy between the two figures.

A second source of differences arises from the nature of the figures. To refer again to the FAO calorie scale, it is derived from what healthy people have been found to eat, and not from any intimate understanding of the relationship between the several nutrients and health. Some nutritionists argue that this puts the cart before the horse; the emphasis should be on goals for fitness and health, rather than on dietary standards (Keys, 1949). Be that as it may, one result is that the figures are liable to change. Earlier FAO committees had few good data for older children; as these have become available since 1950, the figures have been progressively reduced.

In basing their scales on what well-fed Westerners eat, the committees deliberately chose to leave out of account all that is known about nutritional adaptation. Yet as Dubos notes

> immense numbers of human beings all over the world remain healthy and vigorous on diets that are considered grossly deficient by nutritionists. . . . This paradoxical state of affairs can be explained in part by more efficient use of foodstuffs in underprivileged populations. . . . In addition . . . there are biological adaptations such as the biosynthesis of essential growth factors. . . . Of greater interest and importance probably is the fact that man and animals can develop truly metabolic adaptations to a wide range of nutritional changes, both qualitative and quantitative. (Dubos, 1965, pp. 81–82)

(See Dubos, especially pp. 81–85 and p. 475 for further references.) It would obviously be absurd to class such adjustments as malnutrition.

Perhaps the most important aspect of calorie "requirements" that limits their use as a standard for measuring the adequacy of diets is that they are average figures. The biological needs of individuals of the same size and activity differ. For example, the calorie "requirement" of the moderately active FAO reference man is 3000, but it would be possible to find a man A who fits the specifications regarding size, activity etc. but who needs, say, 2500 calories, and another B who needs 3500 calories. The fact that they regularly eat food with these amounts of energy but do not put on weight indicates their needs. The "requirements", therefore, refer only to groups, not to individuals. If A and B each ate food providing the mean 3000 calories, both would be malnourished; A would be eating too much and B too little, and we would expect the excess or deficiency to show up in changes in weight. Obviously, their mean consumption would be the same whether A and B were ingesting 2500 and 3500 calories, respectively, or whether both were taking in 3000 calories. In other words, a mean can mask excesses and deficiencies, so that a community equally divided between overfed and starving individuals could consume the "requirement" specified for it. Only examination of the individuals would reveal their nutritional status.

Turning now to protein "requirements", scales for international use follow a different approach. The FAO/WHO committees base these on average physiological needs, which are estimates of intakes required to maintain nitrogen balance and normal growth. However, no harmful or beneficial effects have been demonstrated if the amount of protein eaten is far above the probable need. Consequently, the committees have tended to err on the generous side. Instead of recommending average figures, as for calories, they estimate the mean plus twice the standard deviation, enough to cover practically everybody in the population. In the most recent report (1973) these are called the "safe levels of protein intake", and are intended to exceed the actual physiological need of all but a small minority of people. Hence, they are a different type of "requirement" from the figures for calories, but like them may also be changed to conform with advances in knowledge. Rappaport seems to have taken as his standards the average protein "requirements" suggested by the 1965 FAO/WHO committee, but for children over ten years of age and for adults these now exceed the most recently suggested "safe levels". In other words, what the 1965 report considered the "requirement" of only about half the adults in a population, is now suggested as more than adequate for most of them.

Moreover, both 1965 and 1973 figures are expressed in terms of a specified standard type of protein. The 1965 report used the concept of a "reference protein", a hypothetical protein assumed to be 100% utilizable. Members of the 1973 committee rejected this because humans do not use even high quality protein with such efficiency, and they expressed their safe levels of intake in terms of egg or milk protein, to both of which they gave a score of 100. The reasons for adopting some type of standard are that proteins vary in quality, and the foods in which they occur differ in digestibility. Proteins are made up of amino acids, of which the human body needs at least 22. Provided the necessary components are available it can synthesize all but eight, the so-called essential amino acids, that have to be supplied from outside sources. (Infants may also need an additional amino acid.) They are, moreover, needed simultaneously but in different amounts. Most food proteins contain all of them, but often one or more is present in a smaller amount than the body needs. This is particularly true of vegetable proteins, which are less like our own than those from animals. Thus, rice is short of lysine and isoleucine whereas beans are short of the amino acids that contain sulphur. The component present in smallest amount limits a protein's use—known as its biological value or quality—since it imposes a ceiling to the amount the body can synthesize of its own particular type. Fortunately what one lacks another may provide; thus, rice and beans complement each other, and the mixture has a higher value than either alone. Hence, an evaluation of the protein in a whole diet rather than in individual foods is needed, but so far as I know none has been determined for any New Guinea diet. In the absence of such information we must make do with a guess. Rappaport chose the figure of 70, and by multiplying the FAO/WHO standards by $\frac{100}{70}$ he estimated their equivalent in this type of protein. But however well informed the guess may be, it introduces a further element of uncertainty.

It is unfortunately true that earlier FAO/WHO reports left some doubts about the use of scales of "requirements" for measuring the adequacy of diets, but the most recent one states clearly.

> The safe level of protein intake can ... be used to obtain preliminary information on the adequacy of the protein intake of individuals as well as groups of persons, but should never be used as the sole basis for the evaluation of nutritional status. For the latter purpose other criteria, such as clinical and biochemical examinations, are also needed. The energy requirement, being an average value, is of limited use in the appraisal of dietary intakes of small groups; appraisal of the adequacy of energy intake is based primarily on clinical and anthropometric examinations. (FAO/WHO, 1973, p. 11)

Already in 1958 the members of the Food and Nutrition Board of the National Research Council, Washington, had made their view quite explicit regarding their figures when they wrote "it cannot be assumed that food practices are necessarily poor or malnutrition exists because these goals of nutrient intake are not completely met".

C. COMPARISON WITH CHIMBU NUTRITION

1. Surveys

Rappaport seemed to be aware that many different types of clinical, biochemical, parasitological and anthropometric data are needed to assess nutritional status, but he says he was not able to arrange for the appropriate tests. Some such data were available for the Chimbu, as well as the results of dietary surveys, and he would have done better to see how his material tallied with these, rather than simply compare Tsembaga food consumption with "requirements". Venkatachalam (1962) had published the findings of his pioneering study carried out in 1956. Then, in 1961 the Department of Public Health established a Nutrition Research Unit at Kundiawa, and between 1963 and 1965 Bailey, the medical nutritionist, produced at least eight articles reporting his results.

In one of the earlier papers Bailey and Whiteman (1963) gave details of two Chimbu localities, Wandi and Gumine. At the time of the survey food was short at Gumine. Whiteman, a nutritionist with many years experience in New Guinea, weighed food eaten by each person in five families at each locality for 24 hours on five non-consecutive days. Tables IV(A) and IV(B) compare the results for Chimbu adults aged between 21 and 50 years of age with Rappaport's estimates for the Tsembaga. In Table IV(A) the calorie and protein intakes, calculated from food composition tables, are listed in the columns headed "observed". From Hipsley's charts (1961) and the FAO Protein report (1957) Bailey estimated the corresponding "requirements" for persons with the body weights specified, and converted the figures for reference protein to the "requirements" for the "actual" type of protein in the diets. He gave the Wandi diets a protein score of 66; they contained a few grams of animal food per day, but sweet potatoes provided 87% of the total calories. He scored the Gumine diets much lower at 59; they contained no animal food, and 94% of the calories were derived from sweet potato. Rappaport, as I have mentioned converted at 70, taking into account the greater variety of foods the Tsembaga eat.

The Chimbu men and women were considerably heavier than the Tsembaga. Consequently, if their levels of activity were similar, they would require more calories and more protein. Moreover, the Chimbu women in the study were all lactating, and this would increase their needs, too. These differences account for the variations listed under "requirements". The figures in Table IV suggest the Tsembaga diet is more than adequate in calories and protein, whereas the women at Gumine had a low calorie intake and all of the Chimbu appear short of protein. Their intakes did not reach the quantities of reference protein recommended, let alone the amounts authorities consider they need of the type contained in their diets.

Bailey examined the subjects of the Chimbu surveys and concluded that calorie intakes appeared adequate for all adults except the lactating women at Gumine. The others were well built, muscular,

TABLE IV

Comparison of Chimbu and Tsembaga adult diets

A. Chimbu

No. days/ persons	Body wt (kg)	Calories		Protein (g)		
				Observed	Required	
		Observed	Required		Reference	Actual
Men 21–50 years						
W 25/6	59·5	2570	2510	27·7	31·8	48·1[a]
G 22/7	56·0	2810	2410	29·9	30·5	51·7[b]
Women 21–50 years, all lactating						
W 33/6	49·5	3150	2890	33·7	34·2	51·8[a]
G 27/8	44·8	2150	2830	23·1	34·3	58·1[b]

W: Wandi; G: Gumine.

B. Tsembaga

No. persons	Body wt (kg)	Calories		Protein (g)			
				Observed[d]		Required	
		Observed	Required	Min.	Max.	Reference	Actual
Men ? age							
6	43·0	2575	2130	43·2	58·2	25·4	36·3[c]
Women, ? age, ? lactating							
4	38·0	2165	1735	36·3	48·9	22·4	32·0[c]

[a] Diets contained small amount of animal protein, but 87% of calories came from sweet potatoes; converted at 66.

[b] Diets contained no animal protein, and 94% of calories came from sweet potatoes; converted at 59.

[c] Converted at 70; diet more varied.

[d] Vegetable protein only.

strong, physically fit and had no oedema. Skinfold thicknesses were well below the average for Caucasians but did not decrease until after 40 years of age. Ratios of weight to height followed the familiar pattern for New Guinea, beginning to decline from the age of 25 years in women and 30 years in men. This decrease with age in weight per unit of height occurs among many populations in underdeveloped countries. Many nutritionists, including Bailey, suggest it may be due to protein malnutrition. However, the 1947 survey visited three coastal villages—

Busama on the Huon Gulf, Kavataria in the Trobriands, and Koravagi in the Purari Delta—and at the time Kavataria people were each eating on average 110 g (4 oz) of fish a day. It was not possible to weigh the food at Koravagi but these people, too, ate sea foods regularly, yet height and weight data from these two villages did not differ from those inland where animal products were scarce.*

The men Bailey examined had an average protein intake of 29 g, similar to the 30 g Venkatachalam (1962) reported and the 28 g in the study by Oomen and Malcolm (1958, p. 40), but higher than the 20 g Hipsley and Kirk (1963) recorded. (Nutritionists weighed individual food portions in all of these studies of the Chimbu.) Yet it is only 60% of the 50 g of this type of protein recommended by FAO and Hipsley's standards. In view of the men's excellent physique and fitness, later confirmed by Hipsley and Kirk (1965), Bailey wondered if the protein "requirements" had been set too high, or whether the protein scores of the diets may include an unnecessary correction factor. As I have mentioned, the correction from reference to actual dietary protein takes into account the imbalance of amino acids in the diets, in particular the shortage of some that contain sulphur. Perhaps, Bailey suggested, their relative scarcity has no practical metabolic significance. If all the protein in the food could be utilized, the difference between observed and required would be negligible, except for the Gumine lactating women.

Among the other adults in the two villages and at Gembogl in the upper Chimbu valley he found 7% of the men to have mild oedema, which he presumed to be due to a protein deficiency. Comparable figures for the women were 4% at Wandi and Gumine, and 27% at Gembogl; half of them were elderly, and the younger ones were all lactating. At the time, food was scarce at Gembogl following a large pig feast eleven months before (Bailey, 1963c). Another study of lactating women, whose greater protein needs make them more susceptible to oedema, produced much higher figures, up to 80% during the puerperium (Bailey, 1964b).

The picture at Baiyer river and in two villages near Maprik presented a strong contrast. All adults were free of oedema except for two women at Baiyer river and two men in the Maprik area, an incidence of less than 1% at both places. To account for the difference between the Kyaka Enga at Baiyer river and the Chimbu, both on the same sweet potato staple, Bailey suggested in the absence of systematic inquiries that adults at Baiyer ate more game and peanuts. Dietary studies there some years later (Oomen and Corden, 1970, 1971) did

---

* Sinnet *et al.* (1973) present more recent data on changes in body build with age in an Highlands community.

not bear this out, but they were limited in scope and the food supply could have changed in the meantime. Whatever the reason for the higher incidence of oedema among the Chimbu, certain puzzling features remain.*

Village women spend much of their mature lives either pregnant or lactating, and Venkatachalam (1962) found a statistically significant difference between the mean body weight of women with one child and that of women with more than one. He presumed the fall in weight to be due to the deleterious effects of repeated pregnancies and lactation. But differences in mean heights may also contribute, and he did not take these into account. If we do so by calculating weight for height ratios (W/H), mothers with two, three or four children all have approximately the same ratio.

In the Chimbu women Bailey examined, W/H and skinfold thickness both showed a fall between those with no children and those with one or more, but additional pregnancies after the first did not lead to further declines. He noted that most of the non-parous women in his sample were young and unmarried and did little or no gardening, and he speculated that the mature women's strenuous life, rather than successive pregnancies and periods of lactation was responsible for the fall in W/H and skinfold thickness with advancing age. In the light of these Chimbu data, since duplicated,† it seems misleading to speak of the changes as a "maternal depletion syndrome" (Jelliffe and Maddocks, 1964).

In his earlier paper Bailey also gave both dietary and clinical data for the children. Most of them consumed only about 50% of their protein "requirements". The calorie values of the diets of the school age children were also below the "requirements" based on Australian and American children of the same body weight, though, as he comments, some of these are overweight. He considered the Chimbu children to be reasonably well covered, healthy and active. Some were pale but not anaemic, and on average they gained 3·5 kg in a year. Calorie intakes of the toddlers were adequate. They were well covered, even over-

---

* Ivinskis et al. (1956) first drew attention to oedema in pregnant and lactating Chimbu women but it would seem to have disappeared by 1964–65 (Blackburn et al., 1966). Vines (1970) reported an incidence of 5% in Mainlanders, slightly higher in men than in women, compared to 1·5% equally distributed between Highlands men and women. In most cases the causes were not determined, and he recommended the matter be further investigated. Overt signs of malnutrition were not common in Lumi adults, despite their low protein diets (Wark and Malcolm, 1969). Sinnet and Whyte (1963) recorded a low incidence of oedema among a Yandapu-Enga group, but noted that it probably is not nutritional in origin.
† Malcolm (1970) has since duplicated Bailey's findings among Bundi mothers. Vines (1970), too, could discern no association between lactation or higher parity and lower skinfold, body weight, lower W/H or lower serum cholesterol among the women examined in the epidemiological survey that covered all parts of the country except Papua.

weight, and though most of them, too, were pale and had reddish hair, it was not straight, sparse or loose as in patients with kwashiorkor. None were anaemic or showed any other evidence of the disease. During the year they gained an average of 1·5 kg. The infants, he concluded from a comparison of intakes and "requirements", were not getting enough to eat, though he comments that they, too, were well covered.

A mixed longitudinal growth study of children from birth to two years, living in four rural areas and on Kundiawa station (Bailey, 1964a), confirmed what Venkatachalam (1962) had earlier demonstrated, that they grow well for the first three or four months and then begin to fall behind Australian children, and by their second birthday weigh about 3 kg less. Infants of Chimbu parents who were employed on Kundiawa station fared considerably better than their rural cousins; they outstripped Australian babies for the first two months but beyond eight months they, too, gained weight more slowly, due mainly to poor supplementary feeding.

The overall incidence of severe malnutrition was about 3% in the 0- to 5-year age group in Chimbu (Bailey, 1966). Hospital admissions provide the only estimate of how significant it was relative to other diseases of childhood, and may not, of course, reflect the situation in the community. For what it is worth, the figure for Kundiawa hospital in 1961–62 was 13%. Marasmus was five times as common as kwashiorkor, and acute cases were often precipitated by diarrhoea or some other infection. Victims of kwashiorkor tended to share certain characteristics; they were usually the fourth or later child whose mothers almost invariably had either died a short time before, had suffered a severe illness or had become pregnant.

2. *Dietary Supplementation*

Another way of trying to detect a deficiency is to follow the effects of supplementing a diet with the appropriate nutrient, or foods that contain it. Venkatachalam (1962) conducted such a feeding test on 59 Chimbu men aged between 18 and 50 years. Each day for 12 weeks he gave them meat, whole milk or skim milk containing respectively 15 g, 28 g and 35 g of protein and contributing 220, 510 and 370 extra calories. They ate their regular diets, and worked in the gardens as usual. At the end of the experiment the incidence of orolingual lesions usually attributed to a lack of riboflavin was lower, but he could find "no marked changes in the general physique or biochemical values of the subjects" (Venkatachalam, 1962, p. 61).

Becroft and Bailey (1965) designed another trial to test the effect of three protein-rich foods—skim milk powder, peanut butter and soya bean meal on the growth of toddlers. They selected healthy breastfed village infants, aged initially between six and twelve months, living in the Baiyer river area. Mothers were instructed to feed their children as usual, plus enough supplement to double their protein intakes which would then reach the recommended amounts. The doctors do not mention how they checked that mothers followed their instructions, but they eliminated from their final analysis the babies of approximately 50% who did not attend regularly to collect the supplements. At the end of a year Bailey could discern no significant improvements over a control group in weight, length or any other characteristic.

3. Diet, Growth and Health

In brief, then, the Chimbu studies suggested that the children were growing slowly, partly at least because of their diets, and they might become vulnerable to acute malnutrition if they contracted some infection. As they grew older they adjusted to the bulky diet, and in consequence fared better but continued to grow slowly. Most adolescents looked healthy. Men were well built with good muscular development, and the contrast between their diet and their physique often evoked surprise among observers. As Bailey (1963b) remarked "we are in fact dealing with a highly specialized adaptation to a particular way of life". Women began in their late twenties to show signs of their strenuous life of gardening and caring for their families. This, rather than the stresses of child-bearing appeared responsible for the declines in W/H and skinfold thickness with age that were more pronounced in them than in men. Bailey suggested that a mild chronic protein deficiency led to depletion of body tissue, but as Oomen and Malcolm (1958) noted, it remained a "metabolic puzzle" how the women managed to carry and then suckle their children for long periods on such low protein diets.

For some reason that has never been accounted for, the Chimbu—or at least some of them—seem to have been more seriously affected by malnutrition than other Highlanders, such as the Enga, though it is possible that the difference is more apparent than real. Even if it is genuine, any number of factors, singly or in combination, might contribute. The nutritional quality, the proportions or the quantities, both relative and total, of the staple and supplementary foods could all influence nutrient intakes. Then, on a marginal nutritional state, one or more features of the social or physical environment might be superimposed to precipitate acute symptoms of deficiency in some individuals. Without belittling the significance of this ill health, the main impression is rather of a successful adaptation. At the same time, the tentative nature of much of the discussion indicated how little was known about some of these processes, and the negative results of the feeding tests served to emphasize the point. These should also caution us against jumping to conclusions that increased supplies necessarily have the beneficial effects we might expect. They also underline that a set of standards, even one based on the best available knowledge, might not be a reliable measure of what a particular group or individual needs to eat.

It is apparent from the Chimbu and Enga data I have cited that the composition of the staple foodstuff is not an infallible guide to the general state of nutrition of a community, but at a more superficial level, epidemiological studies around the world have shown it to be a clue, particularly if, as is true for many New Guinea villagers, it comprises a very large part of their diet. The protein–calorie ratio—the percentage of calories provided by crude protein—indicates how much of this nutrient a consumer will receive in satisfying his energy needs. Table V lists a range of values for New Guinea staples, and for comparison I have included rice, wheat flour, milk and whole-carcass pork of medium (53%) fat grade. The figures illustrate that people who derive a large proportion of their calories from tubers, especially most varieties of sweet potato, some taro and plantains, will receive in the process only small quantities of protein, especially as 30–40% of the crude protein may be present as non-protein nitrogen.* They are likely to be considered worse off than cereal eaters. Sago is the poorest of all: it contains virtually no protein, but fortunately many who eat it as their staple food are able to supplement it with fish and other aquatic animals and with plants. Communities like those living up-river on tributaries of the Sepik, or in the foothills of the Torricelli mountains, have to depend on supplementary vegetables and occasional small quantities of domestic pork, sago grubs, insects or game to provide all of their protein. Yams, some taro and the Okinawa variety of sweet potato have the highest protein–calorie ratios of the tubers. But clearly, a diet like the Tsembaga's, consisting of 35% by weight of taro and yams, 29% of sweet potatoes and bananas, 27% of fruits, stems and leaves, contrasts markedly in quality with the 80–90% of sweet potatoes in the Chimbu diets, even if Rappaport's weights are overestimated.

* Most proteins contain about 16% nitrogen, and the concentration of protein in food is usually obtained by multiplying the nitrogen content, obtained from chemical analysis, by $\frac{100}{16} = 6\cdot25$. The product is designated "crude protein", and includes a variable quantity of non-protein nitrogen as well as the nitrogen of protein and amino acids. The actual protein content of foodstuffs is rarely known. See FAO (1973, pp. 61ff and 105–106).

TABLE V

Energy and protein values of New Guinea staples and other foods

Food	Crude protein	Calories	Protein (g) per 100 cal	Protein–calorie ratio
Yam[b]	1·9	110	1·7	5
Taro[b]	1·4–2·2	130–145	1·0–1·7	3–5
Sweet potato[b]	0·9–1·3	120–150	0·6–1·1	2–4[a]
Okinawa variety of sweet potato[b]	1·67	93	1·8	5
Plantain[b]	1·3–1·5	127–140	0·9–1·2	3
Sago[b]	0·1	349	—	—
Green leaves[b]	4	44	9	22
White rice[c]	6·7	360	2·1	7
Wheat flour[c]	11·8	365	3·6	15
Cow's milk[c]	3·5	65	5·4	23
Whole-carcass pork[c]	10·2	513	2·0	9
Separable lean pork[c]	17·8	171	10·4	44

[a] Most values fall between 2 and 2·5. Figures cited by Sinnett and Whyte (1973a) average slightly higher at 2·9.
[b] New Guinea Nutrition Survey Report (1953) and Bailey (1968).
[c] United States Department of Agriculture (1963).

4. Protein Adequacy

Let us now return to his argument that the Tsembaga are short of protein. On p. 77 he sets out such evidence as he can muster: "a number of the children had soft and discoloured hair", "the parotids of a few were slightly enlarged", and he thought all of them were probably retarded in growth. He saw no case of acute protein–calorie malnutrition.

I have already implied that Bailey attached little importance to the reddish hair of Chimbu toddlers. By itself, children's hair colour is of no value as an index of protein malnutrition.

Swelling of the saliva-producing parotid glands at the base of the ears has been observed in various undernourished populations. Among the Chimbu, Venkatachalam (1962) noted that its greatest incidence— from 6 to 10 years, then decreasing into adulthood—does not coincide with the peak of overt malnutrition, which occurs in the 1- to 5-year age group and, probably, among pregnant and lactating women. Nevertheless, the swelling disappeared in the few subjects to whom he fed a high protein diet. He suggested that these findings are consistent with the view that it is the end result of continued chronic protein deficiency, though he does not account for it becoming less common in adult life. Hipsley and Kirk (1965) considered enlargement of the parotid glands to be somehow related to malnutrition, but they could not decide from the available evidence whether a shortage of protein, fat or some other nutrient causes it. Bailey did not list it as even an accompanying feature of kwashiorkor. Farago (1964) considered it more likely to be a physiological response to a diet extremely rich in starch. The glands secrete ptyalin, and she suggested that an average sized parotid could not produce enough of this enzyme to begin the digestion of the large bulk of carbohydrate. The swelling, that results from proliferation of the cells, is a response to the increased demand placed upon the gland. She found no sign of swelling in nearly 3000 people living on or near the coast. It seems a plausible hypothesis, but confirmation in the form of controlled experiments is still lacking.*

And while there is no reason to doubt that Tsembaga children grow slowly, probably like most in New Guinea rural areas, it is easy to over-look the fact that it is only in the last century and particularly in the last 50 years, that growth rates began to increase to their contemporary levels in prosperous industrial countries. It is too early yet to know whether quickest is best.

IV. THE AVAILABILITY AND DISTRIBUTION OF PORK

To begin with, however, Rappaport (1968, p. 77) sets out in a reasonable form such information about Tsembaga nutritional status as he has. By the next page, this flimsy evidence has been re-interpreted to "some pathology" which "suggests that the Tsembaga achieve nitrogen balance at a low level", and consequently "the contexts in which the Tsembaga consume the limited amounts of animal protein available to them may be of considerable significance". A few pages on he writes

> given the adequacy of the protein derived from vegetables and non-domesticated animals for maintaining the Tsembaga in nitrogen balance at low levels in the absence of stress, the practice of sacrifice in situations of misfortune or emergency is a highly effective way to utilize the scarce and costly pigs. Individuals who are already traumatized or diseased are provided with high-quality protein, which may go far to offset the nitrogen losses they are already experiencing as a direct result of the injuries to their bodies, and which also assists them in producing sufficient antibodies to

---

* The epidemiological sample survey included some coastal people in the Islands who have enlarged parotids, but otherwise the findings conform to Farago's hypothesis. But as Vines (1970) observed, it remains a mystery why the other salivary glands are not enlarged, too.

resist infection. Those close to the victims also receive protein, which not only may offset the nitrogen loss resulting from the anxiety they may be experiencing but also might possibly prepare their bodies better to withstand the injuries or infections likely to be forthcoming if the victim is suffering from a contagious disease, for example, or was wounded in warfare that must be continued. (Rappaport, 1968, p. 87)

Later on the same page he adds that "until (appropriate physiological tests) are (undertaken) this formulation must remain hypothetical only".

Before we examine some of the assumptions underlying Rappaport's hypothesis, I should perhaps note the mystery of nitrogen metabolism in New Guineans has not yet been solved, but Oomen and Corden (1970) have advanced an interesting suggestion to account for some of the discrepancies between the amounts consumed and excreted.* As a result of their investigations on this topic they concluded that "it is abundantly clear that the formulated protein "requirements" are not applicable to the original New Guinean way of life" (Oomen and Corden, 1971). Consequently, I consider it unprofitable for laymen to speculate on a matter that still baffles authorities who have studied it.

On the surface, Rappaport's hypothesis seems plausible, though in a wider context it might be interesting to examine all occasions of stress and relate them to the incidence of sacrifice. In other words, do the Tsembaga kill a pig in all situations of stress, or only in some? But in his limited version, according to the rules, if, for example, a man is sick and he or his agnates provide the pig to be sacrificed, he receives the liver and only they may consume the flesh. (If a cognate or an affine supplies the pig a larger but still restricted number of people may partake of the meat.) The first assumption—that the victim and all of his agnates are on diets containing marginal amounts of protein—I think we must conclude is not proven. The second step in the argument is that the patient's sickness distresses his agnates (or his cognates if one of them provides the pig) and throws them into negative nitrogen balance. Presumably here he is talking about who ought to be distressed, rather than who is. I do not think, for example, we can take on faith the proposition that in a society where agnates are competitors as

* So great was the excretion of nitrogen in faeces, relative to intake, some subjects even losing more than they consumed, that Oomen and Corden (1970, 1971) suggested that bacteria in the gut of these people may be able to fix gaseous nitrogen. (See also Oomen, 1970.) Strains with this capacity have been identified in human faeces (Bergersen and Hipsley, 1970); whether they actually do so has not yet been established. The joint FAO/WHO *ad hoc* expert committee (1973) convened to consider energy and protein requirements commented that these enteric organisms use organic or ammonia nitrogen in preference to gaseous nitrogen which, committee members considered, they would be unlikely to fix under conditions obtaining in the intestine, but admitted the question is not settled.

well as co-operators, the sickness of one produces stress in the others. Rappaport (1968, p. 131) gives evidence that such antagonisms in fact exist; feelings may be strong enough to prompt residents to kill a clan brother themselves or, alternatively, to provide their enemies with the means of doing so. But even if we assume the rules refer to what should happen, it is hard to see why more people are affected when a cognate or an affine provides the sacrifice than when an agnate does. The third, and possibly most crucial step in the argument is that a share of the meat restores the nitrogen balance of those who are distressed. Obviously, this could be determined only by physiological tests, but to decide if such were warranted we would need to know at what stage of an illness pigs are killed, how much meat each person receives, and how long it lasts relative to the duration of the illness.

Quantities and frequency of consumption are important because the body needs protein regularly. Most of the amino acids produced each day in protein breakdown are used again, but some are lost in urine, faeces, skin etc. The 1965 FAO/WHO Committee on Protein Requirements estimated these losses plus an extra 10% for minor infections and other sources of stress in daily life at about 40 g of protein for a 65 kg man. (The 1973 committee reduced the estimate for losses alone to approximately 25 g.) This is what has to be replaced. Only a small amount of surplus protein is stored in the body. Intake in excess of need is deaminated, the nitrogenous component is excreted in urine, and the residue is converted to carbohydrate or fat. It is the nitrogen that is important. We need it regularly because we store little, and if we consume more than we need it is wasted.

Rappaport does not say when the Tsembaga kill sacrificial pigs but probably, like most people, they delay until a victim is seriously ill; they cannot afford a precious animal every time somebody is indisposed. We would need to know how much liver such a sick person could eat, how long his share lasts and what happens to the left-overs. Considering the lack of storage facilities for food, I suspect the nutritional benefit for the patient might be very short lived, especially if he is sick for any length of time, though according to informants more than one pig may be killed if his illness is protracted. In any case, if anthropologists want to test Rappaport's hypothesis in their analyses of animal sacrifice, they should collect such details as a first step. Preferably, they would also need a physiologist on hand to monitor metabolic changes.

So far we have been considering only the pigs that are killed to meet ritual obligations arising from misfortune or emergency in the years between festivals. It is in reference to the meat from these that he propounds his hypothesis that ritual enhances the value of pork in the diet. It seems that some Maring groups kill additional animals during this intervening period to make affinal prestations, but he gives no details about these and does not say whether he thinks recipients would be under stress at the time. Other groups, including the Tsembaga, appear to postpone many or most of these gifts to their affines until they hold their *kaiko* (Rappaport, 1968, p. 82). Obviously, ritual also dictates the killing of the pigs at the year-long activities associated with this festival, and though he does not mention his hypothesis when he describes the resulting distribution of meat, I can see no reason why it should not apply to this pork, too.

For their *kaiko*, the 200 Tsembaga killed approximately 140 pigs between June 1962 and November 1963. They appear to have eaten about 60 themselves, and presumably they would receive back over the years, as those to whom they gave pork in turn held their festivals, the equivalent of the 80 or so they gave away. I can find no evidence to suggest they consumed any of this meat at times of especial physiological need. Hence, they would have to kill more than these 140 pigs (plus any they gave to affines) during non-festival years to lend even marginal support to the hypothesis. Unfortunately he does not say what fraction of a family's total herd is killed in the years between festivals, though presumably it would be possible to get an estimate from selected informants, whose memories, judging by New Guinea parallels, are usually long on the matter of pig debts and credits.

Even more damaging to his assertion than the fact that the Tsembaga ate meat from approximately 140 pigs on occasions of no particular physiological need, is my deduction that they actually wasted at least 22 of the animals they ate. I arrive at this figure in the following way. He estimated that the local group of approximately 200 persons kept for themselves about one-third of the 96 they killed on the last two days of the *kaiko* (Rappaport, 1968, p. 213). These, he calculates, would provide every man, woman, and child with between 5 and 6 kg of edible meat, which they ate over a period of 5 days. If we exclude the $\frac{1}{2}$ kg per head they gave the ethnographer's household, that leaves between 0·9 and 1·1 kg of meat a day for every individual, including the children—equivalent to a family of seven eating a 68 kg pig in 5 days. From the FAO figures he cites for pork—10·9% protein, 27% fat and 2906 calories per kg—0·9 kg would supply a man's daily calorie needs of 2600 without intake of vegetables, and would provide 98 g of high quality protein, of which less than 30 g would meet the intake FAO/WHO recommend for him. Even if we ignore the suggestion that physiologically he may not need even that much, the surplus 70% would be deaminated. The loss would in fact be higher, because a man's share of the available meat would be closer to 1·4 kg, and if he ate any vegetables at all during the five days they, too, would meet part of his protein needs. Even the minimal estimate that 70% is converted to carbohydrate or fat means that the precious nitrogen contained in the equivalent of 22 of the 32 pigs would be nutritionally wasted. The number would be increased still further if guests, who received large gifts, similarly made less than nutritionally optimal use of them.

Until we understand the nitrogen metabolism of people eating their traditional diets we cannot, of course, be certain that these calculations truly reflect the waste of protein, but there can be no denying that some occurred at Highlands pig festivals such as Luzbetak described.

> To eat 10 pounds of pork in a single day was certainly not something out of the ordinary. Sometimes a native, whose stomach had been filled to capacity, caused nausea by smelling a certain variety of the rhododendron plant and thus emptied his stomach only to be able to fill it again. Much sickness was caused not only by overeating but also by eating dirty, and especially partly decayed pork. (Luzbetak, 1954, p. 113)

Any hypothesis about ritual enhancing the value of pork, if it is intended to have general relevance, cannot afford to ignore such well-documented evidence of the ill effects of gorging at festivals.

V. SALT INTAKE AND FIGHTING

The only other nutrient Rappaport discusses at any length is salt, which the Tsembaga and their Simbai valley neighbours made from spring water, and traded together with plumes and furs to the Jimi valley for stone axes, pigs and shells. He considers the salt and axes were necessary for survival, and suggests that their inclusion in the same exchange system with non-utilitarian valuables stimulated their production and facilitated their distribution. I shall make only a passing reference to this, but first I outline, and then comment on, his account of the effects of salt consumption on fighting.

Before Tsembaga warriors proceed to battle they carry out certain rituals that include eating salt with either pork fat or the special leaves they consider make them wild and bloodthirsty. Until they depart from the fighting ground later that day they may not drink, a prohibition he suggests that is likely to limit the time they can remain out in the sun. While the combat lasts, however, the effects of the salt may increase the intensity of their fighting. Their diet, he argues, is deficient in sodium, and ingestion of large amounts of salt would allow the warriors to sweat normally while maintaining normal blood volume.

Without it, sweating may have produced a reduction in blood volume and consequent weakness. Sabine and Macfarlane also suggested to him that the salt may have played a part in catabolizing the fat, generating energy two hours after the warriors had eaten, and providing them with a "second wind" (Rappaport, 1968, pp. 136–137).

Unfortunately for this argument, many New Guineans have successfully adapted to low sodium intakes, making it unwise to assume their physiological responses would be the same as those of people accustomed to eating much salt. Despite diets that are high in potassium but low in sodium, Oomen (1961) noted that the proportion of the two ions in the blood of Highlanders appeared normal, while values in urine and sweat were not. Hipsley and Kirk (1965) reported a ratio of 0·2 in the urine of adults living in a Papuan coastal village, a figure that is only about 10% of the accepted clinical norm of 1·8. Ample sources of salt and seawater were readily available, but they saw nobody using them, suggesting the imbalance was not caused by a shortage of supply. Since then, Oomen (1967) has recorded a much lower figure of 0·02 for mountain dwellers in West Irian. People living on very low sodium diets are able to conserve supplies and maintain normal blood levels by reducing losses in urine, sweat, and faeces.* Hence, if they sweat as usual, it does not follow that the concentration of sodium in their blood and their blood volume are thereby reduced, though these may well be the reactions of people on high sodium diets.

Either Rappaport misunderstood, or he was misinformed about, the correlation between appetite for salt and the need for sodium. Certainly, depleted organisms consume it, but so do human beings and some animals that are replete (Dahl, 1958; Denton, 1967), making appetite for sodium chloride in man an unreliable guide to physiological need. Moreover, as many mountain villagers never had access to mineral spring salt, it is unlikely the Maring needed it to survive (Rappaport, 1968, p. 107).

The relative concentration of sodium and potassium has a vital role in the maintenance of several physiological processes, and the plausible suggestion that people in countries like New Guinea need the sodium in salt from mineral springs to offset the high concentration of potassium in their mainly vegetarian diets has often been invoked to account for the trade of such salt. If Kaunitz (1956) is correct, the history of this hypothesis might serve as a warning to those who wish to use conclusions reached by other disciplines. According to him, von Bunge, a physiologist, formulated this in 1901 from anthropological studies— but only by "brushing aside" evidence that some African tribes on a

* Blair-West *et al.* (1968) cite Macfarlane's study of Chimbu salt metabolism. McArthur (1972) gives more details.

mainly vegetarian diet use potassium-rich plant ashes rather than sodium salts as a condiment. After experiments in 1918 had shown animals could live on traces of salt, Kaunitz (1956) comments "one might have expected this theory could never have achieved major importance, but curiously enough this has not been so". Likewise, if fieldworkers in New Guinea had looked over the mountains, the chances are they would have found people going to a great deal of trouble to burn vegetable materials to produce a high potassium salt, which they also trade (McKee, 1955). Langley (1953, p. 101) and McKee record a preference for this flavouring over imported salt.

But whether Rappaport's facts are correct or incorrect, he fails to link his discussion of the effects of salt consumption on fighting to the context of Maring warfare. Warriors appear to eat salt only once before an axe fight (perhaps after each resumption? Rappaport, 1968, p. 142) that may continue sporadically for weeks or perhaps months (Rappaport, 1968, p. 140). Changes in blood volume, rate of sweating, development of thirst, and the production of energy from pork fat— even if we grant that they occur—would be unlikely to last longer than a day or two.

VI. THE POLITICS OF THE *KAIKO*

After a brief statement headed "political structure" at the beginning (Rappaport, 1968, pp. 28–31) that deals only with leadership and decision making within a local population, Rappaport makes no mention of political matters until the closing pages of the book. He concludes the penultimate chapter with a three page discussion of the effects of the ritual cycle on the integration of local groups (Rappaport, 1968, pp. 220–223), and in the closing pages he justifies the omission of politics by asserting that "sanctity is a functional alternative to political power among the Maring" (Rappaport, 1968, p. 237). These people, he says, are "without powerful authorities, authorities which have at their disposal men and resources that can be organized to exert force upon the physical and social environment". Lowman-Vayda (1971) gives a different impression. She argues that one type of Big Man, the Ancestor Spirit Man, occupied a political position because he had "the power to affect clan policy on war strategy and the sacrifice of pigs" (Lowman-Vayda, 1971, p. 355). He seems to be the person Rappaport calls a shaman and whom he mentions briefly in his description of the rituals before a fight and prior to the main stage of the *kaiko* festival (Rappaport, 1968, pp. 119, 182). The Ancestor Spirit Man attempts to determine the wishes of the ancestors regarding the number and types of pigs that should be sacrificed, whether fighting should be resumed, and if so, who should be marked for killing. The answers, transmitted through him, give him the opportunity to influence clan policy on these important matters, and as he makes them in the name of the spirits, his pronouncements bear the stamp of legitimacy.

Lowman-Vayda continues

> The viability of the local group as a territorial unit before contact would have depended to some extent on its success in warfare, and on its success in raising a pig herd of sufficient size to use as payments to maintain affinal and cognatic contracts for an exchange of services, including aid in war. (Lowman-Vayda, 1971, p. 355)

The Ancestor Spirit Man (and the shaman) carried out rituals for the clan or the sub-territorial group, of which there are several in each local group. But warfare and festivals are joint efforts of the larger group, and she does not mention how differences between the spokesmen of the subgroups might be resolved. New Guinea ethnography would lead us to expect that they would not always see eye to eye, and the fact that their differences were "sanctified" could conceivably make resolution more difficult, rather than less.

There is plenty of scope in New Guinea rituals for differences of opinion about many points of detail. One of the most crucial for the Maring is when to begin the *kaiko*. The outcome of this festival will determine, in large measure, the reputation of a generation of men. It is the culmination of a decade or more of endeavour, during which they have been building up their pig herds to be able to make a display that will impress their visitors, both human and ancestral. To that end they have postponed killing pigs as obligations fell due, promising instead to fulfil them at the *kaiko*. But for a variety of reasons they are not all equally prepared, and as "the Maring regard especially marked success in pig husbandry or gardening to be associated with witchcraft or sorcery" (Rappaport, 1968, p. 131), it is possible feelings run high. Unfortunately Rappaport did not witness this stage of the preparations, and he gives us no details.

Eventually, he says, some of the women start complaining that their pigs are becoming a burden to them, and when enough join the chorus their husbands decide to begin the *kaiko*. It is surprising to find men leaving such an important decision, in effect, to their wives. After all, more than half of those living in Tsembaga were born elsewhere and, in the context of the ethnography of the New Guinea Highlands might be suspect of not having the best interests of their husbands' group at heart. But I shall resist the temptation of suggesting as evidence of this,

that these women succeeded in making their point with a pig population
only a fraction of that recorded for other Highlands societies (Waddell,
1972, pp. 210–212).

By whatever processes the decision is reached, "the *kaiko* provides . . .
a ritual means for disposing of a parasitic surplus of animals. In somewhat different terms it may also be said that the *kaiko* provides a means
for limiting the amount of calories expended in acquiring animal protein" (Rappaport, 1968, p. 159). Watson (1969) in his review drew
attention to Rappaport's concentration on the festival as a means of pre-
venting pigs becoming parasitic on humans, while ignoring the fact that
it is accumulating them for the ceremony that leads to the parasitism.
Underlying this custom is a very wasteful feature of Melanesian pig
keeping that Rappaport overlooks. He argues that pigs "are a very
expensive necessity" since they "render an obvious nutritional service
to their keepers (Rappaport, 1968, p. 67), but he does not take into
account that an animal once fully grown produces no more meat, however much it eats. That is the time to kill it for maximum return of
protein. Some females must be kept for breeding, and a few for emer-
gencies, but I suspect the Tsembaga, like other Melanesians, may continue to feed fully grown animals for years (Rappaport, 1968, p. 156).
So the *kaiko* limits the energy spent acquiring animal protein only in a
relative sense; it does not limit it to the minimum necessary.

The explanation for this wasteful feature of traditional New Guinea
animal husbandry is, of course, that pigs are a source of prestige as well
as of protein. And the *kaiko*, I suggest, has political aspects akin to fighting. The word *kaiko* refers to the dancing and the Maring say "dancing
is like fighting", an expression Rappaport interprets as meaning that
"to join a group in dancing is the symbolic expression of willingness to
join them in fighting". But there seem to be certain respects in which
the hosts are also "fighting" against their allies—for dancing honours,
women, and the prestige that comes from large presentations of pork
to cancel outstanding obligations (Rappaport, 1968, pp. 184–188, 217).

In other words, it seems to me that a more comprehensive examination of the ecology of pig husbandry raises questions about the relations
between groups to which he only hints. Had he paid more attention to
the harmful or disadvantageous effects of the requirements of ritual,
he might have been led to examine the political aspect of intergroup
relations, though to do so he would also have had to enlarge his view of
politics. For the most part he limits it to hierarchical authority relations, and when he finds these lacking or poorly developed he suggests
the "sacred" conventions of the ritual cycle take their place, by
specifying the courses of action or inaction to be followed at specified
times or during specified periods. This leads him to conclude that

"sanctity is a functional alternative to political power among the Maring".

Nobody would disagree that allegiance to shared religious values can integrate autonomous political groups. But I think those who regard political action, not as a particular form of behaviour but as the aspect of behaviour that deals with competition for the power to determine matters of policy, would not consider sanctity a functional alternative to all political power. Hence they would wish to qualify his equation, not only for local populations but also for relations between the constituent clans or sub-territorial groups of each. Most of what he has to say about these latter relations consists of a list of the measures for resolving conflicts which originate in offences by a member of one group against another (Rappaport, 1968, pp. 110–112). Ritual considerations, in the form of certain taboos on sharing food, constitute one of these forces, but he does not suggest it is the most important, nor would we expect it to be. What is lacking is an account of the competition between individuals and subgroups, of which these occasional outbursts are only the highlights. That rivalry is the essence of local level politics, and in my view, his analysis of the relation between sanctity and political power will be incomplete until he includes it.

VII. CONCLUSIONS

I think it will be clear by now why I doubt that any individual working alone could successfully carry out a study of the scope Rappaport attempted. I have dealt mainly with the nutritional aspect, touched briefly on some of the anthropological points but have not mentioned the horticultural and related material.

To sum up some of the problems for non-specialists in nutrition, surveying food consumption often seems deceptively easy to those who have not tried, but figures are only as good as the methods used to collect and interpret them. A representative sample of the population is likely to be scattered, sometimes over a wide area; weighing all food eaten by a household and following its distribution between members will require a considerable part of an investigator's time throughout the year, and will often conflict with his other interests. To weigh how much an individual eats it is necessary to follow him much of the time, a procedure that obviously imposes considerable strain on both parties. All procedures of data collection should be spelt out in detail.

The next step of converting weights of food into quantities of nutrients from composition tables raises other problems, especially for diets that consist entirely of fresh locally produced products that are likely to vary widely in composition. The alternative method of estimating the nutritional content of a diet is rarely feasible under field conditions. This entails preparing a composite of all foods eaten, in the relative proportion found in the consumption survey, and then chemically analysing an aliquot portion.

By whichever means the figures are obtained they must be correlated with clinical, biochemical and anthropometric data that assess nutritional status. As I have shown, some of the results available from New Guinea are incomplete, inconclusive and even contradictory. To add to the difficulties authors of some of the papers containing this type of information do not discuss the findings of others, leaving laymen open to the temptation to select whatever best suits their argument, a procedure that is likely to provide a shaky foundation. But in addition, the standards commonly accepted for people living in developed Western countries may be irrelevant for groups whose foods and eating habits differ in form, supply and regularity. Human beings have considerable powers of adapting to a range of nutritional regimens, but it is probably safe to say that few of them are understood. This is not the place to speculate upon the reasons, but it emphasizes the nature of the difficulties non-specialists face when they wish to apply the results of another discipline without appreciating the foundations on which its conclusions rest. Unfortunately they may receive little or no guidance from many of the professional practitioners who apply a technology without ever having occasion to question its underlying premises. Finally, unless they are prepared to undertake a thorough search of the relevant medical and biochemical literature—and that can be a formidable task—they should be wary about offering "solutions" to problems that baffle the specialists.

VIII. REFERENCES

Bailey, K. V. (1963a). Malnutrition in New Guinea children and its treatment with solid peanut foods. *J. trop. Pediat.* **9**, 35–43.

Bailey, K. V. (1963b). Nutrition in New Guinea. *Fd Nutr. Notes Rev.* **20**, 89.

Bailey, K. V. (1963c). Nutritional status of East New Guinean populations. *Trop. geogr. Med.* **15**, 389–402.

Bailey, K. V. (1964a). Growth of Chimbu infants. *J. trop. Pediat.* **10**, 3–16.

Bailey, K. V. (1964b). Nutritional oedema in the Chimbu. *Trop. geogr. Med.* **16**, 33–42.

Bailey, K. V. (1965). Quantity and composition of breastmilk in some New Guinea populations. *J. trop. Pediat.* **11**, 35–49.

Bailey, K. V. (1966). Protein malnutrition and peanut foods in the Chimbu. *In* "An

Integrated Approach to Nutrition and Society" (Ed. E. H. Hipsley). *New Guinea res. Bull.* **9**, 2–30.

Bailey, K. V. (1968). Composition of New Guinea Highland foods. *Trop. geogr. Med.* **20**, 141–146.

Bailey, K. V. and Whiteman, J. (1963). Dietary studies in Chimbu. *Trop. geogr. Med.* **15**, 377–388.

Becroft, T. and Bailey, K. V. (1965). Supplementary feeding trial in New Guinea Highland infants. *J. trop. Pediat.* **11**, 28–34.

Bergersen, F. J. and Hipsley, E. H. (1970). The presence of N_2-fixing bacteria in the intestines of man and animals. *J. gen. Microbiol.* **60**, 61–65.

Blair-West, J. B., Coghlan, J. P., Denton, D. A., Nelson, J. F., Orchard, E., Scoggins, B. A., Wright, R. D., Myers, K., and Junqueira, C. L. (1968). Physiological, morphological and behavioural adaptation to a sodium deficient environment by wild native Australian and introduced species of animals. *Nature* **217**, 922–928.

Dahl, L. K. (1958). Salt intake and salt need. *New Engl. J. Med.* **258**, 1152–1157.

Denton, D. A. (1967). Salt appetite. *In* "Handbook of Physiology", Section 6, Vol. 1, pp. 433–459.

Dubos, R. (1965). "Man Adapting". Yale University Press, New Haven.

FAO (1950). "Reports of Committee on Calorie Requirements". Nutrional Studies 5. Food and Agriculture Organization of the United Nations, Rome.

FAO (1957a). "Report of Second Committee on Calorie Requirements", Nutritional Studies 15. Food and Agriculture Organization of the United Nations, Rome.

FAO (1957b). "Report of Committee on Protein Requirements". Nutritional Studies 16. Food and Agriculture Organization of the United Nations, Rome.

FAO/WHO (1965). "Report of Joint Expert Group on Protein Requirements". Food and Agriculture Organization/World Health Organization Nutrition Meetings Report Series 37.

FAO/WHO (1973). "Energy and Protein Requirements", Report of a Joint Food and Agriculture Organization/World Health Organization *Ad hoc* Expert Committee, Nutrition Meetings Report Series 52.

Food and Nutrition Board (1958). "Recommended Dietary Allowances". National Research Council, National Academy of Sciences, Washington.

Hipsley, E. H. and Clements, F. W. (Eds) (1953). "Report of the New Guinea Nutrition Survey Expedition, 1947".

Hipsley, E. H. (1961). *Fd Nutr. Notes Rev.* **18**, 95.

Hipsley, E. H. and Kirk, N. E. (1965). "Studies of Dietary Intake and the Expenditure of Energy by New Guineans". South Pacific Commission Technical Paper 147. Noumea.

Ivinskis, V. (1956). The natives of the Chimbu region. *In* "A medical and anthropological study of the Chimbu natives". *Oceania* **27**, 143–150.

Jelliffe, D. B. and Maddocks, I. (1964). Ecologic malnutrition in the New Guinea Highlands. *Clin. Pediat.* **3**, 432–438.

Kaunitz, H. (1956). Causes and consequences of salt consumption. *Nature* **178**, 1141–1144.

Keys, A. (1949). The calorie requirement of adult man. *Nutr. Abstr. Rev.* **19**, 1–10.

Langley, D. M. (1947). Food consumption and dietary levels. *In* "Report of the New Guinea Nutrition Survey Expedition" (Eds E. H. Hipsley and F. W. Clements).

Lowman-Vayda, C. (1971). Maring Big Men. *In* "Politics in New Guinea" (Eds R. M. Berndt and P. Lawrence). University of Western Australia Press, Nedlands.

Luzbetak, L. J. (1954). The Socio-religious significance of a New Guinea pig festival. *Anthrop. Q.* **27**, 59–80.

Malcolm, L. A. (1970). "Growth and Development in New Guinea—A Study of the Bundi People of the Madang District". Institute of Human Biology mono. 1. Madang.

McArthur, M. (1964). Some factors involved in estimating calorie requirements. *Jl R. statist. Soc.* Ser. A, **127**, 392–408.

McArthur, M. (1972). Salt. *In* "Encyclopaedia of Papua New Guinea". Melbourne University Press, Melbourne.

McKee, H. S. (1955). Salt supply problems in Papua and New Guinea. *Q. Bull. S. Pacif. Comm.* **5** (3), 25–26.

Oomen, H. A. P. C. and Malcolm, S. H. (1958). "Nutrition and the Papuan Child". South Pacific Commission Technical Paper 118. Noumea.

Oomen, H. A. P. C., Spoon, W., Heesterman, J. E., Ruinard, J., Luyken, R., and Slump, P. S. (1961). The sweet potato as the staff of life of the Highland Papuan. *Trop. geogr. Med.* **13**, 55–66.

Oomen, H. A. P. C. (1961). The nutrition situation in Western New Guinea. *Trop. geogr. Med.* **13**, 321–335.

Oomen, H. A. P. C. (1967). Nitrogen compounds and electrolytes in the urine of New Guinea sweet potato eaters. *Trop. geogr. Med.* **19**, 31–57.

Oomen, H. A. P. C. (1970). Interrelationship of the human intestinal flora and protein utilization. *Proc. Nutr. Soc.* **29**, 197–206.

Oomen, H. A. P. C. and Corden, M. W. (1970). "Metabolic Studies in New Guineans: Nitrogen Metabolism in Sweet Potato Eaters". South Pacific Commission Technical Paper No. 163. Noumea.

Oomen, H. A. P. C. and Corden, M. W. (1971). Protein Metabolism in New Guinean Tuber Eaters. Report to the South Pacific Commission (unpublished).

Rappaport, R. A. (1968). "Pigs for the Ancestors". Yale University Press, New Haven.

Rappaport, R. A. (1969). Marriage among the Maring. *In* "Pigs, Pearlshells and Women" (Eds R. M. Glasse and M. J. Meggitt). Prentice-Hall, New Jersey.

Sinnett, P., Keig, G., and Craig, W. (1973). Nutrition and age-related changes in the body build of adults: studies in a New Guinea Highland community. *Hum. Biol. Oceania* **2**, 50–62.

Sinnett, P. F., and Whyte, H. M. (1973a). Epidemiological studies in a Highland population of New Guinea: environment, culture, and health status. *Hum. Ecol.* **1**, 245–277.

Sinnett, P. F. and Whyte, H. M. (1973b). Epidemiological studies in a total Highland population, Tukisenta, New Guinea: cardiovascular disease and relevant clinical, electrocardiographic, radiological and biochemical findings. *J. chron. Dis.* **26**, 265–290.

Sukhatme, P. V. (1961). The world's hunger and future needs in food supplies. *Jl R. Statist. Soc.* Ser. A **124**, 463–508.

United States Department of Agriculture (1963). "Composition of Foods". Agriculture Handbook No. 8.

Venkatachalam, P. S. (1962). "A Study of the Diet, Nutrition and Health of the People of the Chimbu Area". Territory of Papua and New Guinea, Department of Public Health Mono 4.

Vines, A. P. (1970). "An Epidemiological Sample Survey of the Highlands, Mainland and Islands Regions of the Territory of Papua and New Guinea". Department of Public Health, Port Moresby.

Waddell, E. (1972). "The Mound Builders". University of Washington Press, Seattle.

Watson, J. (1969). Review of "Pigs for the Ancestors". *Am. Anthrop.* **71**, 527–529.

CHAPTER VI

Environmental Health Engineering as Human Ecology: An Example From New Guinea

RICHARD G. A. FEACHEM

London School of Hygiene and Tropical Medicine,
London, England

I. INTRODUCTION

The ecologist can be thought of as a scientist seeking to understand the interactions between an organism, or community of organisms, and their environment. This environment may of course include other organisms. The sum total of these interactions will usually be so large and complex that most ecologists will pre-define a subset of inter-actions on which they will then focus attention. This is especially the case for the human ecologist who is typically faced with a massive web of interactions between man and his environment and must seek to disentangle a discrete parcel of these interactions which he hopes he can study without being over simplistic.

Pursuing this view of human ecology one sees a group of scientists from established disciplines who decide that some particular aspect of their discipline is better studied by considering it within the context of man–environment interactions. The first task of such a scientist is then to define the nature of the subset of all possible interactions on which he will focus attention. This process of definition of subject matter will be attempted below in the case of environmental health engineering.

II. ENVIRONMENTAL HEALTH ENGINEERING

Environmental health engineering (otherwise known as public health engineering) is a branch of civil engineering concerned with premeditated man-made changes in the environment designed to improve human health. It has become narrowed in concept so that it is often taken as being simply water supply and waste water engineering and, in certain universities, it is restricted to the purely hydraulic and structural aspects of these branches of engineering. However, there is a growing awareness that the subject must be redefined in much broader terms if it is to be of real value in promoting a more sanitary environment. Thus, environmental health engineers are now increasingly receiving training which includes substantial doses of chemistry, biology, economics and more recently ecology.

Taking a detached view of environmental health engineering, it is apparent that the subject must be studied in the context of human ecology if it is to realise its full potential. The engineer is charged with making carefully planned interventions in the workings of man–environment systems and he clearly can only do this reliably in the light of a broad understanding of the ecological system with which he is interfering. Therefore, the environmental health engineer needs, almost essentially, to be drawn into the broader issues of human ecology and to relate his technical specialization to more fundamental questions of man and his environment. This is particularly true in developing countries because an engineer is likely to be contemplating an intervention the impact of which will be orders of magnitude greater than that of previous interventions in the sanitary environment. In industrialized countries, by contrast, the engineer may simply be contemplating one in a long line of interventions and he will have data from previous schemes on which to base his judgements. Similarly, the ecological approach is more necessary in rural settings than in urban ones because interventions in man–nature systems are more prone to unforeseen negative outcomes than interventions in man–city systems. In general terms, the need for an ecological approach to environmental health engineering is most apparent in rural areas of developing countries where the following conditions often apply.

a. Little or no previous planned improvement to the sanitary environment.
b. A generally insanitary environment and substantial levels of infection directly attributable to this.
c. Delicate and complex man–environment systems which may have little ability to recover from damage caused by major external interventions.
d. A high level of subsistence activity in the agricultural sector, the continued success of which is crucial to community nutrition and well-being.

III. DEFINING THE SUBSYSTEM

Environmental health engineering concerns planned interventions in the sanitary environment and can benefit greatly from the adoption of an ecological approach. It has been suggested that the need for this ecological approach is most marked in rural areas of developing countries. It is now necessary to define what subset of man–environment interactions are the legitimate interest of environmental health engineers. All those concerned with human ecology must define their area of interest and this can most easily be done by selecting certain parameters of individual humans, or of human communities, or of the environment, and then by identifying those interactions which impinge upon the selected parameters. Thus, for instance, the human biologist might select parameters concerned with individual humans on which to build his subsystem of study, the anthropologist might select parameters concerned with human society, and the biogeographer might select parameters concerned with flora in the human environment. This selection of parameters, and subsequent identification of interactions on which to focus attention, is implicit in nearly every chapter in this book although it is often not openly discussed.

Environmental health engineering needs most clear definition of its scope of interest because, in theory, nearly all aspects of the environment affect some aspect of human health. The approach recommended here is to limit the subject by selecting environmental features which have obvious and major effects on health and which are established targets for engineering intervention. These features are—domestic water supply, excreta disposal, refuse disposal, housing and air pollution.

All these not only have gross influences on health but they are also readily altered by the existing range of engineering skills and expertise. The subject may therefore be defined as the study and regulation of those aspects of man–environment systems which include these five environmental features and human health. It is clear that this definition includes many social and cultural matters as the legitimate concern of the environmental health engineer. Matters such as attitudes, beliefs, social organization, sex roles and many others will have obvious bearing on the interactions between a community and, for instance, its excreta disposal practices. The whole question of hygiene, which is a largely sociological attribute, is of central importance. So the engineer, if he is to accept this definition of his subject, must also accept his involvement with social disciplines, some of which have been regarded traditionally with some contempt by the engineering fraternity.

IV. ELEMENTS OF THE SUBSYSTEM

The basic elements of the environmental health subsystem will now be discussed individually with special reference to conditions typically found in the rural tropics and in developing countries.

A. DOMESTIC WATER SUPPLY

The most important single advance in understanding the relationships between water supply and disease is the reclassification by Bradley (1974) of water-related diseases into categories which relate diseases directly to water. A water-related disease is one which is in some way related to water or to impurities within water. We can distinguish between the infectious water-related diseases and those related to some chemical property of the water; as for instance cardiovascular disease is associated with water softness (Shaper et al., 1974) and high nitrate levels are associated with infantile cyanosis (Fish, 1974). This latter type of non-infectious, water-related disease is of major importance only in industrialized countries where infectious diseases have been greatly reduced. In developing countries it is the infectious water-related diseases which are important and so it is only these which will be considered here.

TABLE I

The four mechanisms of water-related disease transmission and the preventive strategies
appropriate to each mechanism

Transmission mechanism	Preventive strategy
Water-borne	Improve water quality
	Prevent casual use of other unimproved sources
Water-washed	Improve water quantity
	Improve water accessibility
	Improve hygiene
Water-based	Decrease need for water contact
	Control snail populations
	Improve quality
Water-related insect vector	Improve surface water management
	Destroy breeding sites of insects
	Decrease need to visit breeding sites

The classification of water-related disease proposed by Bradley (1974) rests upon four distinct mechanisms by which a disease may be water-related. These are shown in Table I, and are related there to the strategies for disease control which are appropriate to each mechanism. Each mechanism will be described.

1. Water-borne Mechanism

A truly water-borne disease is one which is transmitted when the pathogen is in water which is then drunk by an animal or human which may then become infected. Potentially water-borne diseases include the classical, low infective dose infections, notably cholera and typhoid, but also include a wide range of other diseases, requiring larger infective doses, such as infectious hepatitis and bacillary dysentery.

The term "water-borne disease" has been, and still is, greatly abused by public health and water engineers who have applied it indiscriminately so that it has almost become synonymous with "water-related disease". For instance, Pavanello and Mohanrao (1973) remark that "industrial development is leading to more intensive use of water resources often resulting in the spread of some water-borne diseases, such as malaria, filariasis and schistosomiasis". This is a most misleading statement since malaria and filariasis are clearly mosquito-borne and the schistosome trematode, which spends part of its life cycle in an aquatic snail, is not well described as water-borne.

Another source of misunderstanding has been the assumption that, because a disease is labelled water-borne then this describes its usual, or even its only, means of transmission. This is quite incorrect and in fact all water-borne diseases can also be transmitted by any route which permits faecal material to be ingested. Thus cholera may be spread by indirect faecal-oral contact, for instance via contaminated food. It is essential to grasp that water-borne transmission is merely a special case of ingestion of faecal material and that any disease which can be water-borne can also be transmitted by any other faecal-oral route.

2. *Water-washed Mechanism*

There are many infections of the intestinal tract and skin which, especially in the tropics, may be significantly reduced following improvements in domestic and personal hygiene. These improvements in hygiene often hinge upon increased availability of water and the use for hygienic purposes of increased volumes of water. They may, therefore, be described as water-washed diseases and they depend on the quantity of water rather than the quality. The water acts as an aid to hygiene and cleanliness and its quality is unimportant since it is not being drunk. A water-washed disease may be formally defined as one, the prevalence of which will fall following increases in the volume of water used for hygienic purposes, irrespective of the quality of that water.

Water-washed diseases are of three main types. Firstly, there are the infections of the intestinal tract, such as diarrhoeal diseases, which are important causes of serious morbidity and mortality, especially amongst infants in hot climates. These water-washed enteric infections include cholera, bacillary dysentery and other diseases previously mentioned under water-borne diseases. Clearly these diseases are all faecal-oral in their transmission route and are therefore potentially either water-borne or water-washed. Any disease which is transmitted by the pathogen passing out in the excreta of an infected person and subsequently being ingested (a faecal-oral disease) can either be transmitted in a truly water-borne route or by an almost infinite number of other faecal-oral routes, in which case it is probably susceptible to hygiene and is therefore water-washed. Recent publications (Feachem, 1973a; Saunders and Warford, 1974; White *et al.*, 1972) have reviewed a number of investigations which have shown that diarrhoeal diseases, especially shigellosis, decrease with the availability of water and with the volume of water used but do not appear to be strongly associated with the microbiological quality of the water. The conclusion is that, in the communities studied, diarrhoeal diseases, although potentially water-borne, were in fact primarily water-washed and were mainly transmitted by faecal-oral routes which did not involve water as a vector.

The second type of water-washed infection is the infections of the skin and eyes. Bacterial skin sepsis, scabies and cutaneous fungal infections are an extremely prevalent cause of morbidity in many hot climates while eye infections, particularly trachoma, are common and may lead to blindness. These infections are clearly related to poor hygiene and it is to be anticipated that they will be reduced by increasing the volume of water used for personal hygiene. However they are quite distinct from the intestinal water-washed infections because they are not faecal-oral and they can never be water-borne. They therefore relate only to water quantity and are not also potentially related to water quality.

The third type of water-washed infections is also not faecal-oral and therefore can never be water-borne. These are infections carried by fleas, lice, mites or ticks which may be reduced by improving personal hygiene and therefore reducing the probability of the infestation of body and clothes with these arthropods. Mites cause scabies and are also promoters of asthma. Mites, fleas, ticks and lice are all vectors of various forms of rickettsial typhus but it is louse-borne epidemic typhus (due to infection by *R. prowazekii*) which is most likely to be affected by improved personal hygiene. Tick- and louse-borne relapsing fevers (due to infection by spirochaetes, *Borrelia* spp.) may also respond to changes in hygiene linked to increased use of washing water.

3. Water-based Mechanism

A water-based disease is one in which the pathogen spends a part of its life cycle in an intermediate aquatic host or hosts. All these diseases are due to infection by parasitic worms which depend on aquatic intermediate hosts to complete their life cycles. Therefore, the degree of sickness depends upon the number of adult worms which are infesting the patient and the importance of the disease must be measured in terms of the level of infestation as well as the number of people infected. An important example is schistosomiasis in which water, polluted by excreta, contains aquatic snails in which the schistosome larvae develop until infective cercariae are shed into the water and reinfect man through his skin. Another example, especially common in parts of West Africa, is Guinea worm (*Dracunculus medinensis*) the larvae of which escape from man through skin lesions and develop in small aquatic crustacea. Man is reinfected by drinking water containing these crustacea.

4. Insect Vector Mechanism

The fourth and final mechanism is for water-related diseases to be spread by insects which either breed in water or bite near water. Malaria, yellow fever, dengue and onchocerciasis, for example, are transmitted by insects which breed in water while trypanosomiasis (Gambian sleeping sickness) is transmitted by the riverine tsetse fly (*Glossina* spp.) which bites near water.

Table I lists these four water-related transmission mechanisms and links them to the appropriate preventive strategies. In order that these concepts may be employed to assess the impact on health of a water improvement scheme it is necessary first to list the chief water-related diseases and assign them to an appropriate category. Bradley (1974) has proposed that each disease be assigned to a category which corresponds to one of the four mechanisms listed in Table I and described above. However, this leads to the problem of having all the faecal-oral diseases assigned to both the water-borne and the water-washed categories and so the categories cease to be mutually exclusive. The author therefore proposes a revised categorization, shown in Table II, in which faecal-oral infections are all together in a special category which is water-borne or water-washed. Category 2 is reserved for water-washed diseases which cannot be water-borne, in other words the skin and eye infections plus diseases which are associated with infestations of fleas, lice, ticks or mites. All water-related diseases can therefore be

TABLE II

A classification of water-related diseases

Category	Example
1. Faecal-oral (Water-borne or water-washed)	
a. Classical	Cholera
b. Other	Bacillary dysentery
2. Water-washed	
a. Skin and eye infections	Trachoma, scabies
b. Other	Louseborne fever
3. Water-based	
a. Penetrating skin	Schistosomiasis
b. Ingested	Guinea worm
4. Water-related insect vectors	
a. Biting near water	Sleeping sickness
b. Breeding in water	Malaria

TABLE III

Water-related diseases with their water associations and their pathogenic agent

Water-related disease	Category from Table II	Pathogenic Agent
Amoebic dysentery	1b	C
Ascariasis	1b	D
Bacillary dysentery	1b	A
Balantidiasis	1b	C
Cholera	1a	A
Diarrhoeal disease	1b	H
Enterobiasis	1b	D
Enteroviruses (some)	1b	B
Gastroenteritis	1b	H
Giardiasis	1b	C
Hepatitis (infectious)	1b	B
Leptospirosis	1a	E
Paratyphoid	1b	A
Trichuriasis	1b	D
Tularaemia	1b	A
Typhoid	1a	A
Conjunctivitis	2a	H
Leprosy	2a	A
Louseborne relapsing fevers	2b	E
Scabies	2a	H
Skin sepsis and ulcers	2a	H
Tinea	2a	F
Trachoma	2a	B
Flea-, louse-, tick- and mite-borne typhus	2b	G
Yaws	2a	E
Clonorchiasis	3b	D
Diphyllobothriasis	3b	D
Fasciolopsiasis	3b	D
Guinea worm	3b	D
Paragonimiasis	3b	D
Schistosomiasis	3a	D
Arboviral infections (some)	4b	B
Dengue	4b	B
Filariases	4b	D
Malaria	4b	C
Onchocerciasis	4b	D
Trypanosomiasis	4a	C
Yellow fever	4b	B

A: Bacteria; B: Virus; C: Protozoa; D: Helminth; E: Spirochaete; F: Fungus; G: Rickettsiae; H: Miscellaneous.

assigned to one of the four categories in Table II. Table III lists the major water-related infections and assigns them to their category in addition to linking them to their pathogenic agent. This classification is described in more detail elsewhere (Feachem, 1975).

B. EXCRETA DISPOSAL

The manner in which a community disposes of its excreta clearly has a strong influence on the sanitary environment in which that community lives. Hygienic and sensible disposal of excreta can not only greatly reduce the risk of transmission of certain diseases but it can also provide an important source of nutrients for agricultural activity (McGarry, 1977). By contrast, unhygienic excreta disposal will greatly increase the risk of transmission of all diseases in Category 1 cited in Tables II and III, of all diseases in Category 3 except Guinea worm and of certain other helminthic infections listed in Table IV.

Poor excreta disposal may cause pollution of drinking water sources and so interact with the problems outlined in the previous section. Excreta disposal practices are a profoundly cultural aspect of a community and cannot be considered independently of community ethnography.

TABLE IV

Infections not listed in Table III which are promoted by poor excreta disposal

Infection	Pathogen	Transmission cycle
Hookworm	*Ancylostoma duodenale* *Necator americanus*	Ova passed in faeces larvae develop in warm moist soil to reach filariform infective stage On contact with human skin they penetrate and are carried to lungs Ascend to the bronchi Are swallowed and develop in the small intestine reaching maturity in 4–7 weeks
Strongyloidiasis	*Strongyloides stercoralis*	Eggs hatch in bowel Larvae passed in faeces and develop in moist soil Reinfection is then percutaneous
Larva migrans	Various larval nematodes especially *Ancylostoma* *Strongyloides* *Gnathostoma* *Toxocara*	Eggs or larvae excreted by animals and infect humans orally or by skin penetration Symptoms caused by immature worms damaging tissues as they migrate around the body

C. REFUSE DISPOSAL

Poor refuse disposal will encourage fly breeding and flies may carry faecal material and thus promote the faecal-oral infections (Category 1, Table III). Poorly disposed refuse will promote diseases associated with rats, such as rat-bite fever, Q fever, scrub typhus, endemic typhus, plague, some arboviral infections and leptospirosis. Refuse is also a potentially important source of nutrients and may be used as agricultural composting material (Pickford, 1977) or as a food source for domestic animals. For instance, in Papua New Guinea pigs are active in keeping the area around houses clean by eating both refuse and human excreta (Feachem, 1973b) and in Nigeria large herds of goats are maintained in urban areas largely by allowing them to graze on refuse dumps.

D. HOUSING

The interactions between housing and human health are numerous and only three major areas will be dealt with here. Firstly, the manner in which the house design promotes or hinders domestic hygiene will have bearing on all diseases related to domestic hygiene. These are all the faecal-oral infections and all the water-washed infections; in other words Categories 1 and 2 represented in Tables II and III.

Secondly, the manner in which the house promotes or discourages populations of rats, fleas, ticks, mites and lice will influence the prevalence of all infections related to these animals. These infections have been mentioned previously. In addition, poor housing in Latin America encourages infestation with reduviid bugs which are the vectors of Chagas' disease (American trypanosomiasis).

Thirdly, housing has an important influence on airborne infections; measles, mumps, meningitis, diphtheria, all respiratory infections and pneumonic plague. Housing design will affect crowding, ventilation, air temperature, humidity and air quality all of which will greatly influence the transmission of airborne pathogens. A smoke-filled, or otherwise irritating, atmosphere will also influence the susceptibility of individuals to respiratory infection.

E. AIR POLLUTION

Air pollution, other than domestic air pollution referred to above, is not a problem of the rural tropics and it will not be included in this discussion.

V. INTEGRATING THE SUBSYSTEM

The elements of the subsystem have now been individually described. Figure 1 presents a model of the subsystem and indicates a possible structure and the nature of the principal interactions. This model is derived with the rural tropics in mind and therefore excludes elements such as air pollution and industrial water pollution. The model embodies some substantial simplifications. For instance, crowding will potentially affect the transmission of all infectious disease and there are some obvious feedback mechanisms which have not been shown in Figure 1. However, this simplification is justified because it enhances the heuristic qualities of the model without seriously damaging its validity.

VI. A CASE STUDY FROM PAPUA NEW GUINEA

The previous sections of this chapter have culminated in the conceptual model presented in Figure 1. This model seeks to clarify the structure of a discrete part of any man–environment system and it is argued that the subsystem described is the area of interest of an environmental health engineer—especially one who is working in the rural tropics. The engineer's involvement with subsystems of this kind will be of two kinds. Firstly, there will be the process of understanding, of study and of analysis and secondly, there will be the intervention during which changes in some environmental element of the subsystem are made which will cause waves of reactive changes to occur in other elements of the subsystem and will also induce feedback effects at the point of intervention. These two kinds of involvement, the study and the intervention, are fairly distinct and may well be carried out by different individuals. This is quite acceptable providing the intervener can communicate with the analyst and vice-versa. Unfortunately, engineers in general are much more enthusiastic about intervention than about study and the tendency in the past has been completely to omit any adequate study phase and to move straight to intervention based on preconceived concepts and on inappropriate imported ideas and technologies. This is not surprising because the engineer's training is very largely a training in intervention in the natural order and contains little emphasis on ecological investigation.

Section VI includes a case study of an investigation into the subsystem described in Section V which was undertaken by the author between 1970 and 1974 with fieldwork conducted in New Guinea for

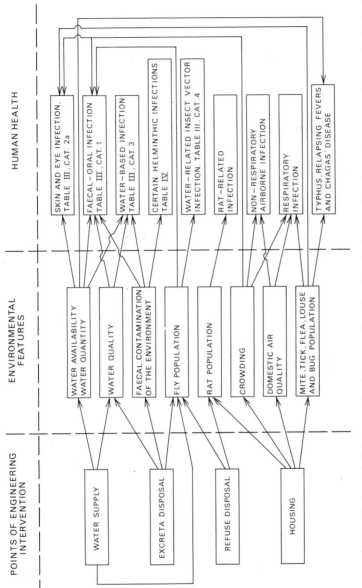

FIGURE 1. A simplified model of the interactions between points of engineering intervention, the environment and human health in the rural tropics.

11 months in 1971–72 and for short periods in 1970 and 1973. It is not suggested that all engineering interventions must be preceded by an investigation of this length and intensity but merely that such an investigation is valuable and can lead to an understanding of the impact of possible interventions which would otherwise be lacking.

A. THE STUDY SITE

A detailed micro-study was conducted on a single clan of Raiapu Enga living in the Saka valley, south-west of Wapenamanda (see Map 1). The Raiapu Enga inhabit the valleys of the rivers Lai, Tare and Minyampu in the Enga district (Map 1). They number approximately 30 000 and are administered from Wapenamanda. Together with the Mae Enga of the Wabag region, they make up the Central Enga, with a population of about 80 000. In many aspects of their culture, social organization and agriculture, the Raiapu are similar to the Mae who have been described in the extensive writings of Meggitt (see particularly 1964 and 1965). Raiapu social institutions are recorded by Westermann (1968) and Feachem (1974b) and their agricultural system has been outstandingly researched by Waddell (1972). Data reported here are drawn from a study of the Tombeakini clan of the Saka valley (the valley of the River Tare). The Saka valley is depicted in Figure 2.

The Raiapu form patrilineal, segmentary, descent hierarchies comprising phratries, clans, subclans and patrilineages. All are named after their putative founders and, in any hierarchy, the founders are agnatically related so that the sons of the phratry founder are usually themselves clan founders. The clan is ideally exogamous (in practice also except in the case of large clans of perhaps 800 people) and clan members reside in a continuous stretch of territory which is deemed to be a clan possession. Population densities often exceed 80 per km² and in some areas rise to over 300 per km² (see Figure 3). Neighbouring clans frequently experience hostile relations (despite the high probability that they belong to the same phratry) and borders are often contested in the courts and ultimately in fierce warfare. The Raiapu scatter their houses about the clan's territory.

The Raiapu staple food is sweet potato grown in large mulched mounds shown in Figure 4. They also cultivate a range of vegetables, sugar cane and bananas which provide them with a fairly varied diet (see Waddell, 1972). Pigs are kept primarily for exchange and ceremonial purposes and pork is not a regular item of Raiapu diet. Feachem (1973b) gives an account of Raiapu pig husbandry and the size of pig

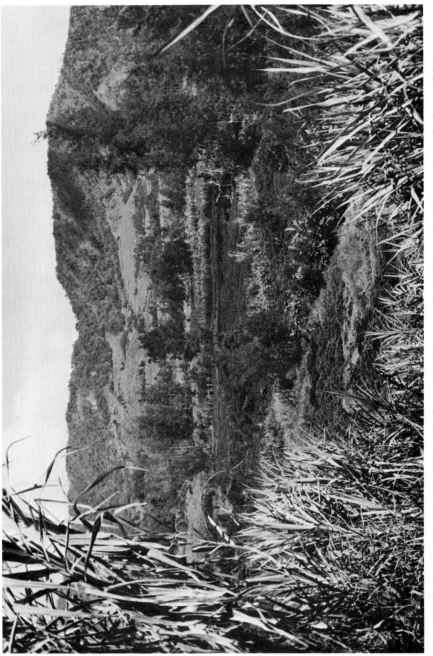

FIGURE 2. The intense cultivation of the Saka valley floor and the large areas devoted to sweet potato mounds are clearly seen. Most houses are concealed in the stands of casuarina trees.

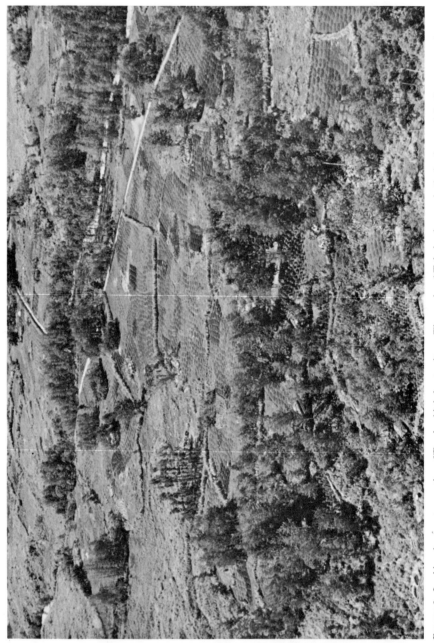

FIGURE 3. Looking down onto a section of Tombeakini clan territory. The road and Tobaka river are in the background. In the centre are large areas of sweet potato mounds and, in front of them, casuarina stands, houses, mixed gardens and coffee can be seen.

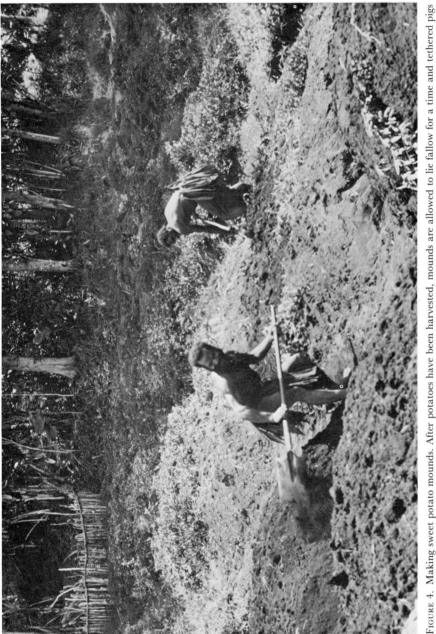

FIGURE 4. Making sweet potato mounds. After potatoes have been harvested, mounds are allowed to lie fallow for a time and tethered pigs forage on them. They are then dug open and remade (as in the photograph) and the centres are filled with old potato vines and other mulch.

herds. In recent years they have turned enthusiastically to the cash cropping of coffee and introduced vegetables, as described by Waddell (1972) and by Meggitt (1971) for the Mae. I (Feachem, 1973c) have described Raiapu religious belief and ritual and have also provided an outline of Raiapu ethnography (Feachem, 1974b).

Map 4 shows the territory of Tombeakini at Lyokote. Lyokote is one of 14 named localities within the territory but, since it includes both the *Tee*-ground (an area for ceremonial activity especially for the *Tee*

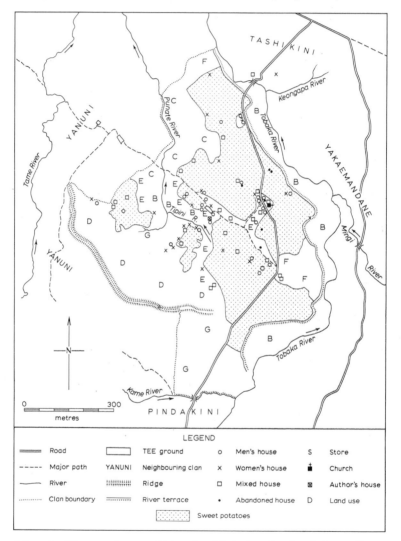

MAP 4. The territory of Tombeakini clan in the Saka valley.

and other pig exchanges) and the cluster of houses round the church, it is often used to refer to the whole clan territory. A vehicular road runs through Lyokote and joins the main Saka road which, in turn, joins the Highlands Highway near Wapenamanda. Various land use

TABLE V

Land use classification of Tombeakini territory[a]

Category	Area (km²)	% of clan area	Description	Utilization
Sweet potato fields	0·21	38	Extensive open fields in which *lpomoea batatas* is cultivated in large mulched mounds	Produces dietary staple and supports pig herds
B	0·09	16	Swampy river flats with casuarina stands and ponds for *kuta* cultivation	*Casuarina oligodon* for timber (*Eleocharis sphacelata* and *E. dulcis*) for women's aprons Pig foraging
C	0·04	7	Grassy swamps	Some taro (*Colocas iaesculenta*) Pig foraging
D	0·07	13	Steep hillside with grass, shrubs and limestone outcrops	*Miscanthus floridus* and *Imperata cylindrica* for house construction A little honey Caves used as retreats in times of war
E	0·08	14	Mixed gardens and coffee gardens	Wide range of traditional and introduced vegetables and coffee Often sold to provide main source of cash income
F	0·03	5	Sweet potato garden lying fallow or with disputed ownership	Pig grazing
G	0·04	7	Steep hillside with cover of trees and scrub Limestone outcrops	Pig foraging and timber A little honey

[a] See Map 4.

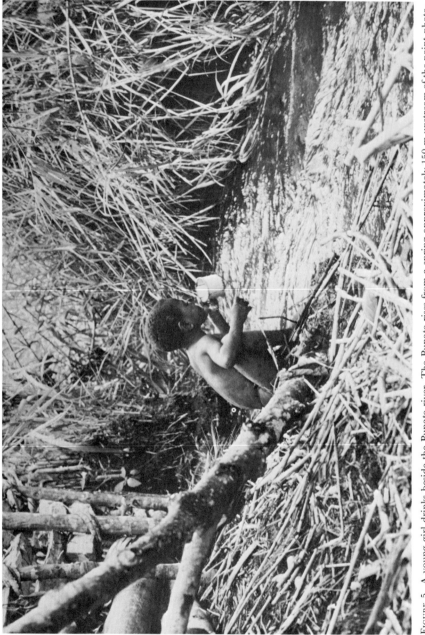

FIGURE 5. A young girl drinks beside the Punate river. The Punate rises from a spring approximately 150 m upstream of the point photographed and is the cleanest water source used by Tombeakini. It has a mean temperature of 15°C, a mean turbidity of 11, and mean faecal coliform and faecal streptococci concentrations of 8/100 ml and 40/100 ml, respectively. It is used as a water source by approximately 250 people and most of its faecal pollution derives from pigs. It has a mean flow of about 0·5 m³/sec.

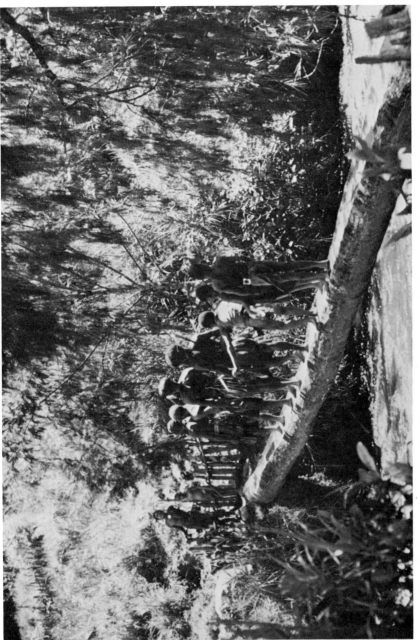

FIGURE 6. Men crossing the Tobaka river. The Tobaka is the third largest river in the Saka with a mean flow of approximately 6·5 m³/sec. It has a mean temperature of 14·4°C, a mean turbidity of 53, and mean faecal coliform and faecal streptococci concentrations of 220/100 ml and 270/100 ml, respectively. It is used as a water source by approximately 1000 people.

categories are indicated on Map 4 by capital letters and these are identified in Table V. Tombeakini has a population of 211 with a density, on the land they claim to be theirs, of 377 persons per km².

Map 4 also indicates the location of various house types which have been described as either "men's", "women's" or "mixed". The men traditionally lived in clubhouses (the men's houses) with older male children, while their wives lived apart with infants, female children and pigs (in women's houses). Today this separation is breaking down and, in 1971, 33% of houses (the mixed houses) in Tombeakini territory were inhabited by nuclear families and their pigs, and contained 48% of the clan population. Meggitt (1964) describes the male–female antagonisms which underlie the sexual segregation of living quarters. This description of housing is relevant to the survey of water use. The normal approach to a water usage survey (for instance White *et al.*, 1972) is to deal with households and household consumption. This is only applicable, however, if the household is a domestic unit with a shared behaviour pattern with respect to water collection, washing, cooking etc. For the Tombeakini mixed household, this is the case. The family is a domestic unit whose members cook and eat together and who share the water which one of them collects. In the case of men's and women's households the situation is more complex and flexible. A woman living with her children in a women's house will cook and eat in that house and may be joined for evening and morning meals by her husband. However, her husband may eat in his men's house or he may join another of his wives (if he is a polygynist) for his meals. An old woman living alone may eat with her daughter-in-law or may join another similar woman. It is also common for old women to be visited by their unmarried, adult sons for meals.

This complex situation necessitates the identification of a "domestic group" for the purpose of the water usage survey. A domestic group is comprised of people who habitually eat their evening (and perhaps their morning) meal together and who share water which has been brought to the house where they gather. They may, or may not, cohabit and they are usually closely related. The size of a domestic group is measured in consumption units which are, somewhat arbitrarily, defined on the basis of children under ten years of age equalling one-half of a unit and all others equalling one unit. All domestic groups sizes are expressed as the mean number of consumption units who belonged to the group during 1971.

Tombeakini have access to two major rivers—the Punate and the Tobaka (shown on Map 4). The Punate rises inside clan territory from a pair of springs at the foot of a limestone outcrop. It is soon joined by the Tipini stream. The Tobaka forms the eastern border of Tombeakini territory and rises at approximately 3500 m many miles to the south on Sugarloaf Mountain. Figures 5 and 6 depict the Punate and the Tobaka respectively.

B. DOMESTIC WATER SUPPLY

1. Attitudes to Water

The Raiapu view of water is generally prosaic. The rivers have never been known to dry up and they are very much taken for granted. Droughts occur (for instance in 1972) but it is the frosts which accompany the droughts that the Raiapu really fear since frosts kill the sweet potatoes. No religious ritual or magic is undertaken to promote rain and people are more concerned with flooding than droughts. The Raiapu perceive the fundamentals of hydrology and are generally uncurious about more complex aspects. They know that rainfall drains into rivers and that heavy rain will lead to floods. They appreciate the power of water to erode and the way in which rivers change their course and eat away their banks. It is now known that the rivers flow down to the sea but before contact, their destination was not known. The source of rain is the *yalyakali* or sky people, who live in a world above the earth and are the creative beings. It is said that rain is caused by sky women (*yalya enda*) swimming in a lake which then spills over the edge and falls to earth. Some say that rain is caused by the sky women urinating. If heavy rain comes it is treated fatalistically and the *yalyakali* are not blamed or appealed to (Feachem, 1973c).

The qualities of water most appreciated by the Raiapu are clearness and coldness and they prefer to drink water of this type. Warm and turbid water will be drunk if that is all which is available, and it is not generally felt that any sickness, or other bad outcome, will result. Some say that drinking very turbid water will lead to a blockage of the small intestine, but this does not worry most Raiapu. If turbid water is collected it is often left to settle before drinking. On a hot day water will be collected in a gourd or bamboo because it is thought (quite correctly) that it stays cooler than in a metal pot or bottle. Water is almost never stored inside a house lest it becomes unpalatably warm. Rainwater is considered good water but it will not be collected from the roof of a house. Roofs are made of thatched *Imperata cylindrica* and water that has run off them contains a heavy load of dust and small grass particles. Rainwater is collected from dripping trees during heavy rain.

The Raiapu are continually apprehensive about the possibility that enemies will introduce menstrual blood, faeces or parts of a corpse into their food or water. To consume these items would mean serious illness or death. The ownership of a spring precludes such a danger but many Raiapu use water which has travelled through the territories of other clans, some of which may well be hostile. This gives rise to accusations and litigations concerning the poisoning of water supplies and may well lead to warfare. Such disputes are not common, however, when compared with other sources of inter-clan strife. Feachem (1973c) should be consulted for an account of Raiapu religious belief, ritual and sorcery.

Males are constantly aware of the contaminating nature of women, which can cause them to become prematurely old and lose their vigour and potency. Meggitt (1964) gives an account of male–female antagonisms amongst the Mae, and the Raiapu case is very similar. Due to this; males will never drink immediately downstream of a place where women are standing or have recently waded. A women, who notices that a man is about to inadvertently drink downstream of a place where she has been standing, will often call out to warn the man of his danger. If she does not do this and is observed by other men, she will be severely chastised for not drawing attention to the hazard.

Generally speaking, larger rivers are regarded as safe from all types of pollution since any contaminants will be quickly carried downstream. Small rivers need to be protected from major pollution (e.g. women), but are acceptable as washing places for pigs' intestines. The smallest rivers are not considered capable of cleansing themselves at all and so they are not used for any washing activities.

2. Choice of Water Source

Typically, the Raiapu use whichever acceptable water source involves the shortest collection journey. Acceptable sources are all streams and rivers, except extremely small and obviously foul trickles, which can be reached without leaving the clan territory. A slight preference is shown for sources which are unusually clear and cool (such as a spring) but only a very few domestic groups will use a spring if there is an alternative source which is closer (Feachem, 1973d). Springs are greatly valued since they not only provide water which is cold and clear but also they are not exposed to the risk of poisoning by upstream enemies or of fouling in floods. Rainwater is popular but can only be collected on days of heavy rainfall. During August 1971 (dry season) only 1·1% of collection journeys were made for rainwater, whereas during December (wet season) the figure was 13·5%.

Since the Raiapu draw their water from natural unprotected sources, and since the area has a high population density of over 100 people and 200 pigs per km², it is not surprising that the water used contains an appreciable load of faecal material. The clan studied used four major streams and the pollution characteristics of these (monitored once a week for 20 weeks) are given in Table VI. There is a clear range from a source which is clean by local standards (river no. 1, Figure 5) to one which has a dangerously high load of faecal material (river no. 2) and will therefore almost certainly contain pathogenic organisms. Details of the microbiological quality of streams in the Saka valley are reported elsewhere (Feachem, 1974a).

TABLE VI

Mean faecal bacterial concentrations, temperatures and turbidities in four Saka rivers during June to December, 1971

River No.	Mean temperature at time of collection (°C)	Mean turbidity	Faecal coliforms colonies per 100 ml	Faecal streptococci colonies per 100 ml
1	15·1	11	8	40
2	20·5	56	1563	1405
3	14·4	53	220	270
4	21·2	29	669	559

3. Water Use

Water use was surveyed by examining the behaviour of 38 "domestic groups". A domestic group meets for its evening and morning meals and its members are usually close relatives. Approximately 40% of domestic groups are also households. The domestic groups surveyed had a mean size of 3·6 consumption units (under 10 years old = $\frac{1}{2}$ unit; all others = 1 unit) and a mean round trip travel time to their nearest water source of 12·5 minutes.

Water is collected at all times except at night; mainly in the late afternoon. Slightly more is collected by females and people of all ages participate; 47% of journeys are made by children or teenagers. It is collected most commonly in gourds or glass bottles but pots, bamboos and tins are often used.

In assessing the benefits which may accrue from a new water supply scheme, it is necessary to know the cost of water in the existing water use system in order that this may be compared to the cost from the proposed new supply. The Raiapu clearly have to make no direct payment for their water. The cost therefore is simply the energy cost of water collection added to the cost of the time spent in water collection which could be otherwise employed. The energy cost is calculated by costing the quantity of staple food required to provide the amount of energy used in water collection. It is not possible to produce a realistic estimate of the opportunity cost of the time spent in water collection. It is assumed, however, that the time is worth at least the cost of food consumed in that time which is calculated by distributing the total caloric intake uniformly over a 24-hour period. The energy cost and the time cost are added to give a value for the total cost of water collection.

Adding the energy cost to the time cost gives 91·75 calories per domestic group per day. This is converted into monetary units by assuming a cost of sweet potato of 1 cent (Australian currency) per pound (the price paid by Waso Ltd of Wapenamanda during 1971) and a caloric content of 150 calories per 100 g of sweet potato (Hipsley and Kirk, 1965, p. 39). Applying these data, costs of 0·134 cents per domestic group daily, 0·037 cents per capita daily and 0·054 cents per litre are obtained.

The pattern of domestic water usage is tabulated in Table VII. It should be stressed that figures refer only to water which is brought to the dwelling and do not include any extra-domiciliary water usage. Seventy-nine per cent of water collected is drunk; of the remaining 21%, 47% is used for cooking, 36% for pigs, 4% for washing, 2% for dogs and chickens and 11% is thrown away. Twenty-nine per cent of domestic groups surveyed used water only for drinking. Per-capita usage is shown in Table VIII.

The most striking feature of the data in Tables VII and VIII is the extremely low level of water use. The Raiapu use little water for purposes other than drinking and they drink little water. This results in low per-capita total usage. The figure of 0·54 litres per capita daily (Table VIII) excludes any water that is drunk away from home and also excludes water drunk in the form of soup (the Raiapu do not typically drink tea or coffee). My impression is that, during days of light work and moderate weather, the Raiapu will drink little or nothing away from home. However, during heavy tasks (clearing new gardens, house building etc.) or hot weather, they will drink heavily while at work. I therefore suggest a mean figure of 0·7 litres per capita daily for water consumed throughout the day. Waddell (1972, p. 121) provides dietary data for a Raiapu clan at the entrance to the Saka valley. Using this, I calculate that the Raiapu consume approximately 1·38 litres per capita daily of water in food and 0·36 litres of water of oxidation (assuming 150 ml of water per 1000 calories of food oxidized).

TABLE VII

Water usage per domestic group

Usage category	Volume used litres per domestic group per day			% of total used	Comments
	Mean	Min.	Max.	(Mean)	
Drinking	1·93	0·60	4·37	79	Mainly drunk with the morning and evening meals
Cooking	0·25	0	2·08	10	Cooking purchased rice, pumpkin leaves and vegetable soups 45% of d.g.s. used no water for cooking
Washing (plates etc.)	0·02	0	0·15	1	84% of d.g.s. used no water for washing
Pigs (for drinking or cooking pigs' food)	0·19	0	1·94	7	Pigs are fed small tubers and leaves normally boiled in water 55% of d.g.s. used no water for pigs
Dogs and/or chickens (for drinking)	0·01	0	0·13	0·5	86% of d.g.s. used no water for dogs or chickens
Thrown away	0·06	0	0·58	2·5	63% of d.g.s. threw none away
Total collected	2·46	0·60	4·99	100	

a d.g.s.: domestic groups surveyed.

TABLE VIII

Per-capita water usage

Usage category	Volume used litres per capita per day		
	Mean	Minimum	Maximum
Total collected	0·68	0·19	1·27
Volume drunk	0·54	0·19	1·16

This gives a total daily water availability of $0.7 + 1.38 + 0.36 = 2.44$ litres which corresponds closely to the clinical norm of 2.5 litres.

The only comparable data from the New Guinea Highlands is provided by Hipsley and Kirk (1965, p. 79) from their data on the Chimbu settlement of Pari and by Oomen and Corden (1969, p. 16) from their study on the Kyaka Enga at Baiyer river. Hipsley and Kirk report extremely low daily fluid intakes of 0.07 and 0.01 litres per capita for men and women respectively. It appears (1965, p. 143) that they obtained these figures by questionnaire and observation and, in the absence of further details, one must view the validity of this data with suspicion. Hipsley and Kirk add to these consumption figures water from food oxidation to obtain total volumes of available water. These are again low when compared with the clinical norm of 2.5 litres for "resting conditions in a moderate climate" (Hipsley and Kirk, 1965, p. 144). The authors discuss this low intake and conclude that it is possibly related to the low protein and low sodium dietary characteristics which lead to a reduced demand for water as a "vehicle for waste nitrogenous products and other solutes" (Hipsley and Kirk, 1965, p. 146).

Oomen and Corden (1969) provide fluid intake data in their study of dietary intakes and nitrogen metabolism among 24 subjects at Baiyer river. They report that between 0.23 and 0.43 litres per capita per day were drunk although these figures may be high because the experimental subjects had water close to hand at all times. Allowing for water in food, but not for food oxidation, Oomen and Corden compute a total daily per-capita intake of 1.56 litres for adult males and 1.95 for adult females. The authors suggest that these low fluid intake figures may relate to the low sodium nature of the diet caused partially by extremely limited salt use and the apparent absence of salt hunger. They note that traditional salt is used mainly on ceremonial occasions (see Meggitt, 1958) and that, in any case, this type of salt is primarily potassium based. Oomen and Corden do not comment on the recent development of purchasing packaged salt from local stores and this practice is certainly common in the Saka. It may be that the taste for salt will grow and with it the Enga thirst.*

Tombeakini data (Table VIII) shows a considerably higher level of fluid intake amongst the Raiapu than the Chimbu. If Hipsley's

* Enga men relish sugar cane (*Saccharum officinarum*) and will eat large quantities when it is available. It is considered to be extremely thirst quenching and the Raiapu say that it is their substitute for water. It contains 82% water by weight (Hipsley and Kirk, 1965, p. 40) and its consumption may dramatically increase the figure of 1.38 litres given here. However, women eat little or no sugar cane and men who are old, or who are not prosperous, will eat little because they have none and are unlikely to receive any from other men. Sugar cane water cannot therefore be included in any generalizations concerning Raiapu water intake.

explanation of the low Chimbu water consumption is correct we should expect the Raiapu to have a diet richer in protein than the Chimbu. This appears to be the case. Waddell (1972, p. 126) reports 29·5 g and 34·7 g of protein daily during his two survey periods while the mean Chimbu figure is only 21 g of daily protein (Hipsley and Kirk, 1965, p. 146). It is likely that other Enga groups have a diet which is lower in protein than the Raiapu and indeed Sinnett (1972) reports a protein intake of 25 g per day for an Enga clan near Laiagam. It may be anticipated therefore that these Enga will require less water than the Raiapu.

A notable feature of Table VII is that, with the exception of the 1% of water used for washing utensils, water is not utilized for hygienic purposes within the home. Most Raiapu households own a few metallic eating and cooking utensils but only 16% of domestic groups surveyed carried any water to the house for the purpose of washing these. The Raiapu never wash their bodies at their houses and this is probably true throughout the Enga region and indeed for most of the New Guinea Highlands. The Enga pay little attention to personal hygiene of any sort, but do occasionally bathe all or parts of their bodies in rivers. This river bathing only occurs on hot days and is practised very rarely by adults of either sex.

4. Water-related Disease

Data on water-related disease is now presented to establish any possible connections between domestic water use and disease. Table III lists the principal water-related diseases and it is necessary to relate these to the situation in the New Guinea Highlands and, in particular, to the situation in the Saka valley. Table IX lists water-related disease which is of importance in the New Guinea Highlands and it is immediately apparent that many major diseases included in Table III are absent. The infections included in Table IX will be discussed in turn drawing partly on data from various epidemiological surveys in the New Guinea Highlands (particularly Vines, 1970) and partly on data collected by myself and Zuzana Feachem during a 22-week morbidity survey of Tombeakini clan. This survey was conducted by inviting all members of the clan to attend a weekly interview every week for 22 weeks (on average 68% of the clan attended) at which standardized questions were asked about 13 symptoms (see Figure 7). As a result of this 48 000 items of medical data were collected and these were analysed by computer at the University of New South Wales. The results of this

TABLE IX

Water-related diseases with their water associations and their pathogenic agents of importance in the Highlands of Papua New Guinea

Water-related disease	Category from Table II	Pathogenic agent
Amoebic dysentery	1b	C
Ascariasis	1b	D
Bacillary dysentery	1b	A
Balantidiasis	1b	C
Diarrhoeal disease	1b	G
Enterobiasis	1b	D
Enteroviruses (some)	1b	B
Gastroenteritis	1b	G
Giardiasis	1b	C
Hepatitis (infectious)	1b	B
Leptospirosis	1a	E
Paratyphoid	1b	A
Trichuriasis	1b	D
Typhoid	1a	A
Eye infections	2a	G
Leprosy	2a	A
Scabies	2a	G
Skin infections	2a	G
Trachoma	2a	G
Yaws	2a	E
Malaria	4b	C

A: Bacteria; B: Virus; C: Protozoa; D: Helminth; E: Sporochaete; F: Fungus; G: Miscellaneous.

survey are reported in detail elsewhere (Feachem, 1973a) and only relevant items will be abstracted here.

Category 1. Category 1 in Table IX includes mainly diarrhoea causing infections which are of great importance throughout the tropics and which are major causes of acute morbidity and mortality amongst infants. Gastroenteric infections were the cause of 7·5% of all hospital admissions in the Highlands between 1963 and 1966 (Maddocks, 1974) and are the third priority for the new National Health Plan, coming after respiratory infections and malaria (Hocking, 1974). Vines (1970) reports monthly period prevalences per 1000 of 10 for diarrhoea and gastroenteritis and 3 for dysentery in the Highlands but these data were obtained by monthly recall and it is quite likely that they severely underestimate the prevalence of diarrhoea. Monthly recall

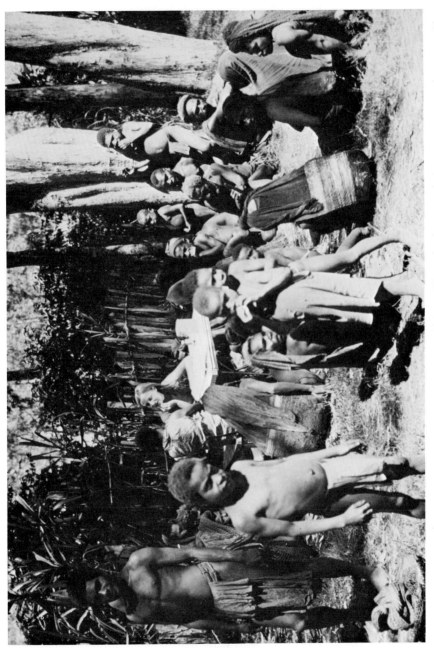

FIGURE 7. The weekly morbidity survey on the *Tee*-ground of Tombeakini clan. The entire clan were asked to report once a week to answer 13 symptomological questions and to be examined for skin disease and trauma.

periods are probably too long for mild symptoms in the U.S.A. (Mechanic and Newton, 1965) and are certainly too long for Papua New Guinea (Feachem, 1973a). Burchett (1966) has reported 46 cases of amoebiasis among the Kyaka Enga of Baiyer river and considers that ameobiasis should be suspected in all cases of infantile diarrhoea not readily responsive to conventional treatment. Vines (1970) reports that 16·4% of stools collected in the Highlands were positive for *Entamoeba histolytica*-like cysts. The presence of salmonella and shigella in water, foodstuffs and the faeces of humans, pigs and a variety of wild and domestic animals and birds have been demonstrated in various parts of Papua New Guinea with obvious implications for the transmission of shigellosis and salmonellosis (Caley, 1972; Egerton and Rampling, 1963; Lane, 1967; Morahan, 1967, 1968a, 1969a, 1969b; Morahan and Hawksworth, 1969a, 1969b; Rampling, 1967; Rampling and Egerton, 1965). My survey of Tombeakini morbidity revealed a weekly period prevalence of 35 per 1000 for diarrhoea and a five monthly period prevalence of 405. In other words, in a five-month period over 40% of the community will suffer at least one attack of diarrhoea while in the average week only 3·5% will be affected. The rates for dysentery (bloody stools) were 3 per week per 1000 and 58 per five months per 1000. Due to the shorter recall period (one week as opposed to one month), and the good rapport between interviewer and interviewee achieved by the participating observer method, these figures are likely to be more reliable than the lower figures of Vines (1970) reported earlier.

Balantidiasis (due to infection by the protozoon *Balantidium coli*) is a prevalent but mild infection in the Highlands (Radford, 1973). Transmission is commonly from pig to man and it is therefore associated with conditions where man lives in close proximity to domestic pigs. Couvee and Rijpstra (1961) report a 28% prevalence in the Highlands of Irian Jaya while Vines (1970) reports 1·7% prevalence in the Papua New Guinea Highlands and none from the lowland or island regions. Walzer *et al.* (1973) report a water-borne epidemic of balantidiasis on Truk.

Infectious hepatitis appears to be prevalent in Papua New Guinea, although often asymptomatic, and water-borne transmission is a clear possibility (Mosley, 1967; Villarejos *et al.*, 1972). Simmons *et al.* (1972) have reported a prevalence of australia antigen of 9·1% among the Raiapu Enga while Woodfield *et al.* (1972) report a national prevalence of 7·5%.

Leptospires have been isolated from rats, pigs, humans and a bandicoot in Papua New Guinea (Babudieri and D'Aquino, 1973; Emanuel, 1959; Kariks and Stallman, 1968; Morahan, 1968b, 1971). Van Thiel *et al.* (1963) report 8% infection among humans and 1·8% among pigs in the Highlands of Irian Jaya. Willis and Wannan (1966) report that 31% of people at Bena Bena had leptospiral antibodies.

Giardiasis (due to infection by the flagellate *Giardia lamblia*) is a prevalent but mild faecal-oral infection in the Highlands, from where Vines (1970) reports a prevalence of 4·6%.

Category 1 contains three helminthic infections. Ascariasis (due to infection by *Ascaris lumbricoides*) is a common parasite of man in New Guinea and Vines (1970) reports a prevalence of 58·9% in the Highlands. *A. lumbricoides* is extremely similar to *A. suis*, a common roundworm in pigs in Papua New Guinea (Talbot, 1972), and it is thus possible that some infection from pigs to man takes place. Trichuriasis (due to infection by the whipworm *Trichuris trichiura*) is a prevalent, but largely asymptomatic, condition in Papua New Guinea. Vines (1970) reports a prevalence in the Highlands of 36·9% and figures from 2% to 85% have been reported from different locations (Ewers and Jeffrey, 1971). Enterobiasis (due to infection by the pinworm *Enterobius vermicularis*) is also common but of "insignificant pathogenicity" (Vines, 1970). Vines (1970) reports that only 8·3% of stools in the Highlands contained *E. vermicularis* ova but that the cellulose tape method showed a prevalence in children under 5 years old of 27·8%.

Finally it is noteworthy that the most serious of all infections in Category 1 of Table III, namely cholera, is not yet reported from Papua New Guinea although it has occurred in Irian Jaya. The world spread of this disease in recent years is alarming (Barua, 1972) and the possible consequences of its introduction into the Highlands, with their dense populations, poor hygiene and poor sanitation are most serious.

Category 2. The water-washed infections in Category 2a (Table III) are common in the Highlands (Table IX). Skin infections are extremely prevalent with Vines (1970) reporting 735 skin conditions per 1000 subjects.

My morbidity survey revealed a weekly period prevalence of 271 and a five monthly period prevalence of 995 per 1000 subjects in the Saka valley. By contrast, Hornabrook *et al.* (1974) report a prevalence of skin disease at Lufa of only 3·8%. The commonest diseases are scabies and sores.

Eye infections are also prevalent and Table X presents data from three morbidity surveys. My survey revealed a weekly period prevalence per 1000 of all eye disorders of 74 which agrees reasonably with data from Lufa (Hornabrook *et al.*, 1974) where a prevalence of eye disease of 6% was found.

Category 3. None of the water-based infections (Category 3—Table III) are found in Papua New Guinea. Blackburn and Ma (1971a) have

TABLE X

Percentages of Highlands populations having eye disorders

Eye disease	Highlands[a]	Lufa[b]	Yandapu Enga[c]	
			Male	Female
Cataract	6·4	1·3	18	10
Corneal opacities	3·8	1·9	7·7	2·4
Pterygium	7·1	4·7	4·5	5·9
Trachoma	8·9	0·2	1·3 of adults	
Conjunctivitis	13·1 (follicular)	0·3	0·5 of adults	

[a] Vines (1970).
[b] Hornabrook et al. (1974).
[c] Sinnett (1972).

reported 11·6% positive skin reactions to an antigen of *Schistosoma mansoni* among the Kyaka Enga. However, there is no human schistosomiasis in this area and the authors consider the reactions were due to infection by other unidentified trematodes.

Category 4. Yellow fever, river blindness and sleeping sickness do not occur in Papus New Guinea. Dengue is found in coastal regions (Chow, 1974; Zigas and Doherty, 1973) but not in the Highlands. Filariasis has not been reported from above 1500 m in the Highlands (Blackburn and Ma, 1971b; Ewers and Jeffrey, 1971). This leaves only malaria from Category 4. Malaria is one of Papua New Guinea's major disease problems and is the second priority in the new National Health Plan (Hocking, 1974). It is hypoendemic in the Highlands with periodic epidemics and accounted for 9·3% of Highlands hospital admissions between 1963 and 1966 (Maddocks, 1974). Overall parasite rates in regions of the Highlands above 1500 m appear to be in the range 0–6%. Vines (1970) reports a Highlands spleen rate of 9·6% although below 1500 m the rate was 53·3% while above that height it was only 6·6%. Vines further reports an overall parasite rate for the Highlands of 11·6% while Hornabrook et al. (1974) give a figure of 1·3% for Lufa.

5. Water and Health

The water-related diseases of the New Guinea Highlands, listed in Table IX, have now been discussed. It has been shown that the main water-related disease problems are in Categories 1 and 2a (in other words they are faecal-oral or water-washed diseases) and that they include some of the most prevalent conditions of the Highlands. It is clear therefore that the engineer, through interventions in the domestic water supply situation, could play a major role in improving community health in this region. The problem is to decide what type of intervention is required and what other complementary inputs are necessary in order that the benefits to health may be realized (Feachem, 1975). All the faecal-oral diseases may be either water-borne or water-washed whereas the water-washed diseases (Category 2) cannot be water-borne. What are the operative transmission mechanisms in the Saka valley? I have formulated a view of the role of water in morbidity causation amongst the Saka Raiapu. This view rests partially on quantitative data and partly on speculation and estimation based on a year's residence in the Saka and on a study of the relevant literature. This view of water and disease in the Saka will be set out below in some detail in the belief that it is a useful and original contribution to understanding in this field. However, it is not proven and parts of it are not supported, or negated, by available data. It must remain therefore for future investigations to add new information which will either support, modify or contradict the view presented here.

a. Although the people of the Saka utilize domestic water sources which are faecally polluted, and in some instances heavily so, the ingestion of this faecal material is not a major influence on their health. There are three main reasons for this. Firstly, all the pathogens which may be ingested in polluted water are also ingested by faecal-oral contact in the domestic situation. The standards of personal and domestic hygiene are so low that direct faecal-oral contact is certainly the primary route for the spread of most infections and the small impact of polluted water is obscured by the overriding factor of poor hygiene. Secondly, the volumes of polluted water which are drunk are extremely small and thus the risk of receiving an infective dose of pathogens is reduced. Thirdly, the great majority of the faecal polluting material is probably of non-human origin and so, although it is potentially pathogenic, it is perhaps less so than an equal amount of human pollution.

b. Following from this is the assertion that water quantity and availability are crucial. If improved availability of water were arranged, coupled with a change of Raiapu attitudes to hygiene which resulted in increased water use, then a dramatic improvement in health is anticipated. This improvement would occur irrespective of the quality of the water being used. In other words, most water-related disease in the Saka today is primarily water-washed rather than water-borne. The important factor is the change in attitudes and habits which would lead to increased water use and increased hygiene. The prevalences of skin infections (presently the most common water-related diseases amongst the Raiapu), eye infections and gastroenteric infections would show the greatest improvement.

c. Following from points a and b above, it is possible to predict the impact of a new water supply installation in a Saka community. Suppose a reticulated supply was installed which provided abundant water at a stand-pipe located centrally in a Raiapu clan territory. If the water was clear and cool, which it probably would be, the Raiapu would welcome it and those who lived nearer to the stand-pipe than to their original source, would use the stand-pipe. If the water supply installation was not accompanied by any supporting health programme,* then the stand-pipe would approximate to the spring in Tombeakini territory. It would provide good quality, but not completely pure, water and those who used it would also drink elsewhere while they were travelling or sleeping with friends. It would not in itself alter Raiapu water use patterns or change the level of hygiene. The effect on the health of those who used this new supply can be predicted to be minute or non-existent. To install a new supply and do nothing else is to change one variable—namely water quality. Since it has been argued that this is the variable of least importance, it follows that a new supply of this type will not cause a marked improvement in the health of its users. However, the installation of a supply which promoted increased use of water for hygienic purposes might well have a substantial impact on disease, irrespective of the quality of water supplied. For instance, if a considerable number of stand-pipes were scattered around the clan territory, so that the mean distance from dwelling to water source was greatly reduced, then increased water use might be promoted. This would be further encouraged by the provision of facilities for clothes washing at the stand-pipe which might cause the water source to become a new focus of female gossiping.

This view of water and disease is based on my perception of the situation in the Saka in 1971. It is subject to one important proviso and

---

* The reader may think that to install a new supply without any supporting medical programme is clearly ill advised and is not likely to be contemplated. However, it is precisely what occurs with most new water supply installations.

that is the unknown effect of the introduction of a new water-borne pathogen into the Saka to which the people have little or no immunity. In other words, the risk of a water-borne epidemic—perhaps of cholera if it were ever introduced. Whether these comments regarding the unimportance of using faecally contaminated water would remain valid in the face of a cholera outbreak is most doubtful. It could be that water pollution would then become an important mechanism for spreading the epidemic and that those people using the imaginary new supply would enjoy a measure of protection. It is notable that the Enga residence pattern of dispersed, and sometimes quite isolated, houses is naturally resilient to epidemics. The classical situation which is conducive to epidemics is that of many people living in crowded and unhygienic conditions and sharing a common water source. The Enga are scattered and use many water sources, but there is always the danger that the faecal material in the rivers will spread the outbreak to downstream populations.

The only evidence available to judge the impact of a water-related epidemic amongst the Raiapu is information on the dysentery outbreak which occurred in the Highlands between about 1938 and 1945. Unfortunately, there are no reliable or comprehensive accounts of this outbreak and one must reconstruct the story from casual references to it (Gitlow, 1947; Simpson, 1954) and from the oral histories of the Highlanders themselves. The first prolonged contact between white men and the Saka Raiapu was in 1938–39 when the Hagen–Sepik Patrol established a camp in the Saka (Taylor, 1940). Soon after this, in about 1941,* a dysentery epidemic swept through the area and caused much mortality.

The Saka Raiapu associate the disease with the white man's arrival. They say that there was never an epidemic like this before or since and that this type of disease was unknown before 1941. It seems most probable that dysentery did spread through the Highlands in early European times due to the introduction of a new pathogen to which the people had little resistance. Bowers (1971) describes the possible impact of the dysentery epidemic on the upper Kaugel valley, and population depletions in immediately post-contact times have been recorded for the Chimbu (Brown and Winefield, 1965), the Maring (Rappaport, 1968), the Siane (Salisbury, 1962) and the Fore and Gimi (McArthur, 1964).

The amount of mortality caused by these post-contact epidemics can be only estimated but the authors cited above indicate that the death rate could have been as high as 20%. Tombeakini claim confidently

---

* I believe that the epidemic occurred in 1941 or 1942 based on interviews with middle-aged Saka men who still clearly remember it.

that 15 of their clan died in the 1941 dysentery epidemic. This is about 7% of the clan population and, if typical of the Saka, gives a figure of 700 deaths in the valley.

Supposing this figure is accurate, how did these 700 people (and the many more who were sick but did not die) become infected? Was the dysentery spread entirely by faecal-oral contact or did water pollution play a part? The dispersed living patterns of the Enga might lead to a belief that water pollution must have been an influence because isolated living mitigates against spread by person-to-person contact. However, the Raiapu response to a death is firstly to gather in large numbers to cry and wail, then to gather in selected houses to live and sleep, thereby causing overcrowded conditions, and finally to gather again in a large ceremonial wealth distribution. All these aspects of the *kumanda* (the Raiapu response to death) facilitate the rapid spread of an epidemic and destroy the advantages gained from dispersed dwelling patterns.

This doubt about the impact and mode of transmission of a new epidemic must remain as an important proviso to what was said earlier on the insignificance of water pollution. If 7% of the Saka population died in the 1941 dysentery epidemic, how many would die in a cholera epidemic tomorrow? More particularly, would the Saka population resist that epidemic any better if they were equipped with clean water sources or would the lack of hygiene and the *kumanda* behaviour be the dominant epidemiological factors?

C. EXCRETA DISPOSAL

1. Excreta Disposal Practices

Defecation takes place at any convenient private location: usually in some thicket or in long grass. The Raiapu are extremely modest and will not defecate unless completely unobserved by others of either sex. At night defecation will take place near the house (Raiapu are afraid to venture far from their houses in darkness; see Feachem, 1973c) but not so close that a bad odour might develop in the dwelling. The faeces may be covered but are not buried. The fairly steady rainfall (73% of days had some rain during May to December, 1971) ensures that no appreciable accumulation of human faeces occurs. Efforts have been made by the government to promote the construction and use of pit latrines and a few pit latrines are seen in the Saka. However, these are either unused or, where in use, they are in a revolting state and constitute a gross health hazard, especially to children.

2. Excreta Disposal and Disease

It has been explained that poor excreta disposal will promote all infections in Categories 1 and 3 in Table III and also infections listed in Table IV. In the case of the New Guinea Highlands, these infections are limited to the Category 1 list in Table IX and to those in Table IV. Table IX infections have already been discussed at length and so it will be necessary here only to discuss Table IV.

Hookworm is the most prevalent nematode infection in Papua New Guinea and Vines (1970) reports a prevalence of 73·8% in the Highlands. Various Highlands data reviewed by Ewers and Jeffrey (1971) show prevalences between 61% and 100%. Kelly and Avusi (1974) record a hookworm prevalence of 98·3% in a Papua mountain village in which ascariasis was rare (1·6%). *Strongyloides* is a rare parasite of man in Papua New Guinea.

3. Excreta Disposal and Health

There is clearly a close interaction in the Saka between poor hygiene, poor excreta disposal and low volumes of water used for washing which promote the Category 1 infections in Table IX and hookworm. It is therefore evident that any programme seeking to combat these diseases will have to focus on all three aspects and not merely deal with improving levels of water use.

D. REFUSE DISPOSAL

Refuse disposal by the Saka Raiapu is not a cause of significant ill health and, in fact, has no discernible influence on the subsystem being considered here (Figure 1). The Raiapu produce very little refuse of any kind. Organic refuse is fed to pigs or chickens while such items as used tins and bottles all find new uses as containers or as raw materials for some new object. In short, there is very little refuse and nearly all put to some productive use.

E. HOUSING

1. Raiapu Enga Housing

Neither the Raiapu, nor the Central Enga, reside in villages but rather they scatter their houses over the clan territories. Houses are typically located on terraces or slightly elevated locations and are often in dense groves of casuarina trees. They occur singly, in pairs, or recently in small groups which form hamlets around a focal point such as a church, a store or a *Tee*-ground. These modern hamlets are often found on, or near, a vehicular road.

Four basic types of Raiapu house can be distinguished. Firstly, the "men's house" (*akaryanda*) is the male clubhouse in which an adult male will live with his brothers, his older male children and possibly several male friends from the same sub-clan or patrilineage. His wife lives in a "women's house" (*endanda*) with her female, and young male, children and the family's pigs. The men's house is circular and approximately 3 m high at the centre and 1·5 m high at the circumference. It is one roomed, although a portion furthest from the door is often partitioned off as a sleeping area. The women's house is rectangular, with one bay end, and measures approximately 10 m in length and 3·7 m in width. It contains three rooms; an outer sitting, cooking and eating room; a room with stalls for the family pigs; and an inner sleeping room. Both types of houses have a small doorway through which the visitor has to crawl, and the women's house also has an emergency (fire and attack) escape exit at the back. Neither house type has any ventilation except for the door and the natural ability of the grass roof to allow smoke to pass out. Meggitt (1957) has described the houses of the Mae Enga. The Mae women's house is identical to that of the Raiapu except that the Mae favour an inclined roof apex whilst that of the Raiapu is horizontal. The Mae men's house is different from the Raiapu circular house but some Raiapu men live in small rectangular houses, similar to those of the Mae.

A man will probably locate his wife's house within easy walking distance of his own and they may be almost adjacent. A polygynist will build separate, widely spaced houses for his wives to minimize the fighting that is common between co-wives, and to exploit efficiently his scattered sweet potato fields. A polygynist's pig herd will be divided between his wives.

In recent years, a new type of house has appeared and this I have called a "mixed house". It is occupied by a complete elementary family and its pigs and structurally it is identical to the traditional women's house. A fourth type of house, called a *nai anda* by the Raiapu, is also found today and is a mixed house which is constructed in a European style (copied from the bush material houses used on mission stations as classrooms) and not in the style of the traditional *endanda*. They are usually square, with one room, and have a large door and adequate ventilation from small windows. The family pigs are stalled in a separate outhouse.

All Raiapu houses are constructed from the same materials. The basic frame is made of casuarina (*Casuarina* spp.) poles. The walls are split logs (*Casuarina* spp.), bark and grass (*Miscanthus* spp.) and the roof is a thick thatching of grass (*Imperata* spp.). The floors are of beaten earth covered with a layer of masticated sugar cane pith, which provides an ideal habitat for many members of the phylum Arthropoda. Of special public health significance are members of the class Insecta such as cockroaches, fleas, beetles, bed-bugs and lice. Houses are also infested with mites and ticks (order Acarina) and particularly with *Sarcoptes scabiei* which give rise to the high prevalence of scabies in the area. All houses are dry and dark and, when a fire is burning in the fireplace, extremely smoky. Table XI presents a summary of the features which distinguish the four Raiapu house types discussed here.

Three types of house (men's, women's and mixed) are marked on Map 4 and abandoned houses are also shown. The house types are defined in accordance with Table XI, except that Tombeakini's

TABLE XI

A typology of Raiapu houses

Type	Enga name	Dimensions	Usual Occupants	Comments
Men's	*Akáryánda*	Circular— Diameter 5 m Height 3·5 m Rectangular— Height 2·5 m Length 6·5 m Width 3·4 m	Adult males with their male children over 8 years old	Mostly circular Traditional
Women's	*Éndánda*	Rectangular with one bay end— Height 2·7 m Length 11 m Width 3·8 m	An adult woman with female and young male children plus pigs	Traditional
Mixed	*Kitisenánda*[a]	Identical to women's house	An elementary family plus pigs	Encouraged by mission Recent
Nai Anda	*Nai Ánda* or *Kitisenánda*	Square, high roof and woven *Miscanthus* walls Copy of Administration resthouse or school classroom	An elementary family	Pigs usually kept in separate outhouse Recent

[a] Literally "christian house" (*ánda*: house).

nai anda is classed as a mixed house and not separately marked. Table XII shows that 69% of Tombeakini houses contain between one and three people and that 45% of clansfolk live in these houses. The maximum number of residents per house is 8. Table XIII shows that 48% of the clan now live in the new mixed houses, whereas traditionally a man would nearly always live in a separate house from his wife. Mixed houses are seen to have nearly twice as many occupants per house as either men's or women's houses. Table XIV shows that 64% of Tombeakini houses (containing 79% of the clan population) contain three generations of occupants. No house contains more than three generations and indeed there are no Tombeakini families in which more than three generations are alive. The 211 members of Tombeakini live in 70 houses and thus have a mean household size of three. Table XV shows the floor areas per person for the different types of houses. The overall mean of 6·0 m² (64·6 ft²) of floor area per resident is high for the Highlands. Vines (1970) shows that only 24·9% of his sample have more than 5·6 m² (60 ft²) per resident and

TABLE XII

Tombeakini household sizes

No. of residents per house	No. of houses	% total no. of houses	No. of residents	% clan population
1	14	20	14	7
2	21	30	42	20
3	13	19	39	18
4	5	7	20	9
5	10	14	50	24
6	5	7	30	14
7	0	0	0	0
8	2	3	16	8
All houses	70	100	211	100

TABLE XIII

Residence pattern of Tombeakini by house type

Type of house	No of houses	% total no. of houses	No. of residents	% clan population	Average no. of residents per house
Men's	26	37	56	27	2·1
Women's	21	30	54	25	2·5
Mixed	23	33	101	48	4·3
All houses	70	100	211	100	3·0

$51 \cdot 1\%$ have less than $3 \cdot 7$ m² (40 ft²). It is notable that the mixed houses are nearly twice as crowded as the traditional housing types.

2. Housing and Hygiene

Raiapu Enga housing style has certain advantages in that it is warm, compact, easily constructed from available materials and it is hard for an attacker to enter rapidly. Data in Chapter IV showed that Enga housing was also efficient in maintaining stable indoor temperatures and humidity with indoor diurnal fluctuations being only 5°C and 10% compared to outside fluctuations of 11°C and 40%. But Enga housing is not conducive to good hygiene. Raiapu hygiene is very poor and this is not helped by the crowded and dirty domestic conditions. The floor is impossible to keep clean because it is a litter of sugar cane pith and rubbish and children will often excrete there if not closely supervised. Housing styles thus encourage the transmission of all infections in Categories 1 and 2 of Table IX.

TABLE XIV

Residence pattern of Tombeakini by generation

No. of generations per house	No. of houses	% total no. of houses	No. of residents	% clan population	Average no. of residents per house
1	22	32	32	15	1·4
2	45	64	167	79	3·7
3	3	4	12	6	4·0
All generations	70	100	211	100	3·0

TABLE XV

Floor areas per occupant in different house types

Type of house	Average no. of residents per house	Floor area for humans (m²)	Floor area per resident (m²)
Men's	2·1	15	7·1
Women's (Excluding pig stalls)	2·5	20	8·0
Mixed (Excluding pig stalls)	4·3	20	4·6
All types	3·0	18	6·0

3. Housing and Pests

Raiapu houses contain large populations of insects and rodents, mainly *Rattus exulans* with some *R. rattus* (Willis and Wannan, 1966). The fleas, bed-bugs, lice and mites are undoubtedly important promoters of various dermatoses. Mites are of particular interest because, in addition to *Sarcoptes scabiei* which causes scabies, there are many other mite species which may cause human dermatosis (Taylor and Murray, 1946).

In order to clarify the public health importance of Raiapu house flooring, in July 1973 I collected eight samples of flooring material from Tombeakini houses. Flooring was collected from houses of different types (Table XI) and of different ages. There was much varied animal life present in all houses sampled and there was appreciably more life in the floors of the older houses. Samples were returned to the University of New South Wales, and with the assistance of the School of Zoology, large numbers of mites were recovered from all samples. Due to the methods of collection and mite recovery, the specimens were of poor quality and generally had legs, or other body parts, missing. Only very tentative identifications were possible but, with the aid of acarologist Dr Phyllis Robertson, the following picture of the mite population was obtained.

a. A large mite population is present and it includes members of the major groups, Oribatei, Sarcoptiformes and Tombidiformes.
b. The dominant mite is the genus *Chortoglyphus*. Other Sarcoptiformes may be Acaridae and Glycyphagidae.
c. The Trombidiformes mites may include the families Cheyletidae and Pyemotidae.

This identification is extremely tentative, but it appears certain that the floors do contain large mite populations, that older houses have a greater infestation and that mites from many different families are present.

Mites are also important in the aetiology of asthma (Anderson, 1974b, 1974c; Turner *et al.*, 1975). Anderson and Cunnington (1974) found large numbers of these mites (pyroglyphid species) in Papua New Guinea houses and they also found species from the families Acaridae, Glycyphagidae and Cheyletidae which were also found in my Saka valley survey. In summary therefore, there are large mite populations in Raiapu houses and they are strongly implicated in the causation of asthma and dermatosis, especially scabies. Dermatosis is by far the most common disorder among Tombeakini with 99·5%

experiencing some skin disease in a five-month period. Analysis of skin disease on a house-by-house basis revealed a significant correlation between skin disease and the number of occupants of a house and a significantly higher prevalence of skin disease in mixed houses (with an average of 4·3 occupants and 4·6 m² of floor space per person) than in other house types (with an average of 2.3 occupants and 7·5 m² of floor space per person) (Feachem, 1973a).

4. Housing and Respiratory Disease

Respiratory disease is the foremost medical problem in Papua New Guinea and has been allocated first priority in the National Health Plan (Hocking, 1974). Hocking (1974) writes that "pneumococcal pneumonia, the leading cause of mortality and bed occupancy, has an annual incidence of up to 10% in babies and 2% in young men and carries a hospital fatality rate of about 3%". Pneumonia was responsible for 16% of hospital admissions in the Highlands between 1963 and 1966 (Maddocks, 1974) and an increased resistance to penicillin in ten pneumococcal serotypes has been reported (Hansman et al., 1974).

There is much acute respiratory disease in the Highlands and chronic lung disease is very prevalent among the older age groups. Master (1974) reports 78% of people over 40 years of age at Lufa having pulmonary disease while high levels of chronic lung disease among older people have also been reported for the Chimbu and the Kyaka Enga (Woolcock and Blackburn, 1967; Woolcock et al., 1972). Woolcock and Blackburn (1967) found an overall coughing prevalence of 28%, with an age specific prevalence for males over 50 years of 41%, among 707 Enga and 148 Chimbu subjects. My survey of Saka Raiapu showed a weekly period prevalence of coughing of 142 per 1000 and a five monthly period prevalence of 899 per 1000. The prevalence of coughing rose markedly with age (Feachem, 1973a).

There is general agreement in the literature that respiratory disease in the Highlands is promoted by a complex interaction of factors which include protein–calorie deficiencies, overcrowding, climate, smoking, smoky houses, the passage of the larvae of intestinal parasites (especially *Ascaris*) through the lungs and possibly sensitivity to certain moulds found in the thatch of Highlands houses (Anderson, 1974a; Blackburn and Green, 1966; Blackburn and Woolcock, 1971; Cleary and Black-burn, 1968; Master, 1974; Woolcock and Blackburn, 1967; Woolcock et al., 1970, 1972). Ignoring the mould possibility, there are therefore two main factors which are directly related to housing; overcrowding and smoky atmosphere.

Firstly, overcrowding encourages the transmission of airborne pathogens and the Saka survey showed a correlation (significant at the 5% level) between coughing among 0–4 year olds and the number of people with whom they cohabit (Feachem, 1973a). However, no significant correlations were found for other age groups and there was no significant difference between coughing prevalences in mixed houses (crowded) and those in other less crowded house types (Feachem, 1973a). Therefore it seems likely that the influence of crowding is overshadowed by the effect of other variables; such as nutrition and helminthiasis.

Secondly, Raiapu Enga houses are extremely smoky and poorly ventilated and there is evidence that this promotes respiratory disease. Cleary and Blackburn (1968) found high concentrations of aldehydes, formaldehydes and particulate matter in the air within houses of the Highlanders and they also report significant levels of carbon monoxide. Levels of these pollutants were highest soon after a fire had been started and were higher in houses at greater altitude because the increased cold and dampness necessitated larger and more smoky fires. Master (1974) has reviewed this and similar work and has reported his own findings on chronic pulmonary disease at Lufa. By relating pathological evidence to atmospheric pollution data he states "air pollutants are the most important factor in the development of lung disease in New Guinea". Later he concludes that "among the multiplicity of factors related to the prevalence of lung disease, air pollutants from smoky fires in poorly ventilated huts remain the major and most preventable factor". These are sweeping assertions and will doubtless prove controversial, but they do highlight the possible importance and preventability of air pollution within houses as a cause of lung disease in the Highlands. Vines (1970), in analysing data from his epidemiological survey, has reached different conclusions and comments that "domiciliary smoke has not been implicated in the aetiology of chronic obstructive lung disease in New Guinea".

It must of course be noted that housing styles in the Highlands, and elsewhere in Papua New Guinea and the Pacific, have distinct benefits. In the Highlands, crowding into smoky houses at night is essential to keep warm and dry in the very cold and damp climate. The housing styles of the Highlands are also of importance in protecting the inhabitants from surprise attack by enemies and presumably crowding in houses boosts the confidence of those who fear attack by hostile humans or hostile ghosts (Feachem, 1973c). Crowding in smoky houses in coastal regions is an important method of escape from mosquito attack and on Ontong Java life would be intolerable without this defence (Bayliss Smith, pers. comm.).

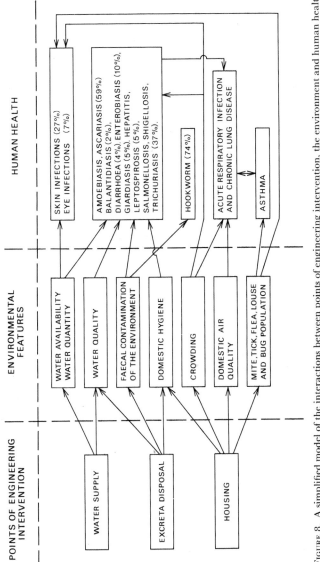

FIGURE 8. A simplified model of the interactions between points of engineering intervention, the environment and human health in the Highlands of Papua New Guinea. Percentages in brackets refer to the prevalence of these conditions in the Highlands (Feachem, 1973a; Vines, 1970).

F. CONCLUSIONS

Based on the data presented on environmental health in the Saka, it is possible to adapt the model shown in Figure 1 so that it describes the Saka situation. This adaptation is shown in Figure 8. It was maintained in the early parts of this essay that the study of the interactions between certain environmental features and health, in an ecological context, was of value in guiding the actions of the environmental health engineer. If this is correct, then it must be possible to rework the data on environment and health in the Saka into a form which is of use to the engineer contemplating a programme of environmental modification in the New Guinea Highlands. Further, if it is to be argued that the Saka study was more than an expensive academic exercise (and a means to a higher degree), then it is necessary to show that the insights gained might guide the engineer into a course of action which he otherwise would not have taken. In other words the insights gained must not be self-evident.

Figure 8 embodies the main conclusions to be drawn from the Saka study. It contains, like Figure 1, some gross simplifications which are necessary if the model is to provide a useful tool for the engineer. Figure 8 shows only the interactions between certain environmental features, which were previously selected as being the legitimate focus of the engineer's intervention, and certain diseases. There are clearly many other causal and contributing factors in the aetiology of these diseases which are not shown in Figure 8. However, taking Figure 8 in conjunction with a basic appreciation of environmental health and of the social and environmental circumstances of the Raiapu Enga (Feachem, 1974b; Waddell, 1972), it is possible to derive a rational set of policies for engineering intervention in the sanitary environment of the Raiapu Enga. These policies are now listed and related to the groups of infections shown in Figure 8.

1. Skin and Eye Infections

Skin and eye infections are the most prevalent complaints in the Saka. They are promoted by a combination of poor water availability, low levels of water use for hygienic purposes, overcrowded and unhygienic housing and very poor personal and domestic hygiene. Any piecemeal approach towards environmental prevention of these infections will not succeed. A combination of improvements to water availability, water quantity, water use, housing and attitudes to hygiene are required.

2. Faecal-oral Infections

This group of infectious diseases are the most serious morbidity problem in the Saka after respiratory disease. Again piecemeal approaches will not be affective. A combination of improved water availability, improved water quality (of least importance), improved excreta disposal, improved housing and a new perception of hygiene are needed. Even excellent excreta disposal will not prevent the transmission of these infections in the absence of improved personal and domestic hygiene and it will, of course, have no effect on the transmission of faecal-oral infections from animals (notably pigs) to man.

3. Hookworm

Hookworm is the one infection which could, in theory, be prevented by a single measure; namely sanitary disposal of excreta. However, this begs the question of how sanitary excreta disposal is achieved. It is not achieved by providing everyone with a latrine nor by encouraging everyone to build their own latrine. Sanitary excreta disposal depends on attitudes and on motivation and it is necessary to provide a reason for, or an advantage from, correct excreta disposal. At present no such reasons or advantages are perceived by the Raiapu Enga and therefore hookworm prevention must await a major change in local perceptions.

4. Respiratory Disease

Respiratory disease is the outstanding disease problem of the Saka, and indeed of Papua New Guinea. In terms of the variables considered in Figure 8, respiratory disease is promoted by overcrowded, smoky and mite infested houses, by the migration of *Ascaris lumbricoides* through the lungs and by the prevalence of all other infections listed in Figure 8 which produce a generally debilitated state.

5. Policy Summary

In summary therefore, there is a need to do several things at once or to do nothing. Piecemeal environmental engineering measures are likely to show very poor returns on investment. A planned programme which stressed the importance of water supplies and excreta disposal and hygiene and housing would have a substantial impact on the infections listed on Figure 8. Single measures, or ad-hoc improvements, are likely to achieve nothing. Changes in basic attitudes towards personal and domestic hygiene form the essential core of any such programme and action would need to be phased over many years to allow time for perceptions to modify and change. It is also essential that all engineering interventions be planned and designed in collaboration with the Raiapu Enga, or preferably, by the Raiapu Enga.

This policy is not one which would normally be arrived at by the environmental health engineer. The conventional response of the engineer to the Saka situation would be to design a programme concentrating solely on water supply and excreta disposal measures. The water supply designs would emphasize improved quality, and might even seek compliance with the stringent World Health Organization drinking water quality standards (Feachem, 1977; WHO, 1971), and would avoid improved water availability because of the high cost of reticulating water in a dispersed community. Excreta disposal measures would emphasize the construction of numbers of latrines (the designs of which would be taken from some standard text) and it would be optimistically hoped that the latrines would be culturally acceptable to the Raiapu and would be used. If this indeed describes the conventional response then the conventional response would be a failure.

VII. ACKNOWLEDGEMENTS

The work in Papua New Guinea reported here was made possible by generous financial support from the Nuffield Foundation, the Wenner-Gren Foundation, the Frederick Soddy Trust, the Australia and New Zealand Association for the Advancement of Science and the University of New South Wales. I am indebted to my former colleagues at the School of Civil Engineering at the university and to the numerous people who assisted and encouraged me while in the field. I owe two very special debts; first to the people of Tombeakini clan for their hospitality and friendship and secondly to my wife Zuzana, who assisted with all aspects of my fieldwork and was entirely responsible for conducting the weekly interview morbidity survey.

VIII. REFERENCES

Anderson, H. R. (1974a). Smoking habits and their relationship to chronic lung disease in a tropical environment in Papua New Guinea. *Bull. Physiopathol. Respir.* (Nancy) **10**, 619–633.

Anderson, H. R. (1974b). Allergic aspects of asthma in the Highlands of Papua New Guinea. *Clin. Sci. mol. Med.* **47**, 12P–13P.

Anderson, H. R. (1974c). The Epidemiological and Allergic Features of Asthma in the New Guinea Highlands. *Clin. Allergy* **4**, 171–183.

Anderson, H. R. and Cunnington, A. M. (1974). House dust mites in the highlands of Papua New Guinea. *Papua New Guin. med. J.* **17**, 304–308.

Babudieri, B. and D'Aquino, A. (1973). Systematics of Leptospirae Strains Isolated in the Sepik District, Papua New Guinea. *Med. J. Aust.* **1**, 701.

Barua, D. (1972). The Global Epidemiology of Cholera in Recent Years. *Proc. R. Soc. Med.* **65**, 423–428.

Beral, V. and Read, D. J. C. (1971). Insensitivity of the respiratory centre to carbon dioxide in the Enga people of New Guinea. *Lancet* **2**, 1290.

Blackburn, C. R. and Green, W. (1966). Precipitins against extracts of thatched roofs in sera of New Guinea natives with chronic lung disease. *Lancet* **2**, 1396–1397.

Blackburn, C. R., Green, W. F. and Mitchell, G. A. (1970). Studies in chronic non-tuberculous lung disease in New Guinea populations: the prevalence of *Hemophilus influenzae* precipitins. *Am. Rev. resp. Dis.* **102**, 567–574.

Blackburn, C. R. and Ma, M. H. (1971a). Skin reaction of natives in the Western Highlands of New Guinea to a *Schistosoma mansoni* antigen. *Trop. geog. Med.* **23**, 278–281.

Blackburn, C. R. and Ma, M. H. (1971b). Skin reactions of natives in the Western Highlands of New Guinea to an antigen prepared from *Dirofilaria immitis*. *Trop. geog. Med.* **23**, 272–277.

Blackburn, C. R. and Woolcock, A. J. (1971). Chronic Disease of liver and lungs in New Guinea. *J. R. Coll. Physicians. Lond.* **5**, 241–249.

Bowers, N. (1971). Demographic problems in montane New Guinea. *In* "Culture and Population: A Collection of Recent Studies" (Ed. S. Polger), Carolina Population Centre Mono. 9. Chapel Hill, North Carolina.

Bradley, D. J. (1974). Water Supplies: the consequences of change. *In* "Human Rights in Health." Ciba Foundation Symposium 23 (new series), Elsevier, Amsterdam, pp. 81–98.

Brown, P. and Winefield, G. (1965). Some demographic measures applied to Chimbu census and field data. *Oceania* **35**, 175–190.

Burchett, P. M. (1966). Amoebiasis in the New Guinea Western Highlands. *Med. J. Aust.* **2**, 1079–1081.

Caley, J. E. (1972). Salmonella in pigs in Papua New Guinea. *Aust. vet. J.* **48**, 601–604.

Chow, C. Y. (1974). *Aedes aegypti* surveillance and control in the South Pacific. *Papua New Guin. med. J.* **17**, 309–315.

Cleary, G. J. and Blackburn, C. R. (1968). Air pollution in native huts in the Highlands of New Guinea. *Archs. envir. Hlth.* **17**, 785–794.

Couvee, L. M. J. and Rijpstra, A. C. (1961). The prevalence of *Balfantidium coli* in the central highlands of Western New Guinea. *Trop. geog Med.* **13**, 284–286.

Egerton, J. R. and Rampling, A. M. (1963). Salmonellosis in Guinea-Pigs due to serotype weltevredon. *Papua New Guinea Agric. J.* **16**, 55–56.

Emanuel, M. L. (1959). Leptospiral infections in Papua. *Papua New Guin. med. J.* **3**, 76.

Ewers, W. H. (1974). *Trypanosoma aunawa* sp. N. From an insectivorous bat, *Miniopterus tristris*, in New Guinea, which may be transmitted by a leech. *J. Parasit.* **60**, 172–178.

Ewers, W. H. and Jeffrey, W. T. (1971). "Parasites of Man in Niugini." Jacaranda Press, Brisbane.

Fish, H. (1974). Nitrate and London's public water supply. *Civ. Engng.* December, 31–37.

Feachem, R. G. A. (1973a). "Environment and Health in a New Guinea Highlands Community Ph.D. dissertation, School of Civil Engineering, University of New South Wales, Sydney. Held in the libraries of ANU. (Canberra); UNSW (Sydney); School of Public Health and Tropical Medicine (Sydney); UPNG (Port Moresby); Faculty of Medicine (Port Moresby); Institute of Medical Research (Goroka); Ross Institute (London).

Feachem, R. G. A. (1973b). The Raiapu Enga pig herd. *Mankind* **9**, 25–31.

Feachem, R. G. A. (1973c). The religious belief and ritual of the Raiapu Enga. *Oceania* **43**, 259–285.

Feachem, R. G. A. (1973d). "Domestic Water Use in the New Guinea Highlands: The Case of the Raiapu Enga." Water Research Laboratory, Report 132. University of New South Wales, Sydney.

Feachem, R. G. A. (1974a). Faecal coliforms and faecal streptococci in streams in the New Guinea Highlands. *Wat. Res.* **8**, 367–374.

Feachem, R. G. A. (1974b). Ethnographic notes on the Raiapu Enga of the New Guinea Highlands. *Asian Pacif. Q.* **6**(3), 9–24.

Feachem, R. G. A. (1975). Water Supplies for low-income communities in developing countries. *Journal of the Environmental Engineering Division, ASCE* **101**, 687–702.

Feachem, R. G. A. (1977). Water Supplies for Low-Income Communities: resource allocation, planning and design for a crisis situation. *In* "Water, Wastes and Health in Hot Climates" (Eds R. Feachem, M. McGarry and D. Mara). John Wiley and Sons, London and New York.

Gitlow, A. L. (1947). "Economics of the Mount Hagen Tribes, New Guinea". University of Washington Press, Seattle.

Hansman, D., Devitt, L., Miles, H. and Riley, I. (1974). Pneumococci relatively insensitive to penicillin in Australia and New Guinea. *Med. J. Aust.* **2**, 353–356.

Hocking, B. (1974). Health problems and medical care in Papua New Guinea. *Int. J. Epidemiol.* **3**, 9–13.

Hornabrook, R. W., Crane, G. G. and Stanhope, J. M. (1974). Karkar and Lufa, an epidemiological and health background to the human adaptability studies of the International Biological Programme. *Phil. Trans. R. Soc. Lond. Ser. B.* **268**, 293–308.

Kariks, J. and Stallman, N. D. (1968). Human leptospirosis proven by culture in the Territory of Papua New Guinea. *Med. J. Aust.* **2**, 20.

Kelly, A. and Avusi, M. G. (1974). A parasitological survey of a village in a mountain district of Papua. *Trop. geogr. Med.* **26**, 178–181.

Lane, A. G. (1967). New Guinea village water supplies, a comparison of faecal pollution levels in wells and traditional supplies. *Med. J. Aust.* **1**, 385–389.

McArthur, N. (1964). The age incidence of Kuru. *Ann. hum. Genet.* **27**, 341–352.

McGarry, M. J. (1977). Domestic wastes as an economic resource. *In* "Water, Wastes and Health in Hot Climates" (Eds R. Feachem, M. McGarry and D. Mara). John Wiley and Sons, London and New York.

Maddocks, I. (1974). Patterns of disease in Papua New Guinea. *Med. J. Aust.* **1**, 442–446.

Master, K. M. (1974). Air pollution in New Guinea. Cause of chronic pulmonary disease among stone-age natives in the Highlands. *JAMA* **228**, 1653–1655.

Mechanic, D. and Newton, M. (1965). Some problems in the analysis of morbidity data. *Journal of chron. Dis.* **18**, 569–580.

Meggitt, M. J. (1957). House building among the Mae Enga, Western Highlands, Territory of New Guinea. *Oceania* **27**, 161–176.

Meggitt, M. J. (1958). Salt manufacture and trading in the Western Highlands. *Aust. Mus. Mag.* **12**, 309–313.

Meggitt, M. J. (1964). Male–female relationships in the Highlands of New Guinea. *Am. Anthrop.* **66** (No. 4, Pt 2), 204–224.

Meggitt, M. J. (1965). "The Lineage System of the Mae Enga of New Guinea". Oliver and Boyd, Edinburgh and London.

Meggitt, M. J. (1971). From tribesman to peasants: the case of the Mae Enga of New Guinea. *In* "Anthropology in Oceania" (Eds L. Hiatt and C. Jayawardena). Angus and Robertson, Sydney.

Morahan, R. J. (1967). Salmonella and shigella isolations at the Boram Corrective Institution. *Med. J. Aust.* **1**, 437–438.

Morahan, R. J. (1968a). Salmonella, shigella and enteropathogenic *Escherichia coli* isolations in the East and West Sepik Districts, TPNG *Med. J. Aust.* **2**, 438–440.

Morahan, R. J. (1968b). Isolations of leptospires in the Tarassovi (Hyos) serogroup from a bandicoot (*Marsupiala peramelidae*) from Koil Island, TPNG *Med. J. Aust.* **2**, 18–19.

Morahan, R. J. (1969a). Salmonella isolation in rats in the East Sepik District, TPNG *Med. J. Aust.* **1**, 979–981.

Morahan, R. J. (1969b). Salmonella isolations made at the Commonwealth Serum Laboratories Research Unit, Wewak, 1964–1968. *Papua New Guin. med. J.* **12**, 96–99.

Morahan, R. J. (1971). Further leptospiral isolations in the Sepik District, TPNG *Med. J. Aust.* **1**, 276–277.

Morahan, R. J. and Hawksworth, D. N. (1969a). Isolation of salmonellae from New Guinea streams and waterholes using an elevated temperature technique. *Med. J. Aust.* **2**, 20–23.

Morahan, R. J. and Hawksworth, D. N. (1969b). Salmonella isolations from foodstuffs in the East Sepik District Territory of Papua and New Guinea, employing an elevated temperature technique. *Med. J. Aust.* **2**, 593–596.

Mosley, J. W. (1967). Transmission of viral diseases by drinking water. *In* "Transmission of Viruses by the Water Route" (Ed. G. Berg). John Wiley and Sons, New York and London.

Pavanello, R. and Mohanrao, G. J. (1973). Considerations on water pollution problems in developing countries. *In* "Progress in Water Technology" (Ed. S. H. Jenkins) Vol. 3, Pergamon Press, Oxford, pp. 103–114.

Pickford, J. (1977). Solid waste disposal in hot climates. *In* "Water, Wastes and Health in Hot Climates" (Eds R. Feachem, M. McGarry and D. Mara). John Wiley and Sons, London and New York.

Radford, A. J. (1973). Balantidiasis in Papua New Guinea, *Med. J. Aust.* **1**, 238–241.

Rampling, A. M. (1967). Salmonellosis in animals and birds in Papua New Guinea. *Papua New Guin. agric. J.* **18**, 142–144.

Rampling, A. M. and Egerton, J. R. (1965). Salmonellosis in animals and birds in Papua New Guinea. *Papua New Guin. agric. J.* **17**, 149–153.

Rappaport, R. (1968). "Pigs for the Ancestors: Ritual in the Ecology of a New Guinea People". Yale University Press, New Haven.

Salisbury, R. F. (1962). "From Stone to Steel". Melbourne University Press, London.

Saunders, R. J. and Warford, J. J. (1974). "Village Water Supply and Sanitation in Less Developed Countries". International Bank for Reconstruction and Development, Washington.

Shaper, A. G., Clayton, D. G. and Morris, J. N. (1974). "The Hardness of Water and Cardiovascular Disease". Paper presented to the International Water Supply Association Congress at Brighton, England in August, 1974.

Simons, M. J., Binns, C. W., Malcolm, L. A. and Yap, E. H. (1972). Australia antigen frequencies in two groups of Highland New Guineans. *Papua New Guin. med. J.* **15**, 91–97.

Simpson, C. (1954). "Adam in Plumes". Angus and Robertson, Sydney.

Sinnett, P. F. (1972). "The People of Murapin: A Study in Human Biology". Doctor of Medicine Thesis, University of Sydney, Sydney.

Talbot, N. T. (1972). Incidence and distribution of helminth and arthropod parasites of indigenous owned pigs in Papua New Guinea. *Trop. Anim. Hlth Prod.* **4**, 182–190.

Taylor, J. L. (1940). Hagen–Sepik Patrol, Interim Report. *In* "Report to the Council of the League of Nations on the Administration of the Territory of New Guinea for the Year 1938–39". Government Printer, Canberra.

Taylor, F. H. and Murray, R. E. (1946). "Spiders, ticks and mites including the species harmful to man in Australia and New Guinea". School of Public Health and Tropical Medicine, service publication no. 6. University of Sydney, Sydney.

Turner, K. J., Baldo, B. A. and Anderson, H. R. (1975). Asthma in the highlands of New Guinea, total IgR levels and incidence of IgE antibodies to house dust mite and *Ascaris lumbricoides*. *Int. Archs. Allergy appl. Immun.* **48**, 784–799.

Van Thiel, P. H., Van Der Hoeven, J. A. and Couvee, L. M. J. (1963). Leptospirosis in the Highlands of West New Guinea. *Trop. geogr. Med.* **15**, 70–75.

Villarejos, V. M., Arguedas, J. A., Gutierrez, A., Eduarte, E., Vargas, G. and Osborne, J. A. (1972). Hepatitis epidemic in a hyperendemic zone of Costa Rica, report of a second outbreak within four years. *Am. J. Epidem.* **96**, 361–371.

Vines, A. P. (1970). "An Epidemiological Sample Survey of the Highlands, Mainland and Island Regions of the Territory of Papua New Guinea". Department of Public Health, Port Moresby, Papua New Guinea.

Waddell, E. W. (1972). "The Mound Builders: Agricultural Practices, Environment and Society in the Central Highlands of New Guinea". American Ethnological Society Mono. 53, University of Washington Press, Seattle.

Walzer, P. D., Judson, F. N., Murphy, K. B., Healy, G. R., English, D. K. and Schultz, M. G. (1973). Balantidiasis outbreak in Truk. *Am. J. trop. Med. Hyg.* **22**, 33–41.

Westermann, T. (1968). "The Mountain People: Social Institutions of the Raiapu Enga". Kristen Press, Wapenamanda, New Guinea.

White, G. F., Bradley, D. J. and White, A. U. (1972). "Drawers of Water: Domestic Water Use in East Africa". Chicago University Press, Chicago.

WHO (1971). "International Standard for Drinking-Water". World Health Organization, Geneva.

Willis, M. F. and Wannan, J. S. (1966). Some aspects of the epidemiology of leptospirosis in New Guinea. *Med. J. Aust.* **1**, 129–136.

Womersley, H. (1952). The Scrub Typhus and Scrub Itch Mites (Trombiculidae, Acarina) of the Asiastic–Pacific Region. *Rec. S. Aust. Mus.* **10**, (2 parts).

Woodfield, D. G., Oraka, R. E. and Nelson, M. (1972). Australia Antigen in Papua New Guinea. *Med. J. Aust.* **2**, 469–472.

Woolcock, A. J. and Blackburn, C. R. (1967). Chronic lung disease in TPNG—an epidemiological survey. *Australas. Ann. Med.* **16**, 11–19.

Woolcock, A. J., Blackburn, C. R., Freeman, M. H., Zylstra, W. and Spring, S. R. (1970). Studies of chronic (non-tuberculous) lung disease in New Guinea populations. The nature of the disease. *Am. Rev. resp. Dis.* **102**, 575–590.

Woolcock, A. J., Colman, M. H. and Blackburn, C. R. (1972). Factors affecting normal values for ventilatory lung function. *Am. Rev. Resp. Dis.* **106**. 692–709.

Zigas, V. and Doherty, R. L. (1973). An outbreak of dengue in the Rabaul community. *Papua New Guin. med. J.* **16**, 42–45.

Part 3

Environmental Change and Human Activity

CHAPTER VII

Man's Impact Upon Some New Guinea Mountain Ecosystems

JEREMY M. B. SMITH

University of New England, Armidale, Australia

I. INTRODUCTION

A recurring emphasis in this collection of papers concerns the value of a quantified approach to problems of human ecology. Accurate quantitative accounts of the energy and nutrient relationships of human populations can only refer with precision to present situations. Acceptance of quantitative studies in human ecology should be tempered by the realization that man's adaptability and success have led to considerable changes to his environment and ecological relationships throughout his history. Perhaps one general message conveyed by this article is that the stable and apparently conservationist ecological strategies adopted by many "primitive" human populations are largely illusory. What stability may be discernible today is conditioned by environmental constraints which are in part the results of man's past exploitation of his biotic environment, this impact often having brought about an impoverishment of that environment to man's own detriment.

Considered here are aspects of man's past and present relationship with his biotic environment in an area in Papua New Guinea above the altitudinal limits of horticulture. This area broadly speaking encompasses the headwaters of the Chimbu river, including the south-east slopes of Mt. Wilhelm, and incorporates terrain between 2600 and 4500 m altitude. The upper Chimbu valley below 2600 m is fairly intensively cultivated for a variety of crops with sweet potato as the staple, and supports a human population of 73–231 people per km² (Kingston, 1960; McAlpine, 1970). The numerically and culturally most important domestic animal is the pig.

The general effect of human disturbance of ecosystems, here as elsewhere, is to favour pioneer species of open communities at the expense of those organisms making up the stable climax vegetation, involving reductions in standing crop and in biotic diversity. In the present context the mountain forests provide man with meat, fur and feathers, timber and bark, pandan fruits and other products: the grass-lands to which he degrades the forests, apart from providing some decorative plants and a few small birds, are almost useless. The present series of ecosystems, altered to varying degrees by man, may therefore serve him less well than their more virginal predecessors.

II. THE PHYSICAL AND BIOTIC ENVIRONMENT

Mt. Wilhelm (4510 m) is the highest mountain in Papua New Guinea, situated at the junction of the Bismarck Mountains and the Sepik–Wahgi divide (see Map 1). North-east of the summit the ground falls away steeply to the wide Imbukum valley draining to the Ramu river, and to the north-west the Bendenumbun valley drains into the Jimi river. To the south several valleys lead to the Wahgi river or to its tributary the Chimbu, and so ultimately to the Purari. Present access to the summit is almost exclusively from the airstrip and roadhead at Keglsugl via the Pindaunde valley to the south-east. Beside the lower Pindaunde lake at 3480 m are a visitors' hut, a small research station and a few shelters of timber and grass. Map 5 is a sketch-map of the area.

Mt. Wilhelm has been studied in some detail, especially since the establishment of the research station by the Australian National University in 1965. The valleys of the granodiorite massif were glaciated during the Pleistocene down to about 3200 m (Löffler, 1972; Reiner, 1960) leaving rugged scenery above 3400 m (Figure 1) and moraines below 3500 m. Weathering of both rock and till, and the deposition of layers of volcanic ash and the accumulation of peat, have led to the development of acid soils often more than 1 m deep. At lower altitudes, though relief is generally great, landforms are fluvial and soils usually deeper (Haantjens, 1970).

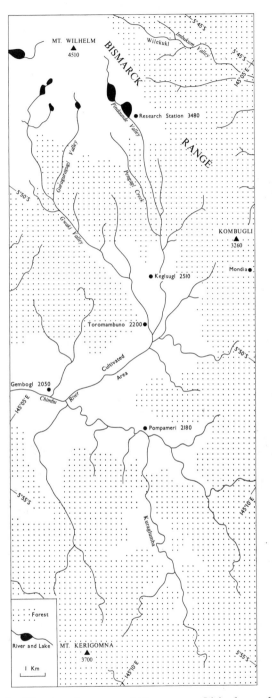

MAP 5. The headwaters of the upper Chimbu valley.

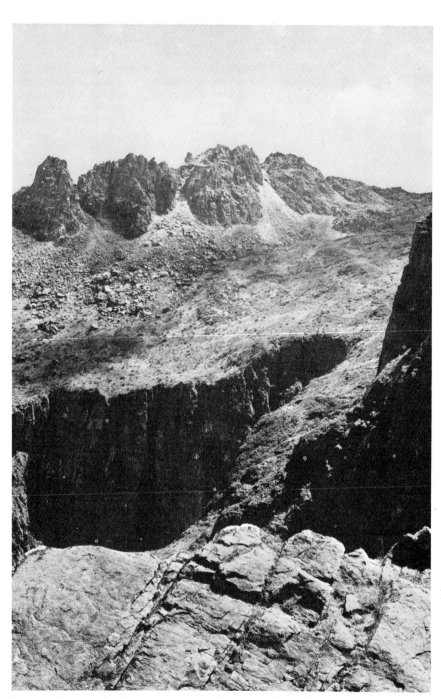

FIGURE 1. Head of the Guraguragugl valley, looking west from 4200 m, showing the glacially eroded valley below the former neve field and the frost-shattered ridgecrest.

The climate is largely non-seasonal (Hnatiuk *et al.*, 1976). Rainfall at 3480 m in the Pindaunde valley is about 3500 mm annually, and is probably less at both higher (4380 m) and lower (3215 m) stations. At Kegslugl (2510 m), mean annual rainfall is 2284 mm, and tends to fall less seasonally than on Mt. Wilhelm. The wettest months are October to May: over 40 consecutive rain days have been recorded in the Pindaunde valley during this season, and periods of up to 22 dry days in the months from June to September. Snowfalls are frequent above 4000 m. Temperatures vary diurnally rather than seasonally. Frosts are frequent in non-forest sites down to 3200 m especially during clear nights in the drier season, and may occasionally occur in the cultivated areas below 2600 m. Mean maximum temperature at 3480 m is 11·3°C and mean minimum 3·9°C. The lapse rate in the area is about 0·55°C/ 100 m.

The upper limit of sweet potato cultivation is determined by the occurrence of frost. Even in the areas currently cultivated, frequent local and occasional widespread loss of this staple crop occurs during clear weather, when ground temperatures are most liable to fall below freezing point (Brown and Powell, 1974). Other crops are less vulnerable to frost and some very local upward extension of cultivation has recently taken place in the upper Chimbu valley with the governmental encouragement of pyrethrum growing. Although I grew radishes successfully at 3480 m on Mt. Wilhelm in 1972 most crops at that altitude, if they survive at all, either grow very slowly (e.g. cabbage, "Irish" potato) or set no seed (e.g. pea, broad bean). Any widescale upward extension of cultivation will only follow a major shift of diet away from sweet potato. In fact there is evidence, for example in the Gwaki tributary of the upper Chimbu valley, of abandonment of gardens at the upper fringe of cultivation during the past few decades, though the reasons for this are not clear.

In the Asian tropics only the mountains of New Guinea support grassland communities above the climatic forest limit. Mt. Kinabalu (Borneo) has a rocky and largely unvegetated summit area, while elsewhere mountains do not reach above the climatic forest limit though some have areas of herbaceous vegetation due to edaphic factors. On Mt. Wilhelm, grasslands areally continuous with those of the summit area extend down to about 3200 m in valley bottoms, and isolated grasslands occur elsewhere in the upper Chimbu catchment, for example on Kombugli hill (3230–3260 m) and at Kuraglumba (2730–2850 m). The remaining area above the zone of cultivation is almost entirely forested, though in places the forest shows considerable disturbance, mainly due to logging and to rootling by domestic pigs, especially below 2750 m.

Twenty-eight plant communities have been defined floristically above 3100 m by Wade and McVean (1969), including 3 forest and 18 non-forest associations below "the upper limit of large shrubs" at 4100 m, and 7 "alpine" associations. A checklist of the vascular plants gives records of 606 species above 2743 m and 387 species above 3200 m (Johns and Stevens, 1971). About 40 further species have been recorded above 2743 m since the compilation of this list (Smith, 1974). Plant nomenclature used here follows Johns and Stevens (1971) for native species, and is provided in Table I for aliens.

A broad classification of New Guinea Highlands vegetation types is provided in Figure 2. Those types delineated by continuous lines are defined on clear physiognomic criteria. Subdivisions of mountain grassland are not so easy to define under field conditions: they differ from each other in their floristics, history or both, but tend to grade into each other and not to present clear mutual boundaries. Problems of nomenclature of New Guinea mountain vegetation have been discussed elsewhere (Smith, 1975).

Tropicalpine tundra occupies the summit ridge of Mt. Wilhelm above about 4300 m, and is characterized by frost-shattered rocky ground supporting open vegetation dominated by non-vascular plants. All vegetation belts below 4300 m, except locally for non-climatic reasons, have closed vegetation completely covering the ground.

Above 3810 m forest growth is probably prevented by climatic factors, and only scattered shrubs occur in the grasslands, the largest species of which is *Drimys piperita* "entity" *subalpina* growing up to 4100 m and sometimes assuming a form describable as a small (up to 3 m) tree. Dominance is usually by the tussock grass *Deschampsia klossii* or a variety of smaller tuft grasses. On Mt. Wilhelm the alpine finger fern (*Papuapteris linearis*) assumes dominance locally and is common in the grasslands above (but not below) the forest limit.

The mountain grasslands shown in Figure 3 include grass-dominated communities at altitudes from 2700 to 4300 m. The occurrence of grasslands below forest limit may be due to edaphic or anthropogenic factors. The former include grass-dominated areas of vegetation on Mt. Wilhelm found on rocky ridges and slopes with shallow soil, and more importantly in ill-drained basin sites, especially the moraine-choked valley bottoms from 3200 to 3400 m. Generally more widespread but not very distinct are anthropogenic grasslands, owing their origin and maintenance to fire.

Mountain forest covered most land below 3800 m prior to disturbance by man. No subdivision is attempted here since there appear to be no clear physiognomic or floristic boundaries within the highland forests. This is not to imply any uniformity however, for the forests become physiognomically and floristically more complex with decreasing altitude. As in other tropical mountain areas, and in contrast to the species-poor forests of temperate zone and arctic timberlines, the forest consists of several tree species even at its altitudinal limit.

In places suffering little human disturbance, tropicalpine mountain grassland and mountain forest interdigitate in a narrow ecotone at the upper altitudinal limit of the forest. For example in the Imbukum valley of Mt. Wilhelm tongues of the higher altitude herbaceous vegetation, dominated by the tussock grass *Deschampsia klossii* and

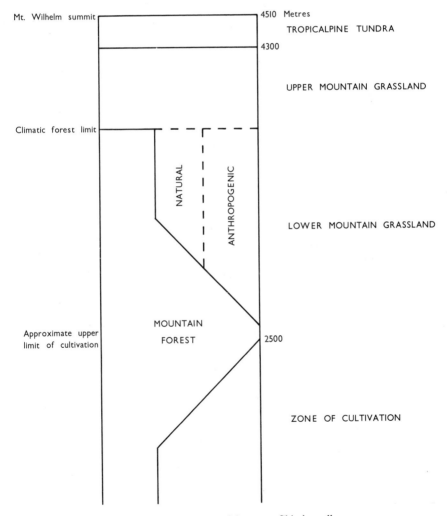

Figure 2. Vegetation types in the headwaters of the upper Chimbu valley.

TABLE I

Plant species alien to New Guinea growing in the Mt. Wilhelm area, 1972

Family	Species	Occurrence at sites													Specimen no.	Earliest collection	Highest record	Frost	Notes
		1	2	3	4	5	6	7	8	9	10	11	12	13					
Gramineae																			
	Eragrostis tenuifolia Hochst. ex Stend.	+		+			+								ANU 15348	1959	2819	?	1
	Lolium rigidum Gaud.			+									+		ANU 15303	1971	3481	H	
	Phalaris tuberosa L.													(+)	NGF 39562	1955	3536	?	
	Poa annua L.	+		+			+		+						ANU 15079	1959	3481	H	2
	Pennisetum clandestinum Hochst. ex Chiov.																		
	Vulpia bromoides (L.) S. F. Gray						+		+				+		ANU 15079	1962	2911	?	
Iridaceae																			
	Tritonia X *crocosmaeflora* Nichols										+				ANU 15301	1972	3481	H	
Liliaceae																			
	Cordyline fruticosa (L.) Gepp.	+	+	+	+	+	+	+	+				+	+	ANU 15302	1953	3481	S	3
		+	+	+	+	+	+	+	+				+	+	ANU 15353	1930	3481	S	4
Caryophyllaceae																			
	Dianthus sp.	+	+	+			+								ANU 15411	1972	2667	?	
	Stellaria media L.	+	+	+	+	+	+	+					+		ANU 15153	1959	3481	H	
Casuarinaceae																			
	Casuarina oligodon Johnson	+					+	+							ANU 15456	1951	2819	?	5
Compositae																			
	Ageratum conyzoides L.	+				+	+	+	+						ANU 15365	1950	2576	?	
	Bidens pilosa L.	+	+	+		+	+	+	+				+		ANU 15205	1953	3490	S	6
	Chrysanthemum cinerariifolium (Trev.) Bocc.	+					+												
	Conyza aegyptica Ait.	+		+		(+)	(+)	+							ANU 15519	1972	2539	?	7
	Cosmos ?*bipinnatus* Cow.	+		+		+	+								Brass 30526	1957	2713	?	
	Crassocephalum crepidioides (Benth.) S. Moore	+				+	+	+	+						ANU 13013	1971	2819	?	
	Erechtites valerianifolia (Wolf.) DC.	+	+	+		+	+	+	+	+				+	ANU 15244	1957	3414	S	8
	Erigeron canadensis L.	+	+	+		+	+	+	+	+	+	+	+		ANU 15373	1953	2880	?	
	Erigeron sumatrensis Retz.	+	+	+		+	+	+	+	+	+	+	+		ANU 15261	1957	3688	H	
	Galinsoga parviflora Cav.	+	+	+	+	+	+	+	+	+	+	+	+		ANU 15148	1950	3688	H	
	Gynura procumbens (Laur.) Merr.	+				+	+								ANU 15253	1959	2966	?	
	Siegesbeckia orientalis L.	+		+		(+)	(+)	+							ANU 15250	1959	2850	?	
	Sonchus asper (L.) Hill			+		+	+	+							ANU 15363	1947	2728	?	
	Sonchus oleraceus L.		+	+		+	+	+							ANU 15201	1963	2911	?	
	Tagetes minuta L.	+	+	+	+	+	+	+	+				+		ANU 15382	1950	3688	H	
	Tagetes sp.	+					+								ANU 15349	1959	2728	?	

Family	Species	ANU no.	Year	Altitude	Frost	Note
	Cardamine hirsuta L.	ANU 15424	1960	3240	?	
	Nasturtium officinale R. Br.	ANU 15357	1960	2667	?	10
	Rorippa sp.					
Labiatae	Coleus sp.	ANU 13011	1971	2661	?	
	Mentha sp.	ANU 15512	1972	3481	H	11
	Stachys arvensis L.	ANU 15342	1957	2966	?	
	Thymus ?vulgaris L.	ANU 15359	1968	2667	?	12
Leguminosae	Cassia tomentosa L.f.	ANU 15351	1959	2713	?	
	Lathyrus ?sativus L.	ANU 15399	1960	2530	?	
	Lupinus sp.	ANU 15249	1959	3481	S	
	Pisum sativum L.	ANU 15300	1972	3481	H	13
	Trifolium repens L.	ANU 15200	1960	2911	?	
	Vicia sativa L.	ANU 7033	1966	3481	?	
Linaceae	Linum usitatissimum L.	NGF 35093	1968	3535	?	
Passifloraceae	Passiflora sp.	ANU 15517	1972	2713	?	
	Tacsonia mollissima Kunth.	ANU 15304	1959	3481	S	14
Plantaginaceae	Plantago lanceolata L.	ANU 15477	1972	3481	H	
	Plantago major L.	ANU 15189	1967	2804	?	
Rosaceae	Fragaria cf. vesca L.	ANU 15078	1971	3484	H	15
Scrophulariaceae	Veronica cf. persica Poir.	ANU 15117	1957	3481	H	
Solanaceae	Centrum ?elegans Schlecht.	ANU 15360	1966	2667	?	16
	Nicotiana tabacum L.	ANU 15455	1961	2633	?	17
	Physalis peruviana L.	ANU 15179	1954	2728	?	
	Solanum nigrum L.	ANU 15352	1956	2713	?	18
Verbenaceae	Verbena bonariensis L.	ANU 15350	1953	3481	S	
Pinaceae	Pinus sp.	ANU 15457	1972	2515	?	19

Sites: 1. Gardens, upper Chimbu valley, 2100–2510 m; 2. Kuraglumba, 2730–2850 m; 3. Mondia road, 2800–2900 m; 4. Clearing on Keglsugl–Kombugli track, 2970 m; 5. Kombugli, 3240–3270 m; 6. Wilhelm summit track (Keglsugl–Komanimambuno), 2510–2710 m; 7. Wilhelm summit track (Pengagl creek: old route), 2710–2900 m; 8. Wilhelm summit track (old route), 2900–3200 m; 9. Banks of Pengagl creek, 2900–3050 m; 10. Gwaki creek and Guraguragugl valleys, 2900–3560 m; 11. Wilhelm summit track (Pindaunde mountain grassland), 3200–3480 m; 12. Near Pindaunde huts, 3480–3490 m; 13. Landslips and other natural habitats, 3200–3700 m.

+ Indicates occurrence during 1972.

(+) Indicates an earlier record not repeated in 1972.

Notes: 1. Probably favoured by trampling; 2. Favoured by pig disturbance of soil below 2750 m; 3. Favoured by pollution at 3480 m; 4. Commonly planted as stem cuttings along paths; 5. Commonly planted as seedlings below 2500 m; 6. Hooked fruits often carried in clothing; 7. Pyrethrum: occasional wild seedlings found near cultivated plots. 8. Very good colonist of newly bared ground; 9. Often grows from discarded cabbage stalks; 10. Watercress: commonly planted as stem cuttings in wet places; 11. Mint: never flowers but reproduces by stolons; 12. Thyme: only found near abandoned home sites; 13. Seeds often carried by children for food; 14. Fruits eaten by man and pigs; seeds germinate in old pig faeces; 15. "Fruits" eaten by man; 16. Ornamental shrub commonly planted near houses; 17. Tobacco: only found near abandoned home sites; 18. Fruits sometimes eaten by man; 19. Pine: planted as seedlings.

All plant specimens quoted are lodged in the Forests Department herbarium, Lae. Earliest and highest records are those represented by collections in Lae from all of Papua New Guinea and from the Mt. Wilhelm area respectively. Altitudes are in metres. H indicates that the species is hardly damaged by frost on Mt. Wilhelm; S indicates that the species is frost sensitive.

Excluded from the table are species growing only below 2510 m (Site 1), and species growing only as deliberately planted specimens near the Pindaunde research station showing no sign of spread or already extinct (including Fuchsia ?magellanica, Petroselinum crispum and various vegetables).

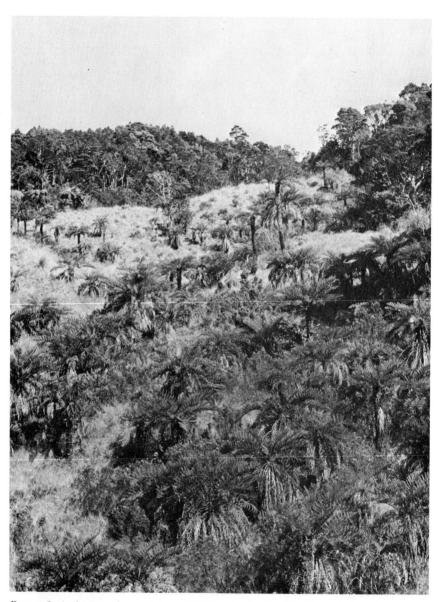

FIGURE 3. Anthropogenic vegetation at 3200 m in the Gwaki valley; the tussock grass *Poa saruwagetica* and tree fern *Cyathea atrox*, fire-tolerant species, are both abundant; unaltered forest in the background.

including small shrubs of *Coprosma divergens, Eurya brassii, Haloragis halconensis* and *Styphelia suaveolens*, extend downward to 3760 m, especially in minor gullies and depressions. Forest vegetation, with emergent conifers (*Dacrycarpus compactus*) and a variety of smaller trees (including *Dimorphanthera microphylla, Olearia floccosa, O. spectabilis, Rapanea vaccinioides* and *Symplocos* sp.) grows on intervening hummocks and small ridges up to 3810 m. Tree ferns, mainly *Cyathea gleichenioides*, are conspicuous along the margins of the two communities (Smith, 1975).

At lower altitudes forest areas tend to have abrupt margins. Sharp vegetation boundaries may have occurred naturally where herbaceous vegetation on ill-drained ground abutted forested slopes, but in the area considered here such situations are uncommon today. Forest margins, whether still in retreat or currently readvancing, are generally the result of fire which has extended the area of combustible grassland at the expense of the generally incombustible and fire-intolerant forest. Repeated fires burning to the edges of forest patches ensure that tree seedlings in the grassland as well as plants of the forest margin are killed.

At least 13 mammal species and 18 bird species are resident in mountain grassland and forest edge habitats above 3215 m, and probably a larger number at lower altitudes. Among the marsupials are the striped bandicoot (*Peroryctes longicauda*), the uncommon carnivore *Satanellus albopunctatus* and a rare species of rock wallaby at high altitudes. The commonest of at least six rodent species is the moss rat (*Rattus niobe*), occurring throughout the areas above 3200 m. Packs of wild dogs may be heard howling at night and kills, tracks and faeces found by day above 3500 m, but the animals themselves are rarely seen. The birds include at least five honeyeaters (Meliphagidae), feeding largely on nectar from a variety of red-flowered ericaceous shrubs. The only two birds common in grasslands above 3200 m, and found above 4300 m, are the pipit *Anthus gutturalis* and the thrush *Turdus poliocephalus*. The duck *Salvadorina waigiuensis* breeds beside the Mt. Wilhelm lakes and may be seen along rivers at lower altitudes. A species of quail is frequent at Kuraglumba. Small microhylid frogs burrow beneath damp tussocks in grasslands between 3200 and 4000 m.

The forests have a richer vertebrate fauna, which has never been fully inventoried. Among the mammals are tree kangaroos (*Dendrolagus*), the cuscus (*Phalanger vestitus*) and the ring-tailed possum (*Pseudocheirus cupreus*); there is a great variety of birds. Cassowaries (*Casuarius ? bennetti*) and feral pigs are present and hunted in the forests of the Imbukum valley but do not occur around the headwaters of the Chimbu.

III. BURNING

The impact of man upon vegetation in highland New Guinea through the medium of fire has been appreciated by many authors. Lane-Poole, writing of a knoll surrounded by forest in the Saruwaged Mountains, states

> This burnt patch is an excellent example of how the destruction starts. The trees had all been killed but the forest conditions not destroyed . . . A few tufts of grass appear . . . There is enough debris from the skeleton conifers above to make a big blaze, and all the natives are waiting for is a spell of dry weather . . . when they will put a fire-stick in. (Lane-Poole, 1925, pp. 175–181)

Describing vegetation at higher altitudes in the same mountains he writes "The annual fires of the natives kill the shrubs, but the grass survives and takes the place of the woody plants". He thought, prior to human interference, "except for the very marshy land and the actual cliffs and outcrops of limestone, the whole of this mountain top was under a forest of conifers and myrtles".

Later observations have confirmed those of Lane-Poole and strengthened his conclusions. Brass (Archbold and Rand, 1935) saw several km² of fire-destroyed forest at 3300 m on Mt. Albert Edward. Paijmans and Löffler (1972) have described the probable sequence of events above 2800 m on the same mountain, the firing beginning in swampy valley bottoms and progressively destroying the forests up-slope. Wade and McVean (1969) describe damage to forest edges by grass fires on Mt. Giluwe, and of the same mountain, Bowers writes

> At the upper limits of montane forest, where environmental conditions are critical for the survival of ligneous species, hunters fell the forest trees more rapidly than colonisation can take place. Both montane forest and alpine shrubbery retreat, while the area occupied by alpine grassland expands. (Bowers, 1968)

During the unusually dry season of 1972 very large areas of grassland above the Mt. Giluwe forests were burned (Brown and Powell, 1974) resulting in local burning of peat to a depth of 5 cm (G. S. Hope, pers. comm., 1973). Grasslands owing their origin and maintenance to fire have been described by Gillison (1969) and by Kalkman and Vink (1970) above 2500 m in the Doma Peaks area.

The general effects of fire are to produce physiognomically and floristically simpler ecosystems by encouraging those species which are both fire tolerant and combustible at the expense of the remaining majority. Forest is degraded to grassland, within which shrubs are uncommon and species generally few if burning is repeated periodically. The tussock grass *Poa saruwagetica* and tree fern *Cyathea atrox* are especially favoured by burning, as are several short-lived herbaceous plants of good dispersal ability, both native and alien, such as species of *Erigeron, Gnaphalium* and *Senecio* (Figure 3).

In the Mt. Wilhelm area, deliberate burning of grasslands above 2600 m is common during dry weather at Kuraglumba, but not on the mountain itself where an Administration ban on grass fires has generally been respected since its imposition in about 1959 (Brass, 1964). Formerly widespread burning is evidenced in the Pindaunde valley, for example, by tree roots, charcoal and charred stumps in grasslands. Forest occurs today in relict patches surrounded by anthropogenic grassland between 3200 and 3800 m in the southern valleys of Mt. Wilhelm. In some grassland areas old trees of the conifer *Dacrycarpus compactus* and less commonly *Pittosporum pullifolium* remain, often with fire-damaged trunk bases, as survivors of the formerly more widespread forest (Figure 4).

At present forest patches are apparently gradually expanding in most areas above 3200 m, mainly by layering (in particular by *Coprosma papuensis* and *Rubus* spp.) as described for the Doma Peaks area by Gillison (1970). In addition shrubs in grasslands have become larger and more common, as shown by comparison of photographs taken before 1960 (Johns and Stevens, 1971; Reiner, 1960) with the same areas in 1972. Amongst the shrubs are young trees, in particular of *Olearia spectabilis*.

Between 3700 and 3800 m, forest does not appear to regenerate in the absence of burning. This may be related to a milder climatic period between 8400 and 5000 years ago. Such a hypsithermal period has been suggested by Hope (1976) as a result of palynological investigations on Mt. Wilhelm showing vegetation belts to be higher than at present during this period. It is possible that forest species can regenerate under the more equable climatic conditions within the forest, but be unable to do so in formerly forested grassland areas at the same altitude (Smith, 1975).

Kuraglumba (2730–2850 m) is a basin of generally gentle topography *c.* 20 km south-east of Mt. Wilhelm summit above Pompameri village. It consists of an area of grassland about 2 km wide and about 5 km long, lying astride an important footpath to Marafunga and Goroka. Over 200 people daily, often with pigs, walk through the area during dry weather along deeply eroded tracks. The central part of Kuraglumba is occupied by an ill-drained alluvial area. The vegetation is mainly composed of plants which can survive or regenerate after

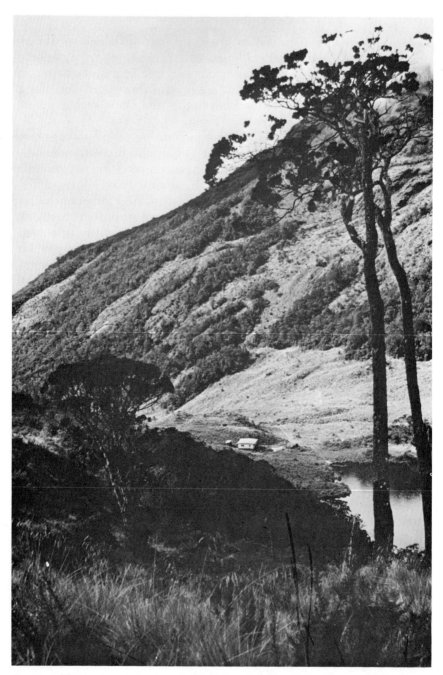

FIGURE 4. Mosaic of vegetation types in the Pindaunde valley; in the foreground isolated trees of *Dacrycarpus compactus* stand as forest survivors in anthropogenic grassland, and on the distant slopes relict patches of forest are surrounded by grassland; the research station (3480 m) is visible on the valley floor near the lower Pindaunde lake.

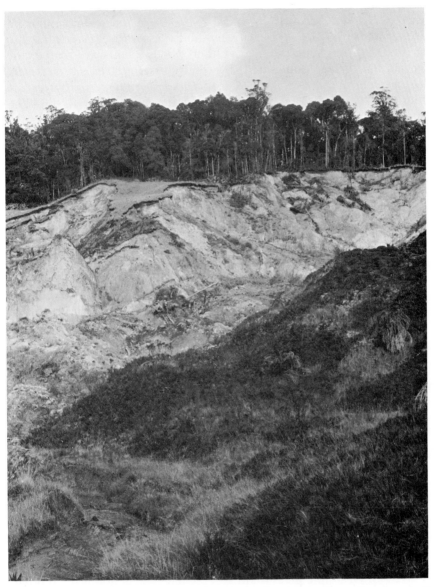

FIGURE 5. Some consequences of repeated vegetation burning in the south-west part of Kuraglumba, *c*. 2800 m; the fern *Gleichenia* cf. *erecta* is locally abundant in the anthropogenic grassland in the foreground; severe accelerated erosion is visible behind; the forest shows an abrupt retreating margin.

fire. Small trees (*Dodonaea viscosa*) grow locally near the river, the shrubs *Hypericum macgregorii* and *Styphelia suaveolens* are common on wetter and drier slopes respectively, and tree ferns (*Cyathea atrox*) are scattered throughout the area. Other woody plants are scarce, the vegetation being dominated by the grasses *Danthonia archboldii*, *Deschampsia klossii*, *Deyeuxia ? brassii*, *Dichelachne rara*, *Imperata conferta* and *Poa saruwagetica*, and the sedge *Cladium glomeratum* R. Br. The surrounding forest presents an abrupt margin marked by much fallen and charred timber. Severe soil erosion has followed vegetation destruction on steeper slopes (Figure 5).

Fire is a dominating ecological factor at Kuraglumba, producing vegetation changes perhaps more marked than those described at Doma Peaks by Gillison (1969). In August 1972, during an unusually dry season, several fires were deliberately lit during a 30-hour observation period. In places grassland fires had reached the margin of the forest killing (or at least severely damaging) trees and shrubs. It is clear that most or all the grasslands at this site owe their origin, maintenance and expansion to human burning.

Local fires have occurred recently on Mt. Wilhelm. A small grass fire beside the main path in the Pindaunde valley at 3380 m in June 1972 caused damage to woody plants up to 2 m inside an adjacent forest patch; seven woody species were recorded as being killed. A larger area, of about 7000 m² at 3550 m in the Guraguragugl valley, was burned an estimated two years prior to observation in May 1972. The area had formerly been dominated by shrubs about 1 m high, mainly *Coprosma papuensis*, *Dimorphanthera keysseri*, *D. microphylla*, *Gaultheria mundula*, *Olearia spectabilis* and *Styphelia suaveolens*. Of these about 90% were dead or only regenerating from the base, the area being dominated by the grasses *Dichelachne rara* and *Poa saruwagetica*.

It is clear then that fire is and has been a potent factor in altering and degrading ecosystems in the area. However, it is probable that natural fire is absent or very rare: the Bismarck range is not volcanic and lightning (though commonly visible from Mt. Wilhelm by evening over the north coast) is unusual in the area and invariably accompanied by substantial precipitation. On the other hand, man continues to light fires where possible and where no authoritative restraint is perceived. Often simple pleasure in spectacular destruction is the motive, but small game killed by fires may be collected, and some fires are lit for warmth.

An early stage in the process of creation through fire of large areas of anthropogenic grassland may be seen at Wilekukl, an area of till-choked valley floor measuring about 200 by 1000 m situated in the Imbukum valley of Mt. Wilhelm between 3300 and 3350 m. It is approximately horizontal in transverse section but slopes gently and consistently downvalley, and is crossed by several braided stream channels. The ground surface is ill-drained, supporting mainly mire vegetation often dominated by *Carex gaudichaudiana*, with small raised "islands" of till on which scattered shrubs grow, mainly *Rhododendron yelliottii*. The slopes at either side of Wilekukl are clothed by almost continuous forest except at the base, where a strip of tussock grassland dominated by *Deschampsia klossii* abuts the mire. Isolated old trees, *Dacrycarpus compactus*, in this strip suggest that it was formerly forested.

Despite the isolation of Wilekukl from permanent human settlements, the presence of a dilapidated grass and timber shelter (in April 1972) showed at least some penetration by man; two local informants who accompanied me on this trip, John Dua and William Nua, confirmed that hunters from both Bundi and the upper Chimbu valley occasionally visit the place. It is very unlikely that the wet ground occupying the majority of Wilekukl (and parts of Kuraglumba and the Pindaunde valley) could have ever supported closed forest. Such places would be far easier to pass through than the adjacent dense forest, and would form natural routes for hunters and travellers. During periods of dry weather, when hunting activity is at a peak, their herbaceous vegetation could easily be fired. Not only would this lead to modification of such vegetation but also to its progressive increase in area at the expense of forest, whose margin is repeatedly killed. Such an anthropogenic and pyrogenic origin can be adduced for the tussock grassland margin at Wilekukl, the bulk of Kuraglumba possibly excepting the central alluvial area, and most of the grasslands on well-drained slopes below 3800 m in the Pindaunde and other valleys of Mt. Wilhelm.

The same anthropogenic origin of mountain grasslands by burning of originally small areas of herbaceous vegetation in mires has been proposed for the Neon Basin and higher grasslands of Mt. Albert Edward by Paijmans and Löffler (1972), for highland grasslands in Java by van Steenis (1968, 1972), and for their lower altitude equivalents in Tasmania by Gilbert (1959).

The forests around Kuraglumba have retreated from the central alluvial area, the nucleus of destruction, by up to 1 km. It was estimated in late August 1972 that one-quarter of Kuraglumba's area had been burned that year. 1972 was an unusually dry year, but at the time of this estimate the dry season, and the fires, had not ended. It seems reasonable to suppose that any forest edge may be burned about once in four years. Grass fires have been seen to penetrate about 2 m into forest vegetation, killing woody plants over this distance. Using these very crude figures it may be calculated that at the present rate of disturbance up to 2000 years were required for the conversion of Kuraglumba to grassland. This does not take into account the possibility of forest fires under extremely dry conditions, such as were noted by Brass (Archbold and Rand, 1935) on Mt. Albert Edward. Nor is the probable increase in human impact over time allowed for. Nevertheless crude as it is this estimate does suggest, not unreasonably, that hunting (with burning) was carried on in the upper Chimbu valley prior to widespread cultivation.

Although gardens may have been present as early as 6500 years ago, a rise in *Casuarina* pollen in Mt. Wilhelm bog and lake sediments beginning 900 years ago probably marks the start of widespread agriculture in the upper Chimbu valley at 1500–2500 m (Hope, 1976). The only species of *Casuarina* in the local area is *C. oligodon*, introduced to sites below 2600 m as a source of timber and firewood, often planted beside gardens or in fallow where it improves soil fertility by nitrogen fixation. The Wahgi valley experienced widespread agriculture from before 5000 years ago (Powell, 1970).

A further aspect of human impact upon vegetation in the area may be illustrated by the observation that the only probable plant hybrids recorded from Mt. Wilhelm, in *Galium, Hypericum, Rhododendron* and *Vaccinium* (P. F. Stevens, pers. comm., 1973), have all been collected only from anthropogenic grassland or its margin with forest. This is in accord with Anderson's (1949) principle that hybridization of plants only follows "habitat hybridization", usually as a result of human activity.

IV. HUNTING AND GATHERING

The oldest record of man in New Guinea, so far unearthed, is at Kosipe in the Owen Stanley range (Papuan peninsula) where White and others (1970) have described human occupation over 23 000 years ago of a site at 2000 m altitude. Considerably older records from Australia indicate the probability of more ancient occupation of New Guinea, as these two areas were not separated by sea during much of the Pleistocene and as recently as 8000–6000 years ago (Jennings, 1972). Pollen analyses of bog and lake sediments in the Highlands of Papua New Guinea (Flenley, 1972; Hope, 1976; Walker, 1970) show that colder conditions prevailed there from before 38 000 to 11 000–10 000 years ago, with forest limit lowered to below 2400 m. Permanent snowline was also lowered, to 3500–3600 m at its lowest (Löffler, 1972; Galloway *et al.*, 1972) and glaciation occurred on Mt. Wilhelm and several other high mountains. These climatic differences resulted in and are in part inferred from far wider expanses of mountain grassland throughout highland New Guinea than exist at present.

Noting the existence of high altitude trading paths and the present usage of high altitude areas for hunting and gathering of plant materials, Hope and Hope (1975) suggest that the earliest men in New Guinea may have included hunters in the formerly more extensive mountain grasslands. Martin (1967) has suggested that the Late Quaternary extinction of large mammals and ground-living birds has been caused or accelerated by hunting man in most parts of the world. Hope and Hope (1975), partly quoting Plane (1967) show that large macropods were present in New Guinea in the Pleistocene and diprotodonts in the Pliocene, some or all of which probably grazed the mountain grasslands and may have been accelerated to extinction by human predation. However as these authors point out, climatic amelioration since 10 500 years ago resulted in upward migration of forest and a reduction in mountain grassland area from about 50 000 km² to about 800 km² in the island of New Guinea. Any grassland animal would therefore become, if not naturally extinct, at least greatly reduced in population and in dietary significance to hunting man due simply to contraction of habitat area.

Whether or not man has reduced his potential range of prey by extinction of species through overhunting, local hunting in the upper Chimbu area of a variety of animals has probably resulted in substantial reductions in their populations. Almost any bird or mammal is regarded as fair game and a welcome dietary addition. Fur of the larger mammals and the plumage of many birds are also of ornamental value. The larger forest mammals including tree kangaroos, possums and phalangers are hunted with the aid of dogs and trapped in snares. Tree kangaroos at least are scarce in the area and the local absence of cassowaries and feral pigs is probably due to hunting pressure.

A rock wallaby was recorded by Wade and McVean (1969) from the area immediately to the north of Mt. Wilhelm summit. Its rarity by comparison with the abundance of this or a similar species on the unhunted Mt. Suckling (P. F. Stevens, pers. comm., 1973) is strongly suggestive of considerable population decrease by the hand of man. Small birds on the other hand, knocked down with three-pronged arrows or thrown stones, seem to have suffered far less. *Astrapia stephaniae*, a black bird-of-paradise much prized for its long tail feathers, is frequently seen in the mountain forests; and the berry pecker *Paramythia montia*, the species most commonly killed above 3215 m as it has a tame and trusting disposition, remains common.

Traditionally the areas above 2600 m in the upper Chimbu valley have been used for various purposes in addition to hunting. Paths cross ridges of Mt. Wilhelm at over 3200 m (e.g. from the upper Chimbu valley south-west towards Kerowagi), across Kombugli hill (to Bundi) and through Kuraglumba (to Marafunga). Walker (1968) records that the vicinity of the Pindaunde lakes was a traditional fighting area for the people of the upper Chimbu valley.

Gathering of plant materials has been and is still important. Though leaves and berries of several species may be eaten, no mountain plants are important as food apart from *Pandanus giulianettii*, growing from below 2600 to 3080 m in the area. Seedlings are favoured by occasional clearance of competing vegetation and the mature trees are said to be owned by individuals or clans. The seasonally available dry fruits are collected and either eaten fresh or stored after being smoked. Another plant formerly very important though less so today is *Pipturus* sp., a small tree of forest-edge and disturbed sites from 2700 to 3600 m whose fibrous bark is pounded to make cloth. *Equisetum debile*, growing in wet places from 2700 to 3700 m, was formerly used as an abrasive in the washing of clothing.

Many plants are used for personal ornamentation, especially of the hair, and some are specifically gathered for use on festive occasions. Most plants collected at high altitudes appear to be used for "second best" self-decoration, as flowers are used in the Mt. Hagen area 80 km west of the upper Chimbu valley (Strathern and Strathern, 1971). Shoots of *Astelia papuana* and *Styphelia suaveolens* and flowers of species of *Anaphalis*, *Dendrobium*, *Dimorphanthera* and *Rhododendron* have been noted as being used in this way. The finger fern *Papuapteris linearis*, only found commonly above 3800 m and up to 4300 m, is valued more highly and used on important festive occasions (see for example Todd, 1974, the lower photograph facing p. 104). Special collecting trips are made to gather fronds of this fern prior to such occasions, and dried fronds are traded throughout the Chimbu district and beyond.

Timber requirements, for housing, fencing and firewood, are largely satisfied by *Casuarina oligodon* planted on fallowed gardens below 2500 m. "Bush timber" is also gathered from forests not far from permanent settlements, although until the acquisition of steel axes, only small trees were probably taken (Meggitt, 1960). Nevertheless this must have led, combined with the impact of domestic pigs, to degradation of the forest near its margin with cultivated ground. With the steel axe, sawmills present in the upper Chimbu valley,* and a demand for heavy timber for purposes such as road bridges, this degradation has greatly accelerated in recent years.

* One at Toromambuno; a second moved in 1972 from the Mondia road (at 2750 m) to a site above Kegslugl (at 2600 m).

V. PLANT AND ANIMAL INTRODUCTIONS

Many introduced plants alien to New Guinea have established themselves in the area being considered, and further species will do so in future. Most of those already present are still spreading and have not realized their full potentials in the area. Fifty-four probably alien plant species have been collected to 1972 above Keglsugl (2510 m), and 24 in non-forest vegetation areally continuous with that of Mt. Wilhelm summit (above 3215 m). These, with local distribution details, are listed in Table I. The degree of certainty of their alien status, probable periods of introduction, uses and external transport by man are given in Table II: only probable aliens are regarded here as introductions, those indicated as possibly alien being regarded as native.

Most species recorded are not abundant and a few are apparently extinct in the area. Of the remainder some are noxious weeds of cultivated ground, including *Bidens pilosa, Crassocephalum crepidioides, Erigeron canadensis, E. sumatrensis, Poa annua, Sonchus oleraceus* and *Stellaria media*. The vegetation of a cultivated area at 2500 m very similar to and less than 170 km west of the upper Chimbu valley has been described by Walker (1966). *Crassocephalum crepidioides* is a notably efficient colonist of sites of disturbance up to 3200 m but is not frost tolerant and has not been recorded above 3414 m. *Erigeron canadensis, E. sumatrensis* and *Sonchus oleraceus* have all been collected on a landslip site at 3688 m, but like most alien plants are only found in such disturbed sites, never in closed, stable vegetation.

Man has introduced many edible plants to New Guinea and several have been recorded growing wild in the upper Chimbu valley. Of these only four can be regarded as being well established. *Fragaria* cf. *vesca*, wild strawberry, said to have been introduced to the area by German missionaries, is abundant from 2500 m to 2800 m along the Mt. Wilhelm track, and has been found occasionally in many other sites in the area including in tussock grassland near the lower Pindaunde lake at 3480 m, and as low as 1585 m beside the Chimbu river. *Nasturtium officinale*, watercress, is widely planted in wet places as cuttings and has become abundant in Gwaki creek up to at least 3055 m. *Tacsonia mollissima*, banana passionfruit, is widespread and frequent in forest edge and degraded forest communities up to over 3000 m, but rarely produces fruit above 2800 m. The fruits of cape gooseberry, *Physalis peruviana*, common below 2700 m, are edible. None of these potential food resources is exploited to more than a limited extent. No other useful alien plants occur commonly above 2600 m.

TABLE II

Times of introduction and uses of alien plants growing in the Mt. Wilhelm area, 1972

Time of introduction	Woody plants	Monocotyledons	Compositae	Other dicotyledons
Possibly pre-European (before about 100 yr ago)		Isachne myosotis Juncus effusus Juncus prismatocarpus Microlaena stipoides[a]	Dichrocephala bicolor[a] Gnaphalium japonicum	Coleus scutellarioides[a] Cynoglossum javanicum Maxus pumilus Oenanthe javanica[b] Oxalis corniculata Polygonum nepalense Wahlenbergia marginata
Probably pre-European	Casuarina oligodon[d] Cordyline fruticosa[d]		Gynura procumbens	Nicotiana tabacum[d] Plantago major Rorippa sp.[b] Solanum nigrum
Probably European (after about 100 yr ago)	Cassia tomentosa[c] Cestrum elegans[c]	Eragrostis tenuifolia Poa annua Tritonia X crocosmaeflora[c]	Ageratum conyzoides Bidens pilosa[a] Conyza aegyptica Cosmos ?bipinnatus[c] Erechtites valerianifolia Erigeron canadensis Erigeron sumatrensis Galinsoga parviflora Siegesbeckia orientalis Sonchus asper Sonchus oleraceus Tagetes minuta Tagetes sp.[c]	Cardamine hirsuta Coleus sp.[c] Lathyrus sativus Lupinus sp.[d] Mentha sp.[b] Nasturtium officinale[b] Physalis peruviana[b] Stachys arvensis Stellaria media Tacsonia mollissima[b] Thymus ?vulgaris[b] Verbena bonariensis Veronica cf. persica
Certainly European	Pinus sp.[d]	Lolium rigidum Pennisetum clandestinum[d] Phalaris tuberosa Vulpia bromoides	Chrysanthemum cinerariifolium[d] Crassocephalum crepidioides	Brassica oleracea[b] Dianthus sp.[c] Fragaria cf. vesca[b] Linum usitatissimum Passiflora sp.[b] Pisum sativum[b] Plantago lanceolata Trifolium repens[d] Vicia sativa

[a] Disseminules cling to clothing. [b] Eaten by man as fruit, herb or vegetable. [c] Planted for decorative qualities.

All alien plants recorded are greatly favoured by disturbance of soil and vegetation and almost entirely restricted to disturbed sites. Such sites include streambanks and landslips, but sites of human disturbance (dug or burned areas, pathsides etc.) or of rootling by domestic pigs are more widespread. It is doubtful whether most of the plants introduced by man could survive in the area in the absence of man-initiated habitat disturbance. Above 3000 m *Sonchus oleraceus* is very characteristic of old fire sites, while *Poa annua* was abundant in 1972 at 3480 m in a section of drain sometimes carrying dirty soapy water, but infrequent in adjacent sections carrying only rainwater. *Tritonia* × *crocosmaeflora* and *Fragaria* cf. *vesca* are especially favoured by pig rootling between 2500 and 2750 m.

Many of the alien plants were carried deliberately by man to New Guinea and probably would not otherwise have arrived, but many others were transported in ignorance and by accident. Human transport of viable disseminules, of both native and alien species, continues in the upper Chimbu valley and is important in enabling some adventive species to reach sites of human habitat disturbance suitable for their colonization.

In both 1971 and 1972, disseminules were collected from footwear and clothing (especially from socks) of climbers reaching the lower Pindaunde lake (3480 m) from Keglsugl (2515 m) or lower in the upper Chimbu valley. Attempts were made to germinate seeds, and in addition the number of disseminules of each species were counted from six individual climbers at various dates during 1972. In this way 12 species (identified as disseminules or as large seedlings) were shown to have disseminules dispersed externally by man, those most commonly so being *Acaena anserinifolia*, *Bidens pilosa*, *Cynoglossum javanicum*, *Microlaena stipoides* and *Uncinia* spp. (see Table III). In addition it is probable that viable seeds of *Fragaria* cf. *vesca* and *Tacsonia mollissima* are carried internally by man: healthy seedlings of *Tacsonia* have been found growing from old pig dung along Pengagl Creek at 2790 m.

An analysis of the distribution of seven species probably commonly transported by man between open sites at 2642–2792 m is shown in Table IV, together with seven common wind-dispersed species for comparison. Sites are grouped under four geographical heads. The Wilhelm path and Mondia road are both commonly used paths along which man may disperse disseminules. Pengagl creek is not now often visited by man, though up to early 1972 part of it was used as a section of the path to the Pindaunde valley. All the sites from Kuraglumba are landslips or streambanks well away from paths. It can readily be seen that the man-dispersed plants, though generally common along Wilhelm path and Mondia road, are infrequent along Pengagl creek

TABLE III

Disseminules carried by man on clothing or footwear from the upper Chimbu valley below 2515 m to the research station, 3480 m, 1971–72

Species	Seeds germinated		Disseminules counted (1972)					
	1971	1972	14/4	14/4	4/5	15/5	12/6	3/7
Acaena anserinifolia	—	+	29	4	59	56	1	11
Bidens pilosa	—	+	2	—	53	51	—	39
Cynoglossum javanicum	—	+	13	—	10	—	—	11
Deschampsia klossii	+	—	—	—	—	—	—	—
Desmodium sp.	+	—	—	—	—	74	—	—
Microlaena stipoides	—	+	—	—	—	—	—	—
Myosotis australis	—	+	11	2	—	—	—	—
Poa annua	+	—	—	—	—	—	—	—
Ranunculus sp.	—	—	—	—	1	—	—	—
Triplostegia glandulifera	—	—	—	—	1	—	—	—
Uncinia spp.	—	?	—	—	—	15	7	5
Unidentified Gramineae	+	+	—	2	25	10	5	8
Unknown	—	?	—	—	—	12	—	2

and absent from the Kuraglumba sites. On the other hand, the wind-dispersed species are common in all four areas as would be expected.

During early 1972 the path from Keglsugl (2510 m) to the lower Pindaunde lake (3480 m) was largely re-routed between 2770 m and 3180 m. Alien plant records in Table I refer to the old path, and it will be interesting to see how the spread of these and other species will be affected by the change. The new route passes through mainly un-disturbed forest in contrast to the old which traversed riverbed and disturbed forest habitats. Only five introduced plants have been recorded above 3000 m on Mt. Kinabalu, all from around a hut at 3353 m (Smith, 1970). This far smaller number in comparison with Mt. Wilhelm can perhaps be partly explained by the fact that the Kinabalu path runs through almost unbroken forest from 1830 m to 3350 m, so providing few "stepping-stone" habitats for invading shade-intolerant plants.

Dogs and pigs were introduced to the upper Chimbu valley before contact with Western man. The earliest record in New Guinea for pig is about 6500 years ago (White, 1972) and for dog less than 2000 years ago (Allen, 1972). The only animal other than solely domestic species subsequently introduced has been the brown trout, in the lower Pindaunde lake. There are no records of any of the four species of deer introduced to New Guinea (Bentley and Downes, 1966) having been

TABLE IV

Distribution of some commonly man-dispersed and wind-dispersed species beside
and away from paths in the Mt. Wilhelm area, 2642–2972 m

Species	Mt. Wilhelm path (used path) 16 sites		Mondia road (used path) 14 sites		Pengagl creek (streambank, occasional path) 27 sites		Kuraglumba (streambanks, landslips away from paths) 10 sites	
Man-dispersed								
Acaena anserinifolia	4	(25%)	0		0		0	
Bidens pilosa	9	(56%)	6	(43%)	3	(11%)	0	
Cynoglossum javanicum	6	(38%)	4	(29%)	1	(4%)	0	
Fragaria cf. *vesca*	5	(31%)	2	(14%)	2	(7%)	0	
Microlaena stipoides	10	(63%)	4	(29%)	3	(11%)	0	
Tacsonia mollissima	6	(38%)	3	(21%)	3	(11%)	0	
Uncinia ohwiana	2	(13%)	0		0		0	
Average	6·0	(38%)	2·7	(19%)	1·7	(6%)	0	
Wind-dispersed								
Anaphalis lorentzii	3	(19%)	5	(36%)	18	(67%)	2	(20%)
Crassocephalum crepidioides	7	(44%)	9	(64%)	15	(56%)	3	(30%)
Epilobium keysseri	2	(13%)	4	(29%)	19	(70%)	9	(90%)
Epilobium ?prostratum	6	(38%)	6	(43%)	20	(74%)	6	(60%)
Erigeron canadensis	2	(13%)	5	(36%)	18	(67%)	0	
Erigeron sumatrensis	10	(63%)	14	(100%)	17	(67%)	6	(60%)
Sonchus oleraceus	7	(44%)	8	(57%)	7	(26%)	2	(20%)
Average	5·3	(33%)	7·3	(52%)	16·3	(60%)	4·0	(40%)

seen in the area, though if they do spread thus far they may be expected to thrive in the less accessible areas of Mt. Wilhelm.

Feral "singing" dogs range in small packs on Mt. Wilhelm, and lairs have been located among rocks in the forest high on the south side of the Imbukum valley (Wade and McVean, 1969). What effects dogs have had upon populations of their prey (probably mainly bandicoots and rats) or of their presumed competitor, the small marsupial "cat" *Satanellus albopunctatus*, are not known. Apart from *Satanellus*, man and some scarce birds of prey, feral dogs are the only large carnivores in the area.

The pig is the most abundant and important domestic animal in New Guinea Highlands. Pigs are generally allowed to run free by day to find for themselves a proportion of their food. This results in considerable disturbance of soil and low vegetation, for example up to 2750 m above Keglsugl. The spread and increase of many adventive herbaceous plants is thereby favoured, and it is probable that regeneration of most forest trees is adversely affected. In addition further forest damage is inflicted by man in order to construct the stout fences necessary to exclude roaming pigs from gardens (Aitchison, 1960). Feral pigs are present in the forests of the Imbukum valley but are probably precluded from the upper Chimbu valley area by hunting pressure. Domestic pigs seldom stray above 2900 m except when led along paths from one area to another, when they may greatly affect local areas by rootling during halts on the journey, as at Kuraglumba and on Kombugli hill.

Brown trout were introduced as fry into the lower Pindaunde lake in mid-1969, it being intended to establish a breeding population from which the Chimbu river could be stocked. Fry were airfreighted from Australia by the Department of Agriculture, Stock and Fisheries, and many did not survive the journey or the temperature change experienced when they were poured into the lake (R. B. E. Smith, pers. comm., 1971). No prior research on lake ecology was undertaken and their impact upon the lake ecosystem is unknown.

By April 1971 several large fish were present, and two netted at that time appeared from growth rings in their scales to be of different age classes, suggestive of successful breeding. They suffered a skin infection however, which may have been caused by the flagellate *Costia necatrix* (R. B. E. Smith, pers. comm., 1971). During August to September 1971 at least 14 large trout died in the lake; several of these showed symptoms of skin infection, but the apparent cause of death of at least half was an inability to shed eggs. In some cases this caused partial extrusion of the viscera through the cloaca or a rupturing of the ventral body wall.

During 1972 trout were seldom seen in the lake, but a juvenile weighing 320 g was captured in the outlet stream in July 1972. It is possible that breeding is taking place in this stream but not in the lake, which may lack suitable sites for oviposition. The largest fish so far recorded, a male killed in the lake in June 1972, weighed 2218 g and measured 52·5 cm to the base of the caudal fin. Despite several attempts no trout have been taken on hook and line. Apart from by nets, fish have been caught using occasional unorthodox techniques involving rocks, bush knives, bows and arrows, or spades. Trout are not a preferred food of the Chimbu, their flavour being regarded as too bland, inferior to that of tinned mackerel.

VI. PRESENT TRENDS

Denglagu Mission at Toromambuno was established in 1934, and a governmental patrol post set up at Gembogl in 1959. The first recorded ascent of Mt. Wilhelm, by L. G. Vial and L. C. Noakes, was in 1938. Since 1946 a steadily increasing number of people has climbed the mountain, almost all using the Keglsugl–Pindaunde route.

During the same period great changes have been wrought in the pattern of Chimbu life (Brown, 1972). These changes have included the introduction of tinned fish, poultry and cattle as alternative sources of protein-rich food within a cash economy, resulting in a decline in hunting activity, which young men generally indulge in today with neither regularity nor skill. Shotguns have not yet been permitted in the densely populated upper Chimbu valley.

One effect of these alterations in human activity is that a single path on Mt. Wilhelm has become well used, and the network of hunting tracks has fallen partly into disuse. Between 17 April and 17 September 1972, about 224 people from outside the area visited Mt. Wilhelm, of whom about 56 were from outside Papua New Guinea, employing about 176 Chimbu as carriers and guides.

The well-used path has become a new habitat for plants. In addition to introduced species finding niches along the disturbed trackside, many native plants benefit from the constant trampling, which excludes shrubs and large herbs. Most of these are small rosette or cushion-forming species. *Plantago aundensis* and, in wet places, *Scirpus crassiusculus* are common on the path from 3200 up to 3500 m, while *Abrotanella papuana*, *Ranunculus pseudolowii* and *Schoenus maschalinus* continue up to 3700 m, and *Gnaphalium breviscapum*, *Monostachya oreoboloides*, *Potentilla foersteriana* and *P. papuana* to 4300 m. *Poa crassicaulis* is a common path plant between 3700 and 4300 m.

Most visitors stay for at least one night beside the lower Pindaunde lake, at 3480 m, either in the hut provided by the local government council, in one of the timber and grass shelters, or camping. This has led to both damage and pollution in the area. The relict patches of subalpine forest have been further reduced by firewood gathering and the cutting of branches to build or repair shelters. Despite the recent provision of signposted rubbish-pits, cans and other refuse continue to be scattered about. However, the greatest single source of solid and visual pollution remains the wreckage of the USAF bomber (nevertheless something of a tourist attraction) which crashed at 3960 m on the Bogunolto ridge (between the Pindaunde and Guraguragugl valleys) in 1943.

A swathe some ten metres wide was cut through the forest between 2900 and 3200 m, along the route of the old path, in late 1969 in a vain attempt to lay a troublefree telephone line to the research station. Secondary forest growth had, in 1972, reached a height of about two metres. More widespread forest damage continues to an increasing extent below 2750 m as a result of the cutting of timber.

Plans for the declaration of a national park to include part or all of the Mt. Wilhelm massif above 2743 m (9000 ft) are under consideration. If these plans reach fruition, a part of the area considered here may, with wise and active management, be preserved in something like its present condition. However, as has been shown this condition is far from virginal as regards human modification. The possible preservation of Mt. Wilhelm's biotic environment and the continued exploitation of neighbouring areas for timber and other resources will be further threads in the complex and changing fabric of man's influence upon his environment; and of the modified environment's reciprocal influence upon man.

VII. ACKNOWLEDGEMENTS

I wish to thank J. S. Womersley and members of his staff at the Forests Department herbarium, Lae, for permission to examine plant collections and for assistance with identifications, and in particular E. E. Henty for his opinions on the native or alien status of plants in the Mt. Wilhelm area. Field observations were made during tenure of an Australian National University research scholarship which I gratefully acknowledge. For discussion of this work and its presentation I would like to thank especially M. J. M. Cooper, W. C. Edmundson, J. Golson, D. A. M. Lea, N. D. Turvey and N. M. Wace.

VIII. REFERENCES

Aitchison, T. G. (1960). The Pig and its Place in the Impact of the New Guinean on Vegetation. In "Symposium on the Impact of Man on Humid Tropics Vegetation". Goroka, sponsored by Admin. Terr. Papua and New Guinea & UNESCO Science Co-operation Office for SE Asia, pp. 158–167.

Allen, F. J. (1972). Nebira 4: an early Austronesian Site in Central Papua. *Archaeol. phys. Anthropol. Oceania* **7**, 92–124.

Anderson, E. (1949). "Introgressive Hybridisation". John Wiley and Sons, New York and London.

Archbold, R. and Rand, A. L. (1935). Results of the Archbold Expeditions No. 7. Summary of the 1933–34 Papuan Expeditions. *Bull. Am. Mus. nat. Hist.* **68**, 527–579.

Bentley, A. and Downes, M. C. (1966). Deer in New Guinea, 1: Notes on the Field Identification of certain Deer Species likely to be encountered in Papua New Guinea. *Papua New Guin. agric. J.* **20**, 1–14.

Bowers, N. (1968). "The ascending Grasslands: an anthropological Study of ecological Succession in a high Mountain Valley in New Guinea", Ph.D. dissertation, University of Columbia.

Brass, L. J. (1964). Results of the Archbold Expeditions No. 86. Summary of the Sixth Archbold Expedition to New Guinea (1959). *Bull. Am. Mus. nat. Hist.* **127**, 145–216.

Brown, M. and Powell, J. M. (1974). Frost and Drought in the Highlands of Papua New Guinea. *J. trop. Geogr.* **38**, 1–6.

Brown, P. (1972). "The Chimbu: a Study of Change in the New Guinea Highlands". Schenckman, Cambridge, Massachusetts.

Flenley, J. R. (1972). Evidence of Quaternary vegetational Change in New Guinea. *In* "The Quaternary Era in Malesia" (Eds P. and M. Ashton). Dept. Geog., Univ. Hull, Misc. Publs 13, pp. 99–120.

Galloway, R. W., Hope, G. S., Löffler, E. and Peterson, J. A. (1972). Late Quaternary Glaciation and periglacial Phenomena in Australia and New Guinea. *Palaeoecol. Africa* **8**, 127–138.

Gilbert, J. M. (1959). Forest Succession in the Florentine Valley, Tasmania. *Pap. Proc. R. Soc. Tasm.* **93**, 129–151.

Gillison, A. N. (1969). Plant Succession in an irregularly fired Grassland Area—Doma Peaks Region, Papua. *J. Ecol.* **57**, 415–428.

Gillison, A. N. (1970). Structure and Floristics of a montane Grassland/Forest Transition, Doma Peaks Region, Papua. *Blumea* **18**, 71–86.

Haantjens, H. A. (1970). Soils of the Goroka-Mount Hagen Area. *In* "Lands of the Goroka-Mount Hagen Area" (Compiler H. A. Haantjens). *Land Res. Ser. CSIRO, Aust.* **27**, 80–103.

Hnatnik, R. J., Smith, J. M. B. and McVean, D. N. (1976). "Mt. Wilhelm Studies II. The Climate of Mt. Wilhelm". Publ. BG/4, ANU Press, Canberra.

Hope, G. S. (1973). "The Vegetation History of Mt Wilhelm, Papua New Guinea". J. Ecol. **64**, 627–663.

Hope, J. H. and Hope, G. S. (1975). Palaeoenvironments for Man in New Guinea. *In* "The biological Origins of the Australians" (Eds R. L. Kirk and A. G. Thorne), Publ. Australian Inst. Aboriginal Studies, Canberra.

Jennings, J. N. (1972). Some Attributes of Torres Strait. *In* "Bridge and Barrier: the natural and cultural History of Torres Strait" (Ed. D. Walker). Publ. BG/3, ANU Press, Canberra, pp. 29–38.

Johns, R. J. and Stevens, P. F. (1971). "Mount Wilhelm Flora. A Checklist of the Species". Division of Botany, Dept. Forests, Lae, *Botany Bull.* **6**.

Kalkman, C. and Vink, W. (1970). Botanical Exploration in the Doma Peaks Region, New Guinea. *Blumea* **16**, 87–135.

Kingston, D. J. (1960). The physical Processes in Subsistence Agriculture and the Necessity therefore. *In* "Symposium on the Impact of Man on Humid Tropics Vegetation". Goroka, sponsored by Admin. Terr. Papua and New Guinea and UNESCO Science Co-operation Office for SE Asia, pp. 232–235.

Lane-Poole, C. E. (1925). "The Forest Resources of the Territories of Papua and New Guinea". Government Printer, Melbourne.

Löffler, E. (1972). Pleistocene Glaciation in Papua and New Guinea. *Z. Geomorph. N.F. Supp. Bd.* **13**, 32–58.

Martin, P. S. (1967). Prehistoric Overkill. *In* "Pleistocene Extinctions: the Search for a Cause" (Eds P. S. Martin and H. E. Wright). Yale University Press, New Haven, pp. 75–120.

McAlpine, J. R. (1970). Population and Land Use in the Goroka–Mount Hagen Area" (Compiler H. A. Haantjens). *Land Res. Ser. CSIRO, Aust.* **27**, 126–146.

Meggitt, M. J. (1960). Notes on the Horticulture of the Enga People of New Guinea. *In* "Symposium on the Impact of Man on humid Tropics Vegetation". Goroka, sponsored by Admin. Terr. Papua and New Guinea and UNESCO Science Co-operation Office for SE Asia, pp. 86–89.

Paijmans, K. and Löffler, E. (1972). High Altitude Forests and Grasslands of Mt. Albert Edward, New Guinea. *J. trop. Geogr.* **34**, 58–64.

Plane, M. D. (1967). Stratigraphy and Vertebrate Fauna of the Otibanda Formation, New Guinea. *Bull. But. Miner. Resour. Geol. Geophys. Aust.* **86**, 1–64.

Powell, J. M. (1970). The History of Agriculture in the New Guinea Highlands. *Search* **1**, 199–200.

Reiner, E. (1960). The Glaciation of Mount Wilhelm, Australian New Guinea. *Geogrl Rev.* **50**, 491–503.

Smith, J. M. B. (1970). Herbaceous Plant Communities in the Summit Zone of Mount Kinabalu. *Malay. Nat. J.* **24**, 16–29.

Smith, J. M. B. (1974). "Origins and Ecology of the non-forest Flora of Mt Wilhelm, New Guinea". Ph.D. dissertation, Australia National University.

Smith, J. M. B. (1975). Mountain Grasslands of New Guinea. *J. Biogeogr.* **2**, 27–44.

van Steenis, C. G. G. J. (1968). Frost in the Tropics. *In* "Proc. Symp. Recent Adv. trop. Ecol." (Eds R. Misra and B. Gopal), pp. 154–167.

van Steenis, C. G. G. J. (1972). "The Mountain Flora of Java". Brill, Leiden.

Strathern, A. and Strathern, M. (1971). "Self-Decoration in Mount Hagen". Duckworth, London.

Todd, I. (1974). "Papua New Guinea. Moment of Truth". Angus and Robertson, Sydney.

Wade, L. K. and McVean, D. N. (1969). "Mt Wilhelm Studies I. The alpine and subalpine Vegetation". Publ. BG/1, ANU Press, Canberra.

Walker, D. (1966). Vegetation of the Lake Ipea Region, New Guinea Highlands. I. Forest, grassland and "garden". *J. Ecol.* **54**, 503–533.

Walker, D. (1968). A Reconnaissance of the non-arboreal Vegetation of the Pindaunde Catchment, Mount Wilhelm, New Guinea. *J. Ecol.* **56**, 455–466.

Walker, D. (1970). The changing Face of the montane Tropics. *Search* **1**, 217–221.

White, J. P. (1972). "Ol Tumbuna: archaeological Excavations in the eastern Central Highlands, Papua New Guinea". Dept. Prehistory, Austr. Nat. Univ., *Terra Australis* **2**.

White, J. P., Crook, K. A. W. and Ruxton, B. P. (1970). Kosipe: a late Pleistocene Site in the Papuan Highlands. *Proc. prehist. Soc.* **36**, 152–169.

CHAPTER VIII

Biomass: Its Determination and Implications in Tropical Agro-Ecosystems: An Example From Montane New Guinea

HARLEY I. MANNER

Bucknell University, Lewisburg, Pennsylvania, U.S.A.

I. INTRODUCTION

In montane New Guinea it is apparent that primitive man, primarily through the agencies of shifting cultivation and fire, has greatly altered the structure and dynamics of his environment. The presence of extensive tracts of grasslands in an otherwise rainforest ecosystem is indicative of the reduction of ecosystem complexity that accompanies the repeated cultivation of sites with insufficient fallow length and the often capricious use of fire.

The conversion of forest to grassland and the resultant decreases in ecosystem biomass and diversity seem significant in defining the stability or instability of the system, as well as the levels of energy required to maintain the general structure of the system (Fosberg, 1965; Clarke, 1969). With the reduction of ecosystem structure and complexity that accompanies the intensive use of land, one can assume that energy levels are decreased such that "the removal of any component must be compensated by addition of energy in a utilizable form" (Fosberg, 1965, p. 162). Furthermore, there is sufficient reason to believe that the nature of the ecosystem is related to the development of a more intensive agricultural system. Indeed, an examination of the literature indicates that there may well exist a close association between the intensification level of agricultural practices and the energy contents of ecosystems prior to clearance for gardening (Brookfield, 1962; Brookfield and Hart, 1971; Clarke, 1966; Clarke, 1969; Deneven and Turner, 1974; Rappaport, 1967; Sorenson, 1972; Waddell, 1972).

For montane New Guinea, ecosystems dominated by high biomass and species diversity and a theoretically low entropy state are often associated with agricultural systems and technologies which require relatively low inputs of human energy. In most cases these extensive and relatively less energy demanding forest-fallow rotation systems are associated with relatively low population densities. On the other hand, those ecosystems that are dominated by low biomass and species diversity and theoretically high entropy are often found in association with agricultural systems which require higher inputs of human energy. Such grass-fallow rotation systems are often found in areas that have higher population densities. To refer again to Fosberg's (1965) argument, the variation in cultivation strategies suggests that, as population densities and pressure on land increase, there is a reduction in ecosystem complexity and viability which necessitates the use of more elaborate techniques of cultivation.

The answer to why ecosystem structure is so important in defining the levels of agricultural intensification, lies partly in the fact that the biomass serves as a storage and regulatory system of nutrients. As most tropical soils are nutrient deficient, the greater proportion of nutrients is to be found in the biomass (Nye and Greenland, 1960; Greenland and Kowal, 1960; Scott, 1973). Also, since grassland soils are nutriently and physically poorer than soils under adjacent forest sites (Kellogg, 1963; Doyne, 1935; Nye and Greenland, 1960; Clarke and Street, 1967), by virtue of the higher biomass in forests, there is a greater amount of nutrients available for production in forest than in grassland gardens. On the basis of experimental sweet potato yield trials conducted in the Bismarck Mountains of New Guinea, Clarke and Street (1967) found that yields from unturned forest garden plots were twice as large as yields from unturned grassland gardens. However, the yields of sweet potato from turned grassland plots were slightly greater than yields from the unturned forest plots. Although tillage of the grassland may improve aeration and nitrification and reduce toxic soil conditions, I infer that the above study underscores the importance of ecosystem structure as a regulator and storage system of available nutrients—as well as a partial determinant of the level of agricultural intensification.

Despite the implications of ecosystem structure and function to the question of agricultural intensification in New Guinea, there are very few detailed studies of ecosystems and how their biomass and flora are affected by shifting cultivation. The lack of this type of information is understandable: a tremendous amount of time and labour is necessary to make such determinations. Furthermore, few researchers have had the time to apply themselves to the dual nature of the problem. The purposes of this paper are: one, to describe relatively simple techniques for estimating biomass in forest, garden and grasslands in order to ascertain the effects of shifting cultivation on ecosystem structure and productivity and two, to present the results of such fieldwork conducted among a group of Mareng shifting cultivators in the Bismarck Mountains of Papua New Guinea.

Basically there are two widely used methods for determining biomass. The choice of method depends mainly on the type of community selected for analysis. The simplest method involves harvesting all of the above and below ground biomass present in a representative plot, or clipping the vegetation at the ground surface and determining its underground component through sub-plot analysis. Usually these harvest methods are best restricted to biomass determinations for grassland, garden, or shrub layer communities, since their simple flora and low biomass content require clearance of relatively small sized plots. For grassland and shrub layer communities (including gardens), clearance of 50 m² and 100 m² plots respectively may be more than sufficient for adequate representation (Ellenberg, 1956). (A detailed discussion of the harvest technique for grassland communities can be found in Milner and Hughes, 1968.)

On the other hand, the application of the harvest technique for the measurement of biomass in a forest formation requires the clearance of much larger areas and a greater expenditure of time and labour. Shimwell (1972) notes that tropical forest may require a minimal area of 256 m², and it is not uncommon to find that plots in excess of 500 m² have been used. For example, in their measurement of an Amazonian rainforest biomass, Fittkau and Klinge (1973) were $5\frac{1}{2}$ months harvesting a total area of 2000 m². Unless the field researcher is blessed with unlimited time and money, the determination of biomass in tropical forests where trees often exceed 30 m in height is a tedious, laborious and time-consuming process.

Fortunately, more rapid methods of biomass estimation are available. These methods, which utilize the relationships between the weight of a tree and its other measurable characteristics, are called allometric relationships. Though first proposed for the determination of temperate latitude forests (Kitteridge, 1944; Ovington, 1957; Ovington and Madwick, 1959a, 1959b; Tadaki and Shidei, 1960; Woodwell and Whittaker, 1968a, 1968b; Whittaker and Woodwell, 1968, 1969), the method of regression analysis has been successfully applied to tropical forest ecosystems (Ogino *et al.*, 1964, 1967; Ogawa *et al.*, 1965; Hozumi *et al.*, 1969; Kira and Shidei, 1967; Scott, 1973; Sabhasri *et al.*, 1968; Kira and Ogawa, 1968, 1971).

The allometric regression equation reads:

$$y = ax^b,$$

or
$$\log_e y = \log_e a + b \log_e x.$$

a and b are empirically derived constants, and y and x are measurable properties of trees. Usually y, the dependent variable, refers to the dry or moist weight of stem, branch, leaf, total above ground or root biomass of a tree, while x, the independent variable, refers to a more readily measured parameter such as diameter at breast height (dbh, 1·3 m above the ground surface), height (h), or a combination of dbh and height characteristics. Very high correlations have been obtained between biomass and dbh^2h (Ogino *et al.*, 1964; Ovington and Madwick, 1959; Ogawa *et al.*, 1965; Sabhasri *et al.*, 1968).

However, in order to determine the regression equation a number of trees need to be harvested, weighed according to component parts and measured for height and diameter characteristics. While the great floristic diversity common to tropical forests suggests the necessity to derive regressions for single species groups, trees having the same life form characteristics (i.e. broadleafs etc.), may be adequately described by a single regression (Kira and Ogawa, 1971; Ogino *et al.*, 1964; Ogawa *et al.*, 1965; Newbould, 1967).

The determination of root biomass in tropical ecosystems is always problematical because of the inordinate amount of time and energy necessary to locate, dig out, and clean and weigh root structures. The application of allometric regressions and root–shoot ratios may adequately define the amount of underground biomass (Newbould, 1967; Bray, 1963; Kira and Ogawa, 1968). (For more detailed information see Newbould, 1967, 1968; Leith, 1968; Jenik, 1971.)

II. FIELD SITE CHARACTERISTICS

The fieldwork was carried out from September 1972 to late August 1973 among the Kauwatyi Marengs, a clan cluster of 771 people at Kompiai (5° 33′S, 144° 38′E), which is located on the southern face of the Bismarck Mountains, Western Highlands, Papua New Guinea (see Map 1). Within an area 31·08 km² and between altitudes of 914 and 1860 m, the Kauwatyi Marengs practise a garden–forest rotation on slopes approaching a 40° incline. Although the area was previously dominated by a broadleaf gymnosperm mixed forest alliance (Robbins, 1958, 1962, 1970), shifting cultivation and the use of fire has converted the area to a mosaic of grassland, forest and gardens in which only about 10% (my estimate) of the primary forest remains. Most of these forests are found above 1860 m, the upper limit of cultivation, and on lower slopes too steep to cultivate. Essentially these forests are two layered with a closed canopy 24–30·5 m high, and a secondary tree layer 12·2–24 m high. The ground flora is exceedingly rich with numerous ferns and forbs occurring in association with young tree saplings.

Approximately 70% of the land is in the form of either gardens or secondary forests of various ages. Usually gardens are created in 10- to 12-year-old secondary forests, though much younger forest sites have been used. Garden clearing operations begin around May, when monthly rainfall totals are lower than 76 mm. Prior to planting, garden site preparation involves the slashing of the undergrowth and the felling of trees at about breast height. Certain trees such as *Casuarina oligodon* are merely pollarded. The felled trees are used for fencing, firewood and garden plot markers. Though larger logs are often left where they have fallen, a concerted effort is made to position the more manageable trunks along the contour. These trunks seem to serve as a form of rudimentary terracing. When the litter is dry, it is fired. The Kauwatyi Marengs try to ensure that the firing is as complete as possible and that all parts of the garden receive some ash. Thus a second or third burn is often necessary.

While some cultigens are planted prior to firing, most of the planting occurs after burning is completed. Gardens are then planted with a variety of crops that seem to duplicate, though in miniature form, the structure and function of the forest. A wide variety of taro (*Colocasia esculenta*), tiem (*Hibiscus manihot*), tiemba (*Rungia klossii*), sweet potatoes (*Ipomoea batatas*), yams (*Discoraceae*), kwiai (*Setaria palmifolia*), mungap, (*Saccharum edule*) and bananas (*Musa* sp.) are propagated. Corns, beans, pumpkins, cucumbers and other leafy greens are planted by seed. Most crop propagules are planted into holes made with a dibble. The time of planting is scheduled so that the ground surface is covered by vegetation before the onset of heavier rains in September.

Five months after planting, corn, cucumbers and leafy greens are ready for consumption. Taro and pumpkins attain consumption size two to four months later. As these crops are harvested, the Kauwatyi Marengs often replant the garden voids with sweet potatoes or bananas, sugar or *mungap*. Approximately 18 months after the initial planting, all of the edible sized taro have been harvested and the garden now consists of a ground covering dominated by sweet potatoes, with sugar cane, *mungap*, and bananas forming an upper canopy.

During the early cultivation period, gardens are assiduously weeded, a labour which may continue for approximately 18 months after initial planting. However, by the time a garden is $2\frac{1}{2}$ years old, weeding has virtually ceased so that these and older gardens may be dominated by a young secondary forest regrowth. The ground cover consists primarily of graminoids such as *Imperata cylindrica, Paspalum conjugatum, Ischaemum digitatum, Setaria palmifolia* and annuals such as *Ageratum, conzoides, Bidens pilosa* and *Emelia* sp.

Because of the high intensity of land use, the secondary forests at Kompiai are relatively species poor and dominated by *Dodonea viscosa, Homolanthus, Maesa* and *Alphitonia incana*. Forested sites on north-facing slopes which have been subjected to repeated cultivation are often dominated by almost pure stands of *Dodonea viscosa*, which seems indicative of intensive environmental degradation (Clarke, 1966).

About 20% of the area is dominated by a grassland dis-climax (Clarke, 1966). While younger and smaller sized grasslands are dominated by an association of *Imperata cylindrica* and *Capillipedium parviflorum* and the fern *Cyclosorus*, the older and more extensive grass-lands sites are dominated by *Themeda australis, Arundinella setosa, Ophioros exaltatus, Eulalia leptostachthys* and *Capillipedium parviflorum*.

Except for a small group of Aerikai clan migrants from the nearby village of Gai, the Kauwatyi Marengs do not garden in these grassland sites. In the case of the Gai migrants, however, their migration to Kompiai occurred at a time after all forested lands had been claimed by the other Kompiai clans. Having little alternative, they were forced to use the grassland sites for cultivation and by turning the soil with dibbles and planting both crops and trees, they have effectively reforested some of these grassland sites such that turning of the soil prior to planting is no longer necessary (Street, 1967).

There are a number of other reasons why the Kauwatyi Marengs do do not use grassland sites for agriculture. In addition to the low fertility of grassland soils (Street, 1966; Clarke and Street, 1967), and the necessity to turn the soil prior to planting, there is a lack of fencing material in grasslands. Fences are necessary as pigs are allowed to forage throughout the Mareng territory. Thus the Marengs feel that the energy expenditures associated with turning of the soils and the transportation of fence materials over relatively long distances would be far greater than those of clearing forest garden plots.

At 1737 m the mean annual temperature averages 18°C. Nights are cool, averaging 15°C, while days are warm. Mean maximum temperatures during the day average 21°C. Average annual rainfall is in excess of 2540 mm. During the 1972–73 fieldwork period, a total of 3324 mm fell for a 10-month gauging period. No month can be considered dry, though in June 1973 only 74 mm were recorded. On the basis of rainfall and temperature data, the climate at 1737 m is classified as a Cfbi, according to Köppen's classification of climates.

III. PROCEDURES

In order to determine the biomass levels along a gradient of increased human interference a series of standardized 25 m² quadrats were located in representative primary and secondary forests (aged 3, 4, 5, 12 and 13 years), gardens (aged 1, 2 and 3 years), and grasslands (new and old). For grasslands, 9 m² and 16 m² plots were also used. The initial plot was located in the approximate centre of the formation and a series of similar plots were then located at right angles and at a distance of 25 m moving towards the site boundaries. Usually, for each field site, the area encompassed by plot analysis amounted to 50 m² in new gardens, 100 m² in grasslands and young secondary forests, 300 m² in 13-year-old secondary forests and 500 m² in primary forests.

Biomass in the grassland formation was determined primarily by clipping the vegetation that had roots situated within the plot. The vegetation was then separated and weighed according to species and sub-sampled for moisture content. In a number of instances, 1 × 1 m² plots were established for root biomass determinations. In such cases all live underground parts were dug up, washed, weighed and dried in a field oven and re-weighed for moisture content. Roots were then compared with above ground biomass for the determination of root–shoot ratios. In other cases individual graminoid or herbaceous species were dug up for similar analysis. The derived root–shoot ratios were then applied to like graminoid or herbaceous species that were out at surface level. In forests and gardens, all herbaceous vegetation was dug up or cut at ground surface and weighed according to species. Moisture contents and root–shoot ratios were determined as previously described. In order to determine the biomass in gardens in various stages of production, $2x$–50 m² plots were bought from their owners. All crop biomass was dug up while the weedy growth was cut at ground surface.

The determination of tree biomass in forest sites necessitated the application of allometric relationships based on the weight to dbh² × h characteristics of individual sample trees. All trees with a dbh greater than 1·28 cm were measured for dbh with a steel tape and, height by triangulation with a Brunton compass and a steel tape. Their biomass was then estimated by applying allometric regression based on a total of 87 trees that were felled at ground surface or dug up entirely.

Of the 87 felled trees, a total of 56 trees were dug up for the measurement of total, above ground, and root biomass and the determination of root–shoot ratios. All felled trees were measured for height and dbh characteristics, separated into component parts (leaves, branches, trunks, roots etc.) and weighed. For large trees, trunks and larger branches were cut into 1 m lengths for more convenient weighing. Component parts were sampled for moisture content.

Regression equations of the form $y = ax^b$ were determined for the following:

a. Total moist weight of primary forest species.
b. Above ground moist weight of primary forest species.
c. Total moist weight of secondary forest species.
d. Above ground moist weight of secondary forest species.

IV. RESULTS OF ALLOMETRIC REGRESSION ANALYSIS

The total and above ground weights (moist), height and diameter at breast height characteristics of 87 primary and secondary forest tree species are presented in Appendices 1 and 2 respectively. The allometric regression for these samples are graphically presented in Figures 1 and 2. The regression equations, correlation coefficients (r), number of samples, and level of significance are also indicated. The allometric regressions between moist weight (kg) and diameter at breast height (cm) squared times height (m) are listed below.

$$y = 0·2599x^{0·82} \quad \text{for total biomass of primary forest trees.} \quad \text{(Eqn 1)}$$
$$y = 0·1094x^{0·91} \quad \text{for above ground biomass of primary}$$
forest trees.   (Eqn 2)

$y = 0.2065x^{0.84}$ for total biomass of secondary forest trees.

(Eqn 3)

$y = 0.1708x^{0.85}$ for above ground biomass of secondary forest trees.

(Eqn 4)

Except for Regression Eqn 1, the correlation coefficients (for Eqns 2, 3 and 4) exceed 0·99 and are highly significant ($p < 0.01$). For Eqn 1, the lower correlation coefficient of 0·92 is essentially due to the smaller numbers (9) of samples, though still highly significant ($p < 0.01$). An increase in the number of samples would probably be accompanied by an increase in the correlation coefficient as well as a change in slope. These high correlations indicate the validity of the technique as an estimator of biomass. Furthermore, the slopes for Eqn 3 and 4 are parallel. Thus, root biomass may be adequately determined for the size classes of sampled trees by subtracting Eqn 2 from 1 and Eqn 4 from 3.

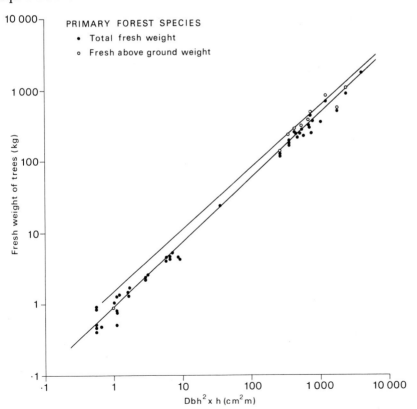

FIGURE 1. The total and above ground allometric relationships between moist weight and Dbh^2 × h for primary forest species.

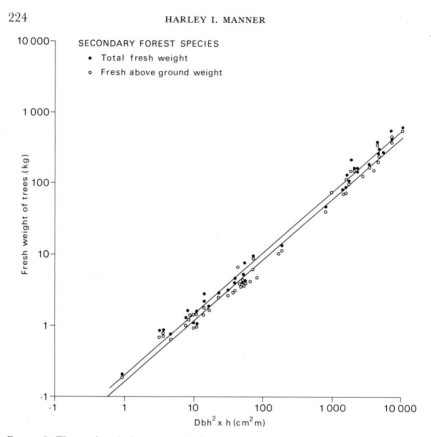

FIGURE 2. The total and above ground allometric relationships between moist weight and Dbh² × h for commonly occurring secondary forest species.

V. RESULTS OF BIOMASS STUDIES

On the basis of harvesting and the application of allometric regressions and moisture content data, the live biomass for a number of Kauwatyi Mareng ecosystems was determined. The results are summarized in Table I. A more detailed description of the data for each site sampled is presented in Appendix 3 and shown graphically in Figure 3. The biomass data in the appendices are grouped into the following biomass categories.

  a. Crop.
  b. Herbs.
  c. Nanophanerophytes (trees, 0–2·5 m in height).
  d. Microphanerophytes (trees, 2·5–8 m in height).

TABLE I

Summary of biomass data for Kompiai ecosystems

Stand type	No. of stands	Site no.	Total area sampled (m²)	Total biomass	Above ground biomass	Root or corm biomass	Total crop biomass/ total biomass	Total taro biomass/ total crop biomass
				(in dry tonnes/hectare)				
1-year-old garden	3	2a 2b 2c	100	7·14	3·18	4·39	0·900	0·599
2-year-old garden	2	3a 3b	50	8·78	7·15	1·76	0·890	0·005
3-year-old garden	1	4	50	13·92	11·26	2·67	0·294	—
4-year-old secondary forest	2	5a 5b	100	16·27	13·87	2·35	—	—
5-year-old secondary forest	1	6	50	27·94	21·03	6·91	—	—
12- to 13-year-old secondary forest	2	7a 7b	375	82·61	72·46	10·15	—	—
Primary forest	2	1a 1b	500	293·09	259·10	33·99	—	—
Imperata grassland	1	8	100	6·18	4·29	1·90	—	—
Themeda grassland	1	9	90	3·56	2·97	0·59	—	—

e. Mesophanerophytes (trees, 8–30 m in height).

f. Megaphanerophytes (trees higher than 30 m).

The trees were categorized by height according to Raunkiaer (cited by Shimwell, 1972).

A comparison of the data indicates the extent of shifting cultivation, fire and fallow length on ecosystem biomass. As expected, biomass is highest in the primary forest (Site no. 1a, 1b) and lowest in the *Themeda* dominated grasslands (Site no. 9).

The average total biomass of 293 tonnes per hectare for Kompiai primary forest agrees well with results from other parts of the tropics. However, a comparison of biomass totals from the two primary forest Sites no. 1a and 1b selected shows a wide range, from 407 tonnes per hectare for Site no. 1a to 179 tonnes per hectare for Site no. 1b. This large difference in biomass may be attributed to the presence or absence of meso- and megaphanerophytes, as well as to site differences. These differences in turn suggest that a larger area of primary forest needs be surveyed, although a more complete statistical analysis is necessary before any conclusions can be made.

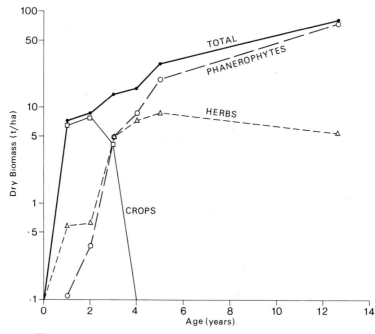

FIGURE 3. The development of total biomass (dry) for a Kauwatyi garden-secondary forest sequence. Data from Table III.

Secondary forests prior to clearance for gardens (Sites no. 7a and 7b) contain an average live biomass (dry wt) of 83 tonnes per hectare or 3·5 times less biomass than primary forests (see Table I). Between-site comparisons of the two stands also indicate a wide range of total biomass; from 63 tonnes per hectare for Site no. 7b, to 102 tonnes per hectare for Site no. 7a. This range may be attributed to the presence or absence of large megaphanerophytes, as well as to the intensity of land use. There are indications that Site no. 7b at Kombitimamp has been more intensively used than Site no. 7a at Nopeyama. Though not indicated in the results, the heavier usage of Site no. 7b may be reflected by the greater abundance of *Dodonea viscosa*, a regrowth species which Clarke (1966) considers to be an indication of more intensive degradation.

A comparison of Site no. 2, 3 and 4 (Table I) indicates changes in biomass, flora and productivity that are consistent with the general process of ecological succession. Kauwatyi subsistence gardens, cleared from previously forested sites, attain their maximum crop biomass between the first and second years of production. In the first year a Kauwatyi Mareng, employing traditional techniques of production, can expect a maximum (total) biomass of 7·14 tonnes per hectare, of which 6·82 tonnes per hectare or 90% is crop biomass.

In one-year-old gardens, taro (*Colocasia esculenta*) is the dominant crop by weight. This dominance is indicated by the ratio of taro biomass to total crop biomass which amounts to 60%. This figure declines rapidly as harvesting of mature corms proceeds and other crops, particularly sweet potatoes (*Ipomoea batatas*), sugar cane (*Saccharum officianarum*) *mungap* (*Saccharum edule*) and bananas (*Musa* sp.) achieve dominance. Thus, at the end of the second year of production the percentage of taro biomass to total crop biomass declines to 0·5.

Total biomass in two-year-old gardens is slightly higher, amounting to 8·78 tonnes per hectare. In addition, total crop biomass is also high, amounting to 7·82 tonnes per hectare, such that the ratio of total crop biomass to total biomass is 0·89. While Clarke (1966) reported that Kompiai gardens remain productive for 18–20 months, the data indicate a lengthening of gardening period to three years—a situation which reflects an increased pressure on land. However, the lengthening of the garden period is accomplished by an increase in energy to counteract the decrease in yields due to insect damage, lowered fertility and increased weed competition. Part of this additional energy expenditure is in the form of weeding, the effects of which are indicated by the relatively low amounts of herbaceous and phanerophyte vegetation in two-year-old gardens. The effect of weeding is shown graphically in Figure 3.

The maintenance of relatively high amounts of crop biomass in two-year-old gardens is also partly accomplished by the transition of crops from taro to sweet potatoes, bananas, *mungap* and sugar cane—crops which according to Mareng informants do better in older gardens. The results of biomass studies in gardens suggest that the higher amounts of weed biomass and the resultant increased competition for nutrients, light and space may preclude the replanting and successful growth of taro in older gardens. On the other hand, bananas, sugar cane, sweet potatoes and *mungap* may be better adapted to the more degraded conditions present in older and weedier gardens.

Between the second and third years of growth there is a rapid decline in crop biomass to 4·10 tonnes per hectare (see Appendix 3). As weeding has all but ceased, the herbaceous and phanerophytic vegetation quickly achieves dominance. In three-year-old garden sites, the ratio of total crop biomass to total biomass falls to 0·29. Though only one three-year-old garden site is presented in this study, the data as well as field observations indicate that there is an overall lengthening of the gardening period among the Kompiai Kauwatyi to almost three years, a situation which reflects an increased pressure on land.

It is conceivable that Kauwatyi gardens with higher inputs of energy and the exclusive production of sweet potatoes may be maintained for even longer cropping periods. However, long-term cropping of garden sites without sufficient fallow may further facilitate the retrogression of forest to grassland ecosystems. As noted earlier there are both *Imperata* and *Themeda* grasslands at Kompiai which reflects a continuum of increasing degradation.

The biomass data for *Imperata* and *Themeda* grasslands amount to 6·18 and 3·56 tonnes per hectare respectively. As biomass is an indicator of the intensity of land use, it is concluded that the *Themeda* grasslands are older and more degraded than the *Imperata* grasslands.

According to Fosberg (1965), successful agriculture in degraded ecosystems requires the addition of energy in a utilizable form. For grassland gardens in montane New Guinea, this input of energy is often in the form of soil tillage. Proof of this relationship is afforded by the previously cited experimental work of Clarke and Street (1967), conducted in turned and unturned grassland soils. While Clarke and Street (1967) note that the primary effect of tillage may be to increase aeration and nitrification and reduce toxic soil conditions, it may be argued that these conditions are determined by ecosystem structure. As ecosystem structure is partly dependent on land use intensity, the experimental work of Clark and Street (1967) lends added support to the relationship between ecosystem structure (biomass) and the level of agricultural intensification.

VI. CONCLUSIONS

Field research was conducted in the Bismarck Mountains of Papua New Guinea to ascertain the effects of shifting cultivation on ecosystem structure, particularly its biomass. Using the harvest technique and regressions based on the allometric relationships between the weight and dbh^2 and height characteristics of 87 primary and secondary forest trees, the biomass for a number of Kauwatyi ecosystems was determined. Primary forests contain an average total biomass of 293 tonnes per hectare, while secondary forests prior to clearance have an average of 83 tonnes per hectare. Maximum crop biomass is achieved during the first two years of gardening and declines rapidly. For the first, second and third years of production, gardens contain a total crop biomass of 6·82, 7·82 and 4·10 tonnes per hectare respectively.

The data and field observations indicate that the Kompiai Kauwatyi are employing longer cropping periods than reported by Clarke (1966). Longer cropping periods may be employed utilizing additional energy inputs and a greater dependence on sweet potatoes. However, the use of longer cropping periods may be accompanied by the retrogression of forest to grassland.

Biomass in *Imperata* and *Themeda* grasslands amounts to 6·18 and 3·55 tonnes per hectare respectively. On the basis of the data, it is concluded that the *Themeda* grasslands are more degraded and older than the *Imperata* grasslands. Despite their low biomass the Kompiai grasslands may become agriculturally productive through the application of more energy intensive forms of cultivation.

The biomass data and field observations from the Kompiai Kauwatyi territory and references to other studies on shifting cultivation, particularly Clarke (1966), Clarke and Street (1967) and Brookfield (1963), indicate that the level of agricultural intensification is related to the biomass levels of ecosystems. Furthermore, since biomass levels are indicative of the extent of land use intensity and capability, I suggest, as have Boserup (1965) and Clarke (1966), that the process of agricultural intensification is a result of and not a cause of high population densities. However, more documentation and experimental studies by students of human ecology are necessary before definite conclusions can be made. The use of the harvest and allometric regression techniques of biomass estimation, though arduous, may prove useful in the analysis of managed terrestrial ecosystems.

VII. ACKNOWLEDGEMENTS

The research in this paper is part of my Ph.D. dissertation, "The Effects of Shifting Cultivation and Fire on Vegetation and Soils in the Montane Tropics of New Guinea", made possible by National Science Foundation Grant No. GB–35098, John M. Street, the principal investigator. I also wish to thank John Wormersley, Chief of Division of Botany, Department of Forests, Papua New Guinea, for the indentification of plant specimens.

VIII. REFERENCES

Boserup, E. (1965). "The Conditions of Agricultural Growth: The Economics of Agrarian Change under Population Pressure". Aldine, Chicago.

Bray, J. R. (1963). Root production and the estimation of net productivity. *Can. J. Bot.* **41**, 65–72.

Brookfield, H. C. (1962). Local study and comparative method: An example from Central New Guinea. *Ann. Ass. Am. Geogr.* **52**, 242–254.

Brookfield, H. C. and Hart, D. (1971). "Melanesia: A Geographical Interpretation of an Island World". Methuen, London.

Clarke, W. C. (1966). From extensive to intensive shifting cultivation: A succession from New Guinea. *Ethnology* **5**, 347–359.

Clarke, W. C. (1969). The Bomagai-Angoiang of New Guinea: The world's most efficient farmers? Paper delivered at 64th meeting Ass. Am. Geogr.

Clarke, W. C. and Street, J. M. (1967). Soil fertility and cultivation practices in New Guinea. *J. trop. Geogr.* **24**, 7–11.

Denevan, W. M. and Turner, B. L. (1974). Forms, function and associations of raised fields in the old world tropics. *J. trop. Geogr.* **39**, 24–33.

Doyne, H. C. (1935). Studies in tropical soils. Increase of acidity with depth. *J. agric. Sci.* **25**, 192–197.

Ellenberg, H. (1956). Aims and Methods of Phyto-sociology. *In* "Introduction to Phytology" (Ed. H. Walter).

Fittkau, E. J. and Klinge, H. (1973). On biomass and tropic structure of the Central Amazonian rain forest ecosystem. *Biotropica* **5**, 2–14.

Fosberg, F. R. (1965). The entropy concept in ecology. *In* "Symposium on Ecological Research in Humid Tropics Vegetation". Djakarta, UNESCO Science Co-operation Office for SE Asia, pp. 157–163.

Greenland, D. J. and Kowal, J. M. L. (1960). Nutrient content of the moist tropical Forest of Ghana. *Pl. Soil* **12**, 154–174.

Hozumi, K., Yoda, K., Kokawa, S. and Kira, T. (1969). Production ecology in south western Cambodia. I. Plant biomass. *In* "Nature and Life in South-east Asia" (Eds T. Kira and K. Iwata). Fauna and Flora Research Society, Kyoto, pp. 1–51.

Jenik, J. (1971). Root structure and underground biomass in equatorial forests. *In* "Productivity of Forest Ecosystems. Proceedings of the Brussels Symposium". UNESCO, Paris, pp. 323–331.

Kellog, C. E. (1963). Shifting cultivation. *Soil Sci.* **95**, 221–230.

Kira, T. and Ogawa, H. (1968). Indirect estimation of root biomass increment in trees. *In* "Methods of Productivity Studies in Root Systems and Rhizisohere Organisms" (Ed. M. S. Ghilarod). Nauka, Leningrad, pp. 96–101.

Kira, T. and Ogawa, H. (1971). Assessment of primary production to tropical and equatorial forests. *In* "Productivity of Forest Ecosystems: Proceedings of the Brussels Symposium". UNESCO, Paris, pp. 309–321.

Kira, T. and Shidei, T. (1967). Primary production and turnover of organic matter in different forest ecosystems of the Western Pacific. *Jap. J. Ecol.* **17**, 70–87.

Kitteridge, J. (1944). Estimation of amount of foliage of trees and shrubs. *J. For.* **42**, 905–912.

Leith, H. (1968). The determination of plant dry matter production with special emphasis on the underground parts. *In* "Functioning of Terrestrial Ecosystems at the Primary Production Level. Proceedings of the Copenhagen Symposium". UNESCO, Paris, pp. 179–186.

Milner, C. and Hughes, R. W. (1968). "Methods for the Measurement of the Primary Production of Grassland". IBP Handbook No. 6. Blackwell, Oxford.

Newbould, P. J. (1967). "Methods for estimating the Primary Production of Forests". IBP Handbook 2. Blackwell, Oxford.

Newbould, P. J. (1968). Methods of estimating root production. In "Functioning of Terrestrial Ecosystems at the Primary Production Level: Proceedings of the Copenhagen Symposium". UNESCO, Paris, pp. 187–190.

Nye, P. H. and Greenland, D. J. (1960). "The Soil under Shifting Cultivation". Technical Communication 51, Commonwealth Bureau of Soils, Farnham, England.

Ogawa, H., Yoda, K., Ogino, K. and Kira, T. (1965). Comparative ecological studies on three main types of forest vegetation in Thailand. II. Plant biomass. In "Nature and Life in South east Asia" Vol. 4 (Eds T. Kira and K. Iwata). Fauna and Flora Research Society, Kyoto, pp. 49–80.

Ogino, K., Sabhasri, S. and Shidei, T. (1964). The estimation of standing crop of the forest of North eastern Thailand. S east. Asia Stud. **4**, 89–97.

Ogino, K., Ongse, D. W., Tsutsumi, T. and Shidei, T. (1967). The primary production of tropical forests in Thailand, S east. Asian Stud. **5**, 121–154.

Ovington, J. D. (1957). Dry matter production by Pinus Sylvestris. Lond. Ann. Bot. **21**, 287–314.

Ovington, J. D. and Madwick, H. A. I. (1959). Distribution of organic matter and plant nutrients in plantations of Scots pine. Forest Sci. **5**, 344–355.

Ovington, J. D. and Madwick, H. A. I. (1959). The growth and composition of natural stand of birch. I. Dry Matter Production. Pl. Soil **10**, 271–278B.

Rappaport, R. (1967). "Pigs for the Ancestors: Ritual in the Ecology of a New Guinea People". Yale University Press, New Haven.

Robbins, R. G. (1958). Montane formations in the Central Highlands of New Guinea. In "Proceedings of the Symposium on Humid Tropics Vegetation". Djakarta, UNESCO Science Co-operation Office for SE Asia, pp. 176–195.

Robbins, R. G. (1962). The anthropogenic grasslands of Papua and New Guinea. In "Symposium on the Impact of Man on Humid Tropics Vegetation". Djakarta, UNESCO Science Co-operation Office for SE Asia, pp. 313–399.

Robbins, R. G. (1970). Vegetation of the Gorka-Mount Hagen Area. In "Lands of the Goroka-Mount Hagen Area Papua-New Guinea". Land Res. Ser. CSIRO, Aust. **27**, 104–118.

Sabharsri, S., Khemnark, C., Aksornkoae, S. and Ratisoothorn, P. (1968). "Primary Production in Dry-Evergreen Forest at Sakaerat Amohoe Pak Thong Chai, Changwat Nakhon Ratchasima. I. Estimation of Biomass and Distribution amongst various organs". Cooperative Research Programme No. 27. Tropical Environmental Data. ASRCT, Bangkok.

Scott, J. (1974). Grassland formations in a tropical rain forest climate and its effects on the soil vegetation nutrient pools and nutrient cycles: A case study in the Gran Pajonal of Eastern Peru. Draft Ms. Ph.D. Dissertation, University of Hawaii.

Shimwell, D. W. (1972). "The Description and Classification of Vegetation". University of Washington Press, Seattle.

Sorenson, R. W. (1972). Socio-ecological change among the Fore of New Guinea. Curr. Anthrop. **13**, 349–383.

Street, J. M. (1966). Grassland on the highland fringe in New Guinea: Localization origin, effects on soil composition. Capricornia **3**, 9–12.

Street, J. M. (1967). Soil conservation by shifting cultivators in the Bismark Mountains of New Guinea. Draft Ms.

Tadaki, Y. and Shidei, T. (1960). Studies on production structure of forests. 1. The seasonal variation of leaf amount and the dry matter production of deciduous sapling stand (Ulmus parvifolia). *J. Jap. For. Soc.* **42**, 427–434.

Waddell, E. (1972). "The Mound Builders: Agricultural Practices, Environment and Society in the Central Highlands of New Guinea". University of Washington Press, Seattle.

Whittaker, R. H. and Woodwell, G. M. (1968). Dimension and production relations of trees and shrubs in the Brookhaven forest, New York. *J. Ecol.* **56**, 1–25.

Whittaker, R. H. and Woodwell, G. M. (1969). Structure, production and diversity of the oak pine forest at Brookhaven, New York. *J. Ecol.* **57**, 155–174.

Watters, R. F. (1960). The nature of shifting cultivation: a review of recent literature. *Pac. Viewpoint* **1**, 59–99.

Woodwell, G. M. and Whittaker, R. H. (1968a). Primary production in terrestrial ecosystems. *Am. Zool.* **8**, 19–30.

Woodwell, G. M. and Whittaker, R. H. (1968b). Primary production and the cation budget of the Brookhaven forest. *In* "Proceedings of Symposium on Primary Productivity and Mineral Cycling in Natural Ecosystems". University of Maine Press, Orono, pp. 151–161.

APPENDIX 1

Regression data for primary forest species

Maregn name	Generic name	Height (m)	Dbh (cm)	Above ground moist weight (kg)	Total moist weight (kg)
Aehuellmai	*Helicia*	5·38	3·43	4·710	
Ambiamtupee	*Urophyllum*	2·79	1·42	0·425	
Ambiamtupee	*Urophyllum*	18·00	18·07	232·618	
Angunuum	*Syzygium*	4·64	2·53	2·497	
Angunuum	*Syzygium*	3·35	1·26	0·909	
Bukko	*Endiandra*	19·00	16·57	224·604	
Bukko	*Endiandra*	5·64	3·44	4·426	
Dawingahn	?	16·00	12·88	130·694	
Dummah	*Trema cannabina* Lour.	10·46	16·00	126·100	130·413
Gawa Kumpf	*Legnephora*	5·94	3·13	4·767	
Gongodemi	*Saurauia*	3·05	1·818	1·078	
Guunsh	*Evodia* c.f. *crispula*	15·99	21·17	455·200	491·227
Kahl	?	3·71	1·81	1·362	
Kalum	?	5·64	3·23	4·426	
Kanjeb	?	16·20	16·12	262·979	297·256
Kina	*Planchonella firima* (Miq) Dub.	2·97	1·77	1·071	
Kulupeng	?	23·00	20·87	360·670	
Kulupeng	?	7·01	3·58	4·426	
Momenah	?	13·87	19·43	284·918	320·298
Momenai	?	17·00	20·18	334·264	
Mopolungum	*Lucinea*	22·72	32·02	906·935	1044·270
Mopolungum	*Lucinea*	3·09	1·92	1·362	
Munneyambo	*Lusianthus* c.f. *papuanus* Wernh.	2·74	1·42	0·511	
Nong	*Castanopsis acuminatissima*	30·82	35·93	1738·249	
Pappah	?	3·28	2·22	1·305	
Puppa	?	14·64	15·51	182·234	

Appendix 1—*continued*

Mareng name	Generic name	Height (m)	Dbh (cm)	Above ground moist weight	Total moist weight (kg)
Puumpf	?	17·00	14·55	184·452	
Rhambai	*Harpullia*	4·83	1·52	0·794	
Rhambai	*Harpullia*	3·81	1·31	0·482	
Tulumoi	*Helicia*	22·71	22·98	742·824	861·664
Tweem	*Sloanea*	3·38	1·82	0·511	
Wombo	?	18·00	20·78	383·802	
Wombo	?	4·34	2·02	1·702	
Wonnum	*Eurya tigang* K. Sch. and Laut.	4·88	2·53	2·667	
Wunya	Lauraceae	16·86	20·95	254·183	290·899
Yamba	*Cryptocarya*	3·23	1·31	0·511	
Yenjek	?	6·70	3·23	5·45	
Yimgurll	?	11·88	17·32	213·305	245·299
Yingua	*Semecarpus decipens* M. and P.	6·09	3·84	4·767	

APPENDIX 2

Regression data for secondary forest species

Mareng name	Generic name	Height (m)	Dbh (cm)	Above ground moist weight (kg)	Total moist weight (kg)
Bokant	*Cladcluvia*	10·44	12·93	94·803	105·689
	celebica	16·73	16·98	187·670	209·008
	(B.L.)				
	Hoogland				
Gant	*Wendlandia*	2·261	1·27	0·793	0·892
	paniculata DC	5·638	2·880	3·802	
		7·163	3·44	4·597	
		6·096	3·49	5·959	
Gongo	*Saurauia*	2·06	2·02	1·289	1·572
		1·63	1·41	0·699	0·869
		2·11	1·92	1·081	1·269
Rokunt	*Saurauia*	1·59	0·95	0·528	0·669
		2·717	2·32	1·880	2·168
		8·00	14·55	106·935	131·203
		6·25	5·25	10·33	
		5·94	3·13	3·86	
Dukambo	*Pipturus*	2·31	1·41	0·652	0·768
		3·023	1·82	0·944	1·094
		2·259	0·635	0·196	0·224
Komukai	*Trema*	17·00	20·919	352·516	373·484
	orientalis	12·69	24·21	436·330	531·954
	(L) Bl.	4·11	3·53	4·109	5·104
		10·74	8·69	39·691	45·248
		9·906	12·243	68·947	79·153
		13·13	16·372	158·365	174·468
Pokai	*Alphitonia*	13·00	18·798	345·823	364·307
	incana	11·75	11·63	70·229	81·796
		12·46	13·54	136·786	146·879
		8·18	15·37	145·266	208·09
		17·61	17·79	241·771	262·523
		20·49	24·00	531·776	583·305
		3·78	3·234	2·936	3·859

Appendix 2—*continued*

Mareng name	Generic name	Height (m)	Dbh (cm)	Above ground moist weight	Total moist weight (kg)
Gra	*Dodonea viscosa*	3·40	1·82	0·9507	0·994
	(L) Jacq.	3·96	1·667	1·469	1·553
		4·42	4·04	8·272	9·207
		10·06	15·09	120·769	152·295
		16·00	17·38	227·310	253·505
		16·00	11·55	147·759	156·038
		4·95	3·34	3·499	4·250
		6·39	5·46	11·319	13·028
		4·57	2·93	3·089	3·546
Rhangahn	*Myristica*	5·10	3·64	4·199	
		2·44	1·92	1·475	
		15·00	16·74	146·926	
Penta	*Macaranga*	3·42	2·22	1·638	1·776
	pleiostamina	4·8006	3·234	3·453	4·136
	Pax and	4·468	2·678	2·643	3·150
	Hoff.	10·516	14·502	141·798	182·715
		2·870	2·223	2·414	2·774
Peiya	*Maesa*	3·40	2·62	2·449	2·889
		4·22	3·59	6·582	7·529

APPENDIX 3

Description and biomass data for Kompiai vegetation formations
sampled (data in dry tonnes per hectare)

Primary forest   Age of stand: —
Location: Kombitimamp   Area surveyed: 200 m²
Altitude: 1859 m   Slope: 30°
Site no.: 1a   Aspect: 187°

Biomass class	Total biomass	Above ground biomass	Root biomass	No. of species/ 25 m²
Herbs	2·329	1·976	0·353	9·12
Nanophanerophytes	0·852	0·756	0·096	20·12
Microphanerophytes	9·552	8·436	1·116	10·75
Mesophanerophytes	394·294	348·742	45·552	2·38
Megaphanerophytes	—	—	—	0
Total	407·028	359·910	47·118	—

Primary forest   Age of stand: —
Location: Kamendabongma   Area surveyed: 300 m²
Altitude: 1920 m   Slope: 35°
Site no.: 1b   Aspect: 185–267°

Biomass class	Total biomass	Above ground biomass	Root biomass	No. of species/ 25 m²
Herbs	0·962	0·844	0·118	6·08
Nanophanerophytes	1·574	1·387	0·187	16·08
Microphanerophytes	10·125	8·944	1·181	11·67
Mesophanerophytes	43·926	38·464	5·462	1·50
Megaphanerophytes	122·560	108·652	13·908	0·167
Total	179·147	158·291	20·856	—

Appendix 3—*continued*

Garden   Age of stand: 1 year old
Location: Mengompf   Area surveyed: 50 m²
Altitude: 1737 m   Slope: 35°
Site no.: 2a   Aspect: 171°

Biomass class	Total biomass	Above ground biomass	Root or corm biomass	No. of species/ 25 m²
Crops	7·028	2·298	4·730	75
Herbs	0·501	0·425	0·076	11·5
Nanophanerophytes	0·414	0·346	0·068	4·5
Total	7·943	3·069	4·874	—

Garden   Age of stand: 1 year old
Location: Tumbepeh   Area surveyed: 25 m²
Altitude: 1725 m   Slope: 30°
Site no.: 2b   Aspect: 190°

Biomass class	Total biomass	Above ground biomass	Root or corm biomass	No. of species/ 25 m²
Crops	6·721	3·348	3·373	7
Herbs	0·898	0·808	0·090	20
Nanophanerophytes	0·026	0·024	0·002	1
Total	7·645	4·180	3·465	—

Garden   Area of stand: 1 year old
Location: Tumbepeh   Area surveyed: 25 m²
Altitude: 1743 m   Slope: 32°
Site no.: 2c   Aspect: 194°

Biomass class	Total biomass	Above ground biomass	Root or corm biomass	No. of species/ 25 m²
Crops	6·710	1·914	4·796	5
Herbs	0·392	0·353	0·039	24
Nanophanerophytes	0·042	0·037	0·005	11
Total	7·144	2·304	4·840	—

Appendix 3—*continued*

Garden
Location: Tumbepeh
Altitude: 1737 m
Site no.: 3a

Age of stand: 2 years old
Area surveyed: 25 m²
Slope: 30°
Aspect: 175°

Biomass class	Total biomass	Above ground biomass	Root or corm biomass	No. of species/ 25 m²
Crops	7·849	6·355	1·494	7
Herbs	0·508	0·403	0·065	18
Nanophanerophytes	0·101	0·091	0·010	6
Total	8·458	6·889	1·569	—

Garden
Location: Mengompf
Altitude: 1706 m
Site no.: 3b

Age of stand: 2 years old
Area surveyed: 25 m²
Slope: 35°
Aspect: 168°

Biomass class	Total biomass	Above ground biomass	Root or corm biomass	No. of species/ 25 m²
Crops	7·792	6·175	1·617	6
Herbs	0·721	0·437	0·284	19
Nanophanerophytes	0·592	0·536	0·056	13
Total	9·105	7·148	1·957	—

Garden
Location: Mengompf
Altitude: 1740 m
Site no.: 4

Age of stand: 3 years old
Area surveyed: 50 m²
Slope: 30–45°
Aspect: 182°

Biomass class	Total biomass	Above ground biomass	Root or corm biomass	No. of species/ 25 m²
Crops	4·101	3·465	0·636	4·5
Herbs	4·896	3·441	1·455	22
Nanophanerophytes	2·696	2·388	0·308	10
Microphanerophytes	2·229	1·962	0·267	4
Total	13·922	11·256	2·666	—

Appendix 3—*continued*

Secondary forest   Age of stand: 4 years old
Location: Kiyonggamp   Area surveyed: 50 m²
Altitude: 1820 m   Slope: 25–30°
Site no.: 5a   Aspect: 4°

Biomass class	Total biomass	Above ground biomass	Root biomass	No. of species/ 25 m²
Herbs	7·662	5·975	1·687	12
Nanophanerophytes	0·507	0·468	0·468	6·5
Microphanerophytes	6·995	6·263	6·263	3·5
Total	15·164	12·706	12·706	

Secondary forest   Age of stand: 4 years old
Location: Rhumakunda   Area surveyed: 50 m²
Altitude: 1798 m   Slope: 20°
Site no.: 5b   Aspect: 50°

Biomass class	Total biomass	Above ground biomass	Root biomass	No. of species/ 25 m²
Herbs	7·368	6·125	1·243	13·5
Nanophanerophytes	0·852	0·745	0·107	5·5
Microphanerophytes	9·149	8·168	0·981	4
Total	17·369	15·038	2·331	—

Secondary forest   Age of stand: 5 years old
Location: Kombeyang   Area surveyed: 50 m²

Altitude: 1850 m   Slope: 30°
Site no.: 6   Aspect: 358–11°

Biomass class	Total biomass	Above ground biomass	Root biomass	No. of species/ 25 m²
Herbs	8·579	7·018	1·741	11·5
Nanophanerophytes	0·394	0·313	0·081	4·5
Microphanerophytes	18·782	12·697	5·085	4
Total	27·935	21·028	6·907	—

Appendix 3—*continued*

Secondary forest   Age of stand: 12 years old
Location: Nopeyama   Area surveyed: 200 m²
Altitude: 1584 m   Slope: 30°
Site no.: 7a·   Aspect: 89–217°

Biomass class	Total biomass	Above ground biomass	Root biomass	No. of species/ 25 m²
Herbs	5·666	4·615	1·051	14·70
Nanophanerophytes	0·130	0·115	0·015	4·88
Microphanerophytes	1·840	1·667	0·173	1·75
Mesophanerophytes	63·735	56·470	7·265	0·75
Megaphanerophytes	30·414	26·586	3·828	0·12
Total	101·785	89·455	12·330	

Secondary forest   Age of stand: 13 years old
Location: Kombitimanp   Area surveyed: 175 m²
Altitude: 1829 m   Slope: 25°
Site no.: 7b   Aspect: 150°

Biomass class	Total biomass	Above ground biomass	Root biomass	No. of species/ 25 m²
Herbs	5·108	4·052	1·056	11·71
Nanophanerophytes	0·054	0·048	0·006	1·875
Microphanerophytes	8·106	7·143	0·963	4·43
Mesophanerophytes	50·166	44·226	7·965	1·29
Megaphanerophytes	—	—	—	0
Total	63·434	55·467	—	—

Appendix 3—*continued*

Grassland: *Imperata* dominated   Age of stand: —
Location: Rhumakunda   Area surveyed: 100 m²
Altitude: 1706 m   Slope: 30–350°
Site no.: 8   Aspect: 350°

Biomass class		Total biomass	Above ground biomass	Root biomass	No. of species/ 25 m²
Herbs		6·184	4·286	1·898	16·12
	Total	6·184	4·286	1·898	—

Grassland: *Themeda* dominated   Age of stand: —
Location: Balambe   Area surveyed: 90 m²
Altitude: 1615 m   Slope: 30°
Site no.: 9   Aspect: 48–326°

Biomass class		Total biomass	Above ground biomass	Root biomass	No. of species/ 25 m²
Herbs		3·558	2·966	0·592	14·8
	Total	3·558	2·966	0·592	—

Part 4

Environmental Exploitation and Human Subsistence

The Ecological Description and Analysis of Tropical Subsistence Patterns: An Example From New Guinea

MARK D. DORNSTREICH

Livingston College, Rutgers University, U.S.A.

I. INTRODUCTION

The anthropological literature is filled with statements but few studies of the way traditional people gain their livelihood. Where conclusions or explanations are advanced for particular food-getting patterns, these are rarely based on an analysis of whole dietary-subsistence systems, and there are a mere handful of societies for which quantitative subsistence data exist. This situation is disappointing for the anthropologist interested in traditional subsistence patterns, especially when it is realized that those societies which retain essentially self-sufficient food production systems are rapidly being forced to relinquish their traditional economic independence.

The information presented in this paper represents one attempt to redress the above situation. It offers a methodology for the description of small-scale subsistence patterns, and then attempts to summarize the pattern of one traditional society—the Gadio Enga of interior New Guinea—in terms of it.* Following this first part of the paper I

* The fieldwork on which this description is based was carried out by myself and my wife during the years 1967–68. Our research was supported by a Dissertation Improvement Grant from the National Science Foundation, a Fulbright grant to the Australian National University, Canberra, and a small grant from the Department of Anthropology, Columbia University, New York.

extend from the Gadio case to consider certain broader questions of interest to ecological anthropologists. In doing this I hope to show that an ecological approach to the description of a subsistence pattern can lead to a better understanding of the relationship between food-getting systems, environmental characteristics, and particular features of small-scale, tropical societies.

II. THE GADIO ENGA PEOPLE

The Gadio Enga are a good example of a small-scale tropical society which follows a highly mixed, or low-energy subsistence pattern. Along with other groups similar to themselves, they live in head-waters of one of the major southern tributaries of the Sepik river of New Guinea (see Map 1). Gadio territory encompasses the entire upper drainage of the Karawari river. It is a mixture of hilly and mountainous terrain, and is covered by an enormous, dendritic complex of streams and small waterways, and a lush carpet of submontane and lower montane tropical rainforest. The forested river valleys in which the Gadio live are located at about 450–900 m above sea level and the entire region is extremely wet, receiving more than 7000 mm of rainfall per year. This territory meets all meteorological and environmental criteria for a true "tropical humid" environment having a "tropical rainforest climate" (see Dornstreich, 1973, pp. 91–113, 534–548, for a fuller discussion of the Gadio physical environment).

The people who have come to be called Gadio are actually a cluster of five small patrilineal clans. Each clan has 15 members (the size range is 5 to 24), and each has its own clan territory, primary hamlet site, and a considerable number of other, active and abandoned garden and living sites. These sites are scattered primarily, but not exclusively, over a clan's own territory. From 5 to 40 people typically reside at a Gadio hamlet and, although the actual number fluctuates daily, there are usually 20 people present at any one time. Through careful genealogical investigations we were able to establish that as of 1967 there were a total of 79 Gadio Enga people. According to existing maps and our own geographical observations, we also determined that Gadio territory is 104–130 km² in areal extent, and that the Gadio people thus live at population density of 0·8 persons per km².*

* "Average density" assumes an equitable distribution of people over land. But since this is not the way people actually live, it becomes a matter of great ecological significance to know by exactly what temporal–spatial pattern they do settle, and what the population density characteristics of different ecological zones or resource areas are. The Gadio population density figure of 0·8 persons per km² is on the low side for small-scale societies generally, but is probably quite characteristic of tropical forest peoples following a highly mixed subsistence pattern (Denevan, 1970b; Miracle, 1973, p. 337; Turnbull, 1972, pp. 295–300; Weiner, 1972, pp. 400–404).

Beyond the level of the local group and the clan-cluster, the Gadio bear close cultural and linguistic similarities to at least five other societies living in this part of New Guinea. These people number about 450 to 550 altogether, and they settle over the entire east–west expanse of the upper Karawari river drainage (and perhaps beyond), an area of some 650 km². I have called this regional population "Outer Enga". This ultimate group can be distinguished from neighbouring populations by the fact that all people belonging to it speak mutually intelligible dialects of the Enga language (there is a major dialect boundary between the Outer Enga and the better known Central Enga peoples of the New Guinea Highlands), and they all participate in a common system of intermarriage, trade, warfare and ceremonialism (Dornstreich, 1973, pp. 475–524).

III. A METHODOLOGY FOR THE DESCRIPTION OF SUBSISTENCE SYSTEMS

If one looks at the way anthropologists have dealt with the subject of subsistence, it is immediately clear that they have never adopted any consistent typology for classifying subsistence patterns, nor is there a standard format for describing them. It is true that familiar terms are used, and that societies are accordingly labelled as "horticultural", "hunter-gatherer", "pastoralist", or something similar, but these terms are superficial and do not bear any definite and detailed relationship to the full range of people's actual subsistence behaviour (see Beals, 1964). Of special importance to the ecologically oriented anthropologist is the fact that they also tell us relatively little about the characteristics of a particular society's ecological adaptation, for instance, about its productive relationship to environmental resources, the input–output energetics of its subsistence pattern (or the individual activities which compose it), the distribution, movement or density of people over the group's territory or a number of similar ecological questions. It seems obvious to me that any subsistence pattern typology or method for description which fails to unambiguously provide us with such information will inevitably produce classificatory inconsistencies and explanatory dilemmas.*

* A classic example of a "problem" created by a superficial classification of subsistence is the apparent enigma of cultural complexity, and high population density of many non-agricultural Native American peoples of the West Coast of the U.S.A. (Beals and Hester, 1956; Heizer, 1958; Zeigler, 1968). As soon as one understands that the wild food staple of these people—acorn flour—has essentially the same productive and nutritional characteristics as some of the best agricultural crops, this classificatory exception is explained.

In our New Guinea fieldwork we decided that an ecological approach to the description of a subsistence system required study of three primary categories of information:

  a. the environmental factors which substantially affect food-getting, and especially the characteristics of food resources and resource areas,
  b. all the food-getting activities which compose the people's subsistence pattern, as well as data about the social implementation, work requirements and the temporal–spatial pattern by which each is followed,
  c. all the foods obtained by these activities, in the form of a quantified account of food returns throughout an entire subsistence cycle.

On the basis of such a description we expect that the Gadio subsistence system could be compared to any other subsistence pattern of comparable scale from the tropics or elsewhere. Although I do not want to give the impression that we were equally successful in documenting each of these categories of subsistence information, we have research results from all of them.

IV. THE GADIO ENGA SUBSISTENCE SYSTEM

Tables I–VI give a comprehensive outline of the Gadio subsistence system. These tables take the three primary components of a subsistence system mentioned above—the environmental resource areas which people utilize, the activities by which food is obtained, and the food items which people eat—and describe how the Gadio system looks. They also show the organizational relationship between many of these different system components. These data clearly show that if the Gadio were to be referred to as "swidden agriculturalists", "tropical mixed horticulturalists", or "hunter-gardeners"—terms which are probably the best available according to current anthropological usage—that major dimensions of Gadio subsistence would be ignored. Some of these dimensions, along with their implications can now be considered.

Table I shows that the different food resource areas which the Gadio utilize span an impressive altitudinal range of territory. This fact suggests that Gadio movement and settlement is dispersed rather than concentrated, and that people are constantly radiating outward, up and down, through the different ecological zones and resource areas of their territory. Interestingly, the Gadio happen to live in a portion

TABLE I

Resource areas of Gadio territory

Resource area	Altitudinal range (m above sea level)	
1 Hamlet site—current	450–750	A
2 Hamlet site—abandoned	450–750	A
3 Living site—current	350–900	A
4 Living site—abandoned	350–900	A
5 Garden—in production (i.e. fenced)	450–750	A
6 Garden—staple foods exhausted	450–750	A
7 Garden—abandoned	450–750	A
8 Fruit tree stands	450–750	A
9 Sago swamp	300–600	N
10 Sago stand	300–900	N
11 Stream or river (lower altitude)	350–600	N
12 Stream (upper altitude)	650–1050	N
13 Streambank	450–750	N
14 Rainforest	450–1050	N
15 Mountains	900–1200	N

A: anthrogenic; N: naturally occurring.

of the New Guinea lower montane rainforest which is more environmentally heterogeneous than either the lower altitude hill country to the north, or the montane valley systems of the New Guinea Highlands proper, to the south.

The considerable environmental diversity found in this part of New Guinea can be partially explained by the fact that a major ecological boundary, the 900 m contour, runs directly through the middle of Gadio territory (Robbins, 1961). This contour separates the lowland tropical rainforest, found predominantly in the lower altitudinal range of Gadio settlement, from the lowland hill forest of the middle and upper ranges. These zones differ in their faunal, as well as their floristic characteristics, and the Gadio have access to, and consistently utilize both of them.* The Gadio pattern of continuous movement between the hamlets, living sites, gardens and resource areas of the different altitudinal ranges of their territory is a central feature of their adaptation. If this pattern were to change in any significant way, it would be reflected by social organization changes at both the local and group level, in various aspects of group demography, in changes in

* Settlement in this transition zone gives the Gadio access to the sago resources, wild pig populations, the lowland cassowary, and betel nut—resources which are more abundant in the lower altitude portion of their territory—along with the other game of their rainforest hunting territories primarily found above their zone of hamlet and garden site location (Hyndman, n.d.; Morren, 1974).

the people's nutritional health status, and perhaps also in the quality of the Gadio resource base.

A picture of the relationship between food resource areas and Gadio food-getting activities, as shown in Table II, shows that certain resource areas (i.e. sago swamps and active and abandoned gardens) are the focus of several different food-getting activities. This means that the Gadio obtain a variety of foods at these localities, but one must be careful not to conclude from this that they are in all ways more important than other resource areas. For example, the tables presented show that many localities which are the site of only one or two food-getting activities continuously provide small quantities of high quality nutrients to the Gadio. This fact is of great nutritional importance, especially for women and children.

Although my figures on the age and sex organization of subsistence work are tentative only, they suggest much about the way the Gadio food-getting pattern is organized (Dornstreich, 1973, pp. 291–297). By and large they support standard anthropological observations about food getting, for example, that men follow activities which require more mobility; that there is a strong association between women and plants, both domesticated and wild (though men are much more involved with tree crops than are women); that the rhythm of male and female subsistence work is quite different, for instance, the work that women do is repetitive and continuous (Figure 2), while men perform more energetically demanding tasks but do not engage in food getting so regularly (Figure 1); that people work most fre-

TABLE II

Activity–resource area associations

Food-getting activity	Associated resource area															
	1	2	3	4	5	6	7	8	9	10	11	12	13	14	15	Total
1 Gardening					×	×	×									3
2 Sago making									×	×						2
3 Silviculture	×	×	×	×	×	×	×	×								8
4 Gathering (plant foods)				×	×		×						×	×		5
5 Animal husbandry	×	×							×							3
6 Trapping	×		×						×			×				4
7 Fishing									×		×	×				3
8 Collecting (animal foods)	×	×	×	×	×	×	×		×	×	×	×	×	×	×	14
9 Hunting														×	×	2
Total no. activities	4	3	3	3	4	3	4	1	5	2	2	3	2	3	2	

quently at those activities which produce the greatest amounts of food—horticulture and sago making; and that non-local people (as defined by kinship and residence history) rely to a much greater extent on those foods which are wild and not "owned" or scarce. One particularly prominent point in this overall activity pattern is that although men and women tend to perform quite different subsistence tasks, and even different aspects of those same activities in which they co-operate, the subsistence work of one sex is no more or less important than that of the other. Reasons for the kinds of activities which each performs can be suggested, but both aspects must be considered in a balanced way (Brown, 1970; Linton, 1971).

Regarding the balance between different activities that contribute to the Gadio diet, some of the major conclusions suggested by Table III are as follows: different food-getting activities make complementary, rather than redundant contributions to the Gadio diet (i.e. certain nutrients are largely supplied by particular food-getting activities); activities which do not account for any significant quantitative part of the Gadio diet are no less important than those which are more prominent and/or productive; women play the primary role in providing most dietary nutrients for the group as a whole, while men perform those activities which supply most of the group's limiting food nutrients—animal protein and fat (the reader is reminded that individual food consumption may considerably complicate this picture); both sexes combine to provide a significant portion of all nutrients; activities which supply animal food provide 25% of the group's dietary protein, and 75% of the dietary fat—calling attention to the importance of the nutritional quality of the plant food portion of the diet.

Table V, on nutrient returns from the various Gadio food-getting activities, presents information of fundamental importance to an analysis of Gadio subsistence. It clearly shows that anthropologists must distinguish, but simultaneously consider, those food-getting activities which provide the bulk of a group's calories and those others by which people principally obtain nutrients which are limiting or scarce. In tropical nutrition, this usually amounts to a distinction between the quantitative and the qualitative aspects of subsistence, especially the role of protein nutrition.* Our information makes a

* The total protein content of tropical food staples is generally much lower than is true for the cereal grains of temperate regions. Whereas the protein content (per 100 g of edible portion) of sweet potato, yam, manioc, taro, bananas and sago ranges from 0·1 to 2·0 g, the grain staples of temperate region agriculture, such as wheat, rice, maize, millet and sorghum, have 2·0 to 4·0 g or more. This difference is extremely important, especially for children (who cannot eat enough of the tropical food staples to meet minimal quantitative protein requirements). In addition, essential amino acids of protein are missing from all tropical root crops, manioc and bananas being especially poor in this respect (Dornstreich, 1973, pp. 352–355; McArthur, 1974, pp. 102–111; Oomen, 1971; Sebrell and Hand, 1957).

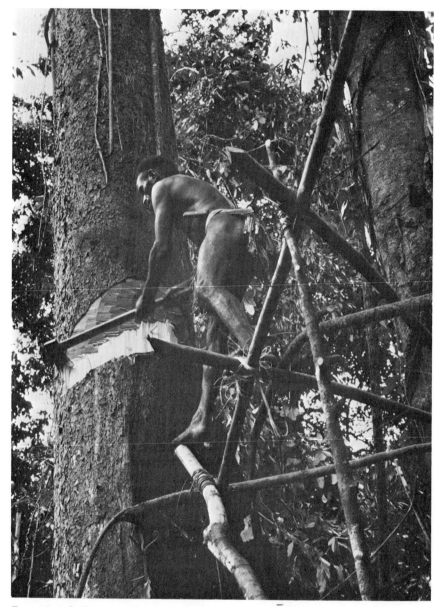

FIGURE 1. A Gadio man making a garden in primary lowland rainforest. In order to cut above the tree buttresses—which flare out 3–5 m at the tree base—a cutting platform is constructed from poles and vines. It takes at least ½ day to fell a tree of this size using a steel axe.

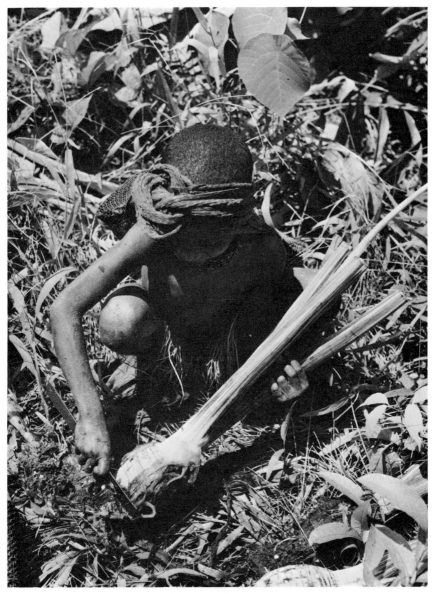

FIGURE 2. A Gadio girl harvests and cleans taro for the evening meal. She scrapes the edible corm, for this is the part to be eaten. The stalk will also be carried back to the hamlet, from where it will be taken to a new garden site for planting the next day. The net bag tied across the head, rather than across the shoulders, marks this child as a girl.

TABLE III

Age and sex organization of Gadio food getting—number of occasions on which various food-getting activities were recorded, 11 June to 20 September 1968

Activity no.			1	2	3		4	7	8		6, 9
					Tree nuts, fruits				Collecting		
Category of person[a]	No. of persons	Total no. of occasions	Gardening	Sago making	Cultivated	Wild	Plant gathering	Fishing	General	Grubs	Hunting, trapping
Residents											
Adult male (18+)	8	341	168	27	25	8	12	26	25	33	15
Adult female (15+)	5	320	186	33	8	16	42	8	17	10	0
Adolescent male (12–17)	1	28	6	2	1	0	3	10	3	2	1
Adolescent female (9–14)	2	56	10	10	2	4	13	11	3	2	0
Boy (6–11)	2	120	20	7	10	3	12	43	9	14	2
Girl (5–8)	0	—	—	—	—	—	—	—	—	—	—
Non-residents											
Adult male		151	51	28	9	3	22	22	5	11	0
Adult female		153	48	22	3	10	45	11	9	5	0
Adolescent male		33	10	6	1	0	5	8	0	1	2
Adolescent female		27	8	5	1	2	4	5	2	2	0
Boy		83	4	8	2	1	15	33	0	7	3
Girl		0	—	—	—	—	—	—	—	—	—

[a] Age in years in brackets.

TABLE IV

Inventory of Gadio foods

No.	Common name or category	Scientific identification
1	Taro	*Colocasia esculenta* L. Schott
2	Sweet potato	*Ipomoea batatas* L. Lam.
3	Manioc	*Manihot utilissima* Pohl.
4	Tapioc*a*	*Pueraria lobata*
5	Yam	*Dioscorea* sp.
6	Banana, plantain	*Musa paradisiaca*
7	Sugar cane	*Saccharum officinarum* L.
8	Cucumber	*Cucumis sativa* L.
9	Pandanus (marita*a*)	*Pandanus conoideus* Lamarck
10	Breadfruit	*Artocarpus incisus, A. altilis*
11	Papaya	*Carica papaya* L.
12	Betel nut, c/w	*Areca catechu* Linn.
13	Grass stem (pit-pit*a*), c	*Saccharum edule* Hassk.
14	Grass stem (pit-pit*a*), c	*Setaria palmifolia* Stapf.
15	Bean	*Phaseolus vulgaris*
16	Pumpkin	*Cucurbita moschata*
17	Ginger	*Zingiber rerumbet*
18	Greens (abika*a*)	*Abelmoschus manihot*
19	Leaves of Cucurbitaceae, c and w	
	Pumpkin, c	*Cucurbita moschata*
	Bottlegourd, c	*Lageneria leucantha*
	Snake gourd, w	*Luffa* sp.
	Ridge gourd, w	*Trichosanthes* sp.
20	Watercress	*Rorippa* sp.
21	Parsley-like green	*Oenanthe javanica*
22	Betel pepper leaf	*Piper betel* Linn.
23	Sago starch	*Metroxylon* sp.
24	Sago heart (growing shoot)	*Metroxylon* sp.
25	Yam, w	*Dioscorea* sp.
26	Tree nuts, w	*Elaeocarpus* sp.
27	Tree fruit, w	*Pangium edule*
28	Mushroom	
29	Lemon grass	*Cymbopogon citratus*
30	Grass stems, w	Urticaceae: *Poulzolzia hirta*
31	Ferns (inc. tree ferns), w	Hypolepsis aff. brooksii, *Thelypteris* sp., *Cyathea* sp., *Lomariopsis* sp., *Diplazium* sp., *Cyathea angiensis, Thelypteris* sp., *Saccoloma* sp.
32	Tree leaves, w	Acanthaceae: *Rungia* sp., Moraceae: *Ficus* sp., *Chisocheton* sp.
33	Tree leaves, c	*Gnetum gnemon* L.
34	Tobacco, c	*Nicotiana tabacum*
35	Pig (domestic and wild)	*Sus scrofa papuensis*
36	Cassowary	*Cassuarius bennetti*
37	Small mammals (bandicoot)	Peramelidae, *Phalanger gymnotis,*
	Phalangers, wallaby	*P. orientalis, P. maculatus,* Macropodidae

TABLE IV—*continued*

No. Common name or category	Scientific identification
38 Rodents	*Rattus* sp., *Hyomys goliath dammermani*, *Mellomys rothschildi*
39 Birds	
40 Bird eggs	
41 Bat, flying fox	*Dobsonia moluccensis*
42 Snakes	
43 Lizards	
44 Fish	
45 Eel	
46 Frogs	
47 Crabs	
48 Turtles	
49 Grubs	? *Monochamus* sp. ? *Scapanes* sp. Cerambycidae
50 Insects (beetle)	
51 Insects (crickets, grasshopper)	
52 Sweat bee honey	
53 Edible stone (clay)	
54 New Guinea salt (black)	57% sodium chloride (NaCl)

C: cultivated; W: wild.
a Pidgin English.

good case for the proposition that anthropologists should be recording information in terms of "nutrient returns" from particular food-getting activities, and not as "food returns" or the "per cent of the diet supplied" by any one of them.

The significance of this distinction can be easily seen by looking at two activities which I believe anthropologists consistently undervalue, especially for tropical rainforest peoples.* Table V shows that the activities called "plant gathering" and "animal collecting" amount to less than 10% of the Gadio diet, by weight. Yet these activities supply more than 20% of the protein (and certainly a much higher percentage of the high quality protein), almost 25% of the fat, and plant gathering alone provides more than 50% of the Vitamin A which the Gadio receive (Figure 3). These figures do not even take into account the fact that it is almost impossible to consistently record food returns from these activities, and also the important point that women and children

---

* For possible examples see Carneiro, 1964, p. 9; Chagnon, 1968, p. 33, 1973, p. 127; Denevan, 1971, p. 513; Siskind, 1973, p. 228. On the other hand, it seems likely to me that anthropologists usually overestimate the importance of hunting, again probably because of the tendency to focus on subsistence behaviour rather than its nutritional results (Carneiro, 1970, p. 331; Denevan, 1971, p. 517).

TABLE V

Percent of nutrients supplied by subsistence activities, 3 June to 20 September 1968

Food-getting activities	Foods (by no.) supplied by activity	Edible grams	Calories	Protein	Fat	Calcium	Iron	Vit. A	Vit. B₂ Thia-mine	Vit. B₂ Ribo-flavin	Niacin	Vit. C Ascorb. acid	Phos-phorus	Potas-sium
								Percent of nutrient supplied						
1 Gardening	1, 2, 3, 4, 5, 6, 7, 8, 13, 14, 15, 16, 17, 18, 19, 20, 21	63·9	42·4	52·6	8·3	72·5	65·1	45·5	70·4	60·1	71·9	74·5	79·6	49·4
2 Sago making	23, 24	23·7	47·4	2·8	1·0	9·9	12·9	0·4	1·8	3·5	1·7	3·3	1·5	30·8
3 Silviculture	9, 10, 11, 12, 34	1·1	1·0	2·2	7·5	0·4	0·3	—	1·4	0·5	1·8	0·6	0·2	—
4 Plant gathering	22, 25, 26, 27, 28, 29, 30, 31, 32, 33	7·1	2·3	14·2	8·2	12·9	17·7	54·1	11·1	14·2	10·4	21·6	11·0	19·7
(Total) Plant food getting	1–34	95·8	93·1	71·8	25·0	95·7	96·0	100·0	84·7	78·3	85·8	100·0	92·3	99·9
5 Animal husbandry	35	0·5	1·5	3·4	19·4	0·1	0·6	—	3·2	1·2	2·6	—	—	—
6 Trapping	36, 37	0·3	0·3	3·1	3·0	0·1	0·3	—	0·5	5·5	2·5	—	0·7	—
7 Fishing	45, 46	0·6	0·4	5·9	1·4	3·4	0·6	—	0·4	2·8	1·9	—	2·4	—
8 Animal collecting	39, 41, 43, 44, 47, 48, 49, 50, 51, 52, 53	1·5	1·6	6·3	14·3	0·4	0·7	—	4·8	6·5	0·4	—	3·6	—
9 Hunting	36, 37, 38, 40, 42	1·3	3·1	9·5	36·9	0·3	1·7	—	6·3	5·6	6·8	—	1·0	—
(Total) Animal food getting 35–53		4·2	6·9	28·2	75·0	4·3	3·9	—	15·2	21·6	14·2	—	7·7	—
Total 1–53		100·0	100·0	100·0	100·0	100·0	100·0	100·0	100·0	100·0	100·0	100·0	100·0	100·0

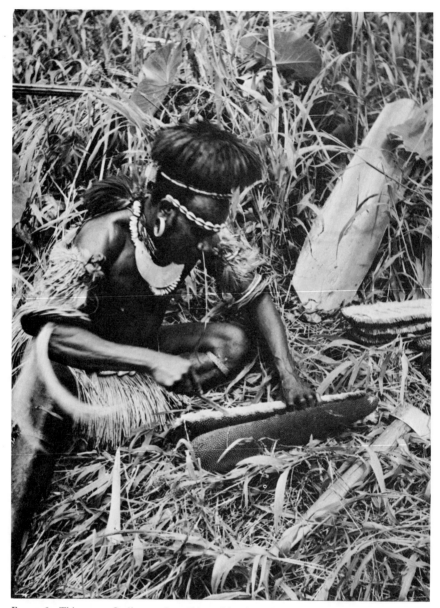

FIGURE 3. This young Gadio man is working with a bone knife to separate the outer part of a pandanus fruit from its core. These outer sections are cooked in an earth oven, after which the many tiny seeds on the husk are washed free of their waxy, red colour. The resulting liquid is eaten, usually with sweet potato, sago or greens. Pandanus is the most important source of vegetable fat in the Gadio diet.

TABLE VI

Comparison of nutrient requirements to nutrient returns for nine nutrients

Nutrient	Days for which nutritional requirements met (of 108-day sample period)[a]	% nutrient supplied by	
		Vegetable food	Animal food
Vitamin C	105	100	—
Vitamin A	73	99 +	—
Vitamin B$_1$ (thiamine)	85	85	15
Iron	100	98	02
Calcium	80	96	04
Calories	55	93	07
Vitamin B$_2$ (riboflavin)	54	78	22
Protein	51	72	28
Fat	11	25	75

[a] Note that this comparison of food returns and nutrient requirements is based on a rather demanding standard of nutrient requirement figures. The figure for total hamlet requirements is arrived at by adding together the requirement for each individual resident in the hamlet on that day, for each nutrient, according to his or her age and sex. This figure is then compared with returns for that nutrient from all the foods obtained on that day. The reader will note that this computation does not take the matter of food distribution into account. It should also be understood that nothing too important is shown by the failure to meet requirements for a particular nutrient on a particular day. This may mean nothing more for example, than a shortfall of a few hundred calories in a total hamlet requirement of 5000 or more calories. A computer program was devised for purposes of making this daily comparison for each nutrient.

get a disproportionately large share of the food returns from them. Clearly, it is impossible to understand the organizational rationale for a particular subsistence pattern unless one is able to talk in terms of nutrient obtainment and distribution.

Finally Table VI shows the relationship between food returns and the "nutritional requirements" of the people living in one Gadio hamlet during 1968.* This is a key subject as far as tropical subsistence systems are concerned, for ecologically-oriented anthropologists have tried to link aspects of group demography, human health, group settlement patterns, population density and distribution, the economy of sex,

* This phrase is put in quotes to indicate that these requirements are necessarily arbitrary. The figures I use are based on a search of the nutritional literature concerned with requirements, together with a consideration of those features of Gadio life which would be expected to affect requirement levels. While the authorities are by no means in agreement on the values to be used, the points of difference and contention between them are too numerous and complex to discuss here. Suffice to say that my requirement figures were separately arrived at for each individual nutrient and that they are not lower than those suggested by any of the authorities I have consulted. Readers interested in a more detailed consideration of this subject are referred to my dissertation (1973, pp. 378–403), and the accompanying tables and references.

and many other ecological concerns to the nutritional limitations of tropical diets (e.g. Brown, 1970; Carneiro, 1964, 1970; Chagnon, 1973; Denevan, 1966; Dornstreich and Buchbinder, 1970; Lathrap, 1968; Meggers, 1971; Morren, 1974; Sauer, 1958; Siskind, 1973; Townsend, 1971).

As a result of our monitoring of Gadio food returns for three months it is possible to state that these people's diet is adequate for all nutrients. This conclusion is based on a daily comparison of (rather demanding) nutrient requirements for all people residing in the Gadio hamlet in which we lived, with the nutritional returns of food obtained during this sample period. There is a noticeable difference however, between how comfortably requirements are met for nutrients supplied almost entirely by vegetable foods (i.e. calories, vitamins A, B_1, and C and calcium), and those for which animal foods are a significant source (i.e. protein, fat and vitamin B_2). For the first group of nutrients, requirements are consistently exceeded, while for the others the Gadio diet seems to be just adequate, but no more than this.

For example, with regard to protein, probably the key nutrient in most tropical diets, the Gadio obtained almost 35 grams per person per day for the entire period of our study (a figure close to the daily adult requirement). Returns also approximated requirements for most days. More important than this however, is the fact that almost 30% of the protein obtained by the Gadio is in the form of animal food (Figure 4). Since some animal protein was available almost every day, it can be safely said that protein returns in this diet are consistently higher in quality than is generally true for other New Guinea societies (Clarke, 1971, pp. 178, 181; Dornstreich, 1973, p. 385; Rappaport, 1968, p. 283; Sorenson, Gajdusek and Reid, 1969, p. 339; but see Morren, 1974, pp. 390–392). Our study emphasizes the general point that in tropical diets composed predominantly of vegetable foods, the amount and distribution of animal food is crucially important.*

The major overall conclusion to be drawn from Tables I–VI is that the Gadio people possess a complex and highly diverse subsistence system. This diversification in all realms of subsistence practice is highly significant from an ecological point of view. It has the primary effect of minimizing the people's impact on their life support system, and thus favours the long-term viability of the Gadio adaptation

---

* It should be remembered that those foods which are limiting in a people's diet are likely to be the same ones about which it is most difficult to get accurate quantitative information. Because these foods also tend to be difficult to obtain, and are also obtained infrequently, they are less likely to be observed and recorded. They may for example, be eaten secretly, as wild game often is among tropical rainforest peoples, or be the subject of special rules regarding their consumption and distribution.

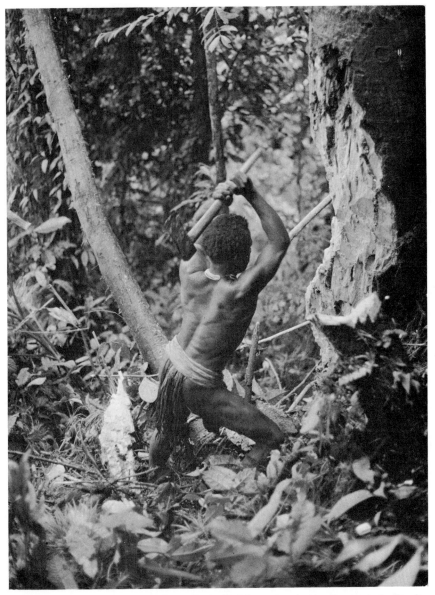

FIGURE 4. A Gadio man chops up the trunk of a dead forest giant looking for tree grubs. Despite the fact that this tree was a three-hour walk from the hamlet where he lived, this tree was well known to him and we travelled to it specifically to collect grubs. On this occasion he obtained 3 kg of grubs, a food high in fat and protein and of very great importance in the Gadio diet.

(Clarke, 1966, p. 357; Rappaport, 1971, p. 130). There is also a positive relationship between subsistence diversity and the maintenance of the good nutritional and health status of the Gadio people—a fact which is especially important when it is realized that present trends in most portions of the world's tropics are moving in very much the opposite direction.

V. IMPLICATIONS OF THE GADIO SUBSISTENCE SYSTEM

This description of Gadio subsistence raises the broader question of how subsistence systems are to be classified. I have called the Gadio system "mixed" or "diverse", and my presentation indicates which factors I think are basic to a consideration of subsistence pattern diversity. Since anthropologists have traditionally focused on sub-sistence behaviour—that is, food-getting activities—it might at least be possible to cross culturally examine subsistence diversity in these terms. The Gadio case illustrates, however, that one must not only enumerate the food-getting activities which people follow, but also determine their relative importance according to some system of actual measurement (preferably by studies of time apportionment, energy expenditure and food productivity). Unfortunately, anthro-pologists have generally failed to collect such information, and without it there is no way of establishing just how "equitably diverse" entire subsistence patterns are (for a consideration of the equitability aspect of diversity, though in another ecological context, see McIntosh, 1967).

I suggest that this concept of subsistence diversity is a particularly useful way to compare the subsistence patterns of different small-scale societies. If this were to be done, it would probably be shown that Gadio food-getting activities are followed in a more balanced way, and that they yield a diet of higher nutritional quality, than is true even for broadly similar tropical societies (e.g. see Chagnon, 1968; Clarke, 1971; Bennett, 1962; Denevan, 1971; Dentan, 1965; Harner, 1972; Holmberg, 1969; Hyndman, n.d.; Meggers, 1971; Nietschmann, 1972; Pospisil, 1963; Rappaport, 1968; Sorenson, Gajdusek and Reid, 1969; Townsend, 1974; Waddell, 1972). As a result of such a compari-son it is possible to gauge the extent of food-getting equitability against other characteristics of these societies, an effort which shows that there is a strong relationship between subsistence extensiveness–intensiveness and group demography, including population density, settlement pattern and structural indicators of population increase (Clarke, 1966).

Analysing subsistence patterns along the lines I have suggested is
not only informative about group demography, but also about the
social features of small-scale societies. In the event of more intensive
food-getting patterns, particular activities tend to be more complex,
and to therefore involve more specialized economic work. Labour
demands also increase, a development which is clearly inconsistent
with overall subsistence diversity. Such a narrowing of a people's
food-production focus implies greater economic productivity (but not
efficiency), and brings along with it such adaptational and social
changes as a general tightening and elaboration of group social
structure, a greater emphasis on political, religious and other means of
social control and leadership, and increased specialization in the realms
of economic, ceremonial and aesthetic life. If the occurrence and extent
of these developments can be related to information about the subsistence diversity, energetic efficiency and nutritional status of a
society, then the detailed study of subsistence patterns has obvious
theoretical importance.

In addition to informing us about such general theoretical questions,
the material I have presented on Gadio subsistence clarifies several
specific points concerning the adaptation of tropical peoples. The
Gadio material suggests that it is useful to look at the subsistence
patterns of these societies in terms of three basic components: a staple
food or calorie-rich component, an animal food or protein-rich
component and a generalized component which, to a greater or lesser
extent, lends subsistence diversity and nutritional quality to the
pattern. An analysis of each of these components, and a consideration
of their overall mix for different societies, gives us important insights
into several hypotheses and propositions of interest to ecological anthropologists. This can be illustrated by looking at small-scale societies
from two of the world's major tropical regions—New Guinea and the
South American Amazon—areas for which anthropologists have collected at least some range of subsistence data.

For both of these regions it can be shown that the higher population
density societies always have a subsistence pattern in which the first
component mentioned above, staple food, is relatively abundant and,
perhaps less obviously, in which the second component involves
reliance on a source of animal food which is both localized and reliable.
Further, a consideration of the geographical distribution of these
societies shows that only particular areas within these large regions
are able to meet both of these conditions (assuming a non-mechanized
technology for all peoples). The key environmental characteristic
which must be present, whether the area be coastal, inland, lowland or
highland, is the availability of relatively flat terrain. This is because only

such environments are conducive to the production of an abundant food staple, a clear precondition for high population density. Usually this involves a productive and sophisticated agricultural system, such as might be found in river deltas or floodplains, on alluvial riverbanks, in valley bottoms, perhaps even on raised lake beds or on terraces cut into the sloping sides of highland river valleys (Armillas, 1971; Brookfield, 1962; Denevan, 1970a; Forge, 1972; Golson, 1970; Lathrap, 1970, pp. 38–39, 171). However, the intensive exploitation of a particularly rich wild food staple—such as the sago palm (*Metroxylon* sp.) of lowland New Guinea—is also a possibility (Forge, 1972; Hyndman, 1973, pp. 73–74; Townsend, 1974).

Apart from a high yielding system of staple food production, the relatively flat environments of the tropics are also the only areas in which a localized and reliable source of animal food can be obtained or produced. The reason that such a source of animal food must be available is that the highly productive systems of staple food obtainment in the tropics are characteristic of subsistence patterns which are low in food-getting diversity and therefore in nutritional quality. As a general rule those tropical agricultural staples which are richest in calories are also the poorest providers of other essential nutrients, and this means that wherever animal food intake is consistently low people begin to develop signs of protein malnutrition.* The limited availability of animal food is especially difficult for pregnant and lactating women (who have elevated protein requirements), for small children (who cannot eat enough food to obtain sufficient protein from lower quality sources), and perhaps in the case of women generally (because the circumstances of food getting and rules governing food consumption often give men greater access to animal food).

If tropical peoples are to obtain localized and reliable sources of animal food, the only possibilities available to them are fish, aquatic or marine animals, domesticated animal stock and perhaps returns from the artificial concentration of non-domesticated animals (e.g. by the construction of fish ponds). Only these sources are sufficiently concentrated to permit dense human settlement. For this reason all

---

* The higher population density groups of lowland Amazonia primarily cultivate bitter manioc (or sometimes corn), as opposed to such alternative staple food possibilities as sweet manioc or bananas. Several reasons for this have been suggested. Thus only bitter, not sweet manioc can be made into storable food (Lathrap, 1970, p. 51), bitter manioc has a very high yield of calories per acre relative to other crops (Lathrap, 1970, pp. 49, 53; Meggers, 1971, p. 117; Miracle, 1973, pp. 340, 341, 343–344; Spath, 1971, p. 10) and this crop has a high tolerance for environmental variation. Similarly, the sago palm starch, on which the dense populations of lowland New Guinea depend, has between two and three times as many calories per unit weight as any tropical root crop (Dornstreich, 1973, pp. 350–351; Townsend, 1974). But both bitter manioc and sago are almost devoid of protein, particularly after all the washing which must be done to make them suitable as food. See also footnote on p. 251.

the large populations of tropical Amazonia—where significant animal domestication never took place—are riverine, lacustrine or maritime in their subsistence orientation (Carneiro, 1970, pp. 3–4; Denevan, 1970b, pp. 63–64, 72; Lathrap, 1970, pp. 20, 35; Meggers, 1971; Sauer, 1958). In lowland New Guinea there is a similar reliance on substantial fish resources. In both regions as soon as one moves away from the larger lowland rivers, the fish are small and few in number (Dentan, 1965, p. 46; Denevan, 1971, p. 499; Dornstreich, 1973, pp. 145–146, 173, 257; Harner, 1972, p. 60; Holmberg, 1969, p. 63; Meggers, 1971, p. 56). Of course it is possible for people to rely on the hunting of wild game for animal food—and even to do so to a significant extent—but such a subsistence emphasis is inconsistent with dense or localized settlement (Morren, 1974).

The Highlands of New Guinea is a classic area for illustrating the practice of intensive animal husbandry, in this case of pigs. In terms of the analysis presented here, there are at least two aspects of this practice which warrant special consideration. First, any significant emphasis on animal husbandry also requires an intensification of the methods by which the animals are to be fed. In New Guinea the only two possibilities in this respect are the cutting of more sago palms or a substantially increased commitment to horticulture (or possibly some combination of the two). One rarely finds intensive pig husbandry in sago areas for the simple reason that at altitudes where the sago palm is really abundant—principally areas below 300 m above sea level— fish resources are similarly so, and fishing is an easier and more productive method for obtaining animal food than pig husbandry.* It is therefore the case in New Guinea that animal husbandry is always accompanied by a system of intensive horticultural production, and that where possibilities for substantial commitment to this type of staple food source are limited, so too is the practice of animal husbandry.

Another important aspect of tropical subsistence patterns is highlighted by New Guinea pig keeping. This has to do with the nature of animal and vegetable food production in the tropics, and the relationship of both to human nutrition. Unlike the obtainment of a food staple, even densely settled human populations do not have a source of animal food which is extremely abundant or a system for obtaining it which is notably efficient. For example, it seems that the energy expended on the maintenance of domestic pigs in New Guinea is often little different from what the people receive back from the animals as food (Rappaport, 1968, pp. 59–63; Waddell, 1972, pp. 117– 121). However, this practice, and perhaps other methods for obtaining

---

* For an interesting case in which horticulture provides the staple food for people, but sago is used to feed pigs, see Hughes, 1970.

animal food, cannot be understood by looking at it in terms of caloric efficiency, or the quantitative side of subsistence. Rather, it must be evaluated according to its effectiveness in converting abundant, calorically rich staple food into food which contains the scarcer, high quality nutrients fat and protein—nutrients which can then be eaten as the people decide (Rappaport, 1968, pp. 67–68; Vayda *et al.*, 1961).

The third component of tropical subsistence patterns, the generalized one which lends diversity and quality to the system, is the most difficult to characterize. It is true that most tropical diets are strongly vegetarian in their emphasis, and that significant amounts of such good quality foods as fruits, nuts, stems, leaves and legumes are often eaten. In those cases where these foods are regularly and rather abundantly available, and where they can also be combined with a food staple which is of relatively good quality (e.g. corn or rice), less emphasis can be placed on the second, or animal food component of the subsistence pattern. A predominantly vegetable food diet which is diversified and carefully composed can be adequate for all essential nutrients (e.g. as one which uses the corn, beans and squash complex of Mesoamerica as a basis). However, if either of the vegetable food components is limited in abundance or reliability, low animal food intake will almost certainly result in nutritional deficiencies.*

It is also possible that within this third component of tropical subsistence patterns there may be a significant emphasis on the intake of a great variety of small sources of animal food. Such resources are numerous in the highly complex ecosystems of the tropics, and the Gadio subsistence pattern in fact exemplifies one in which there is such an emphasis (see Table IV, food Nos 38–52; also Dornstreich, 1973, pp. 232–291, 319, 322–326, 365–416; Deevey, 1968). In some few cases there may even be a major reliance on these otherwise minor foods (Miracle, 1973, pp. 337–338). Considerable and equitable diversification within this third component of tropical subsistence patterns however, is rarely associated with high population density.

From what has been said it follows that unless tropical peoples are either located near substantial fish resources or can intensify produc-

---

* One important implication of this statement is that it is not only the balance between vegetable food and animal food which is important, but the nutritional composition of all the food items which people eat which must be considered. For example, about 14% (by weight) of the Gadio diet is composed of plant stems, fruits and nuts, while animal foods contribute about 5% (by weight) (Dornstreich, 1973, pp. 387–388). If the emphasis on even these high quality vegetable foods were to markedly increase, along with a simultaneous fall in animal intake, nutritional deficiencies might result. For example, among the Tsembaga Maring exactly this situation is found—figures corresponding to those given for the Gadio are 35% and 1%—and nutritional stress is in fact said to occur (Rappaport, 1968, pp. 72–73, 84–87).

tivity of their food staple, they will follow a diversified subsistence system tending toward the Gadio type. If this generalization is true it raises the important issue of the productivity potential of small-scale tropical agriculture. As far as this possibility is concerned, the crucial environmental variables are the slope of the terrain, the amount and distribution of rainfall, and soil fertility.

A survey of the types of societies living in the hilly or mountainous country of the tropics will verify the proposition that unless there is a significant dry season as well as the presence of either natural or artificially created flat terrain, the possibilities for a semi-permanent agricultural system are extremely limited. In these areas the combination of a continuously wet climate and sloping terrain confer a marked potentiality for erosion and the leaching of soil nutrients, and even the burning off of rainforest vegetation can be difficult (Denevan, 1970b, p. 72; Dornstreich, 1973, pp. 114–116, 189–191; Harris, 1971, p. 474; Holdridge, 1959, p. 279; Hyndman, n.d., p. 8; Jen Hu Chang, 1968, p. 352; Rappaport, 1971, pp. 121–127). This means that the agricultural land of certain tropical environments cannot be continuously cultivated, even though it may be abundant and initially productive. This in turn implies a long fallow cycle, dispersed settlement, low population density and a diversified subsistence pattern. In such environments it is not the amount of agricultural land which limits either productivity of the food staple or the duration of permanent settlement, but the fact that marked intensification of horticulture is not possible under the prevailing technoenvironmental circumstances.*

As a final point it should be noted that agricultural intensification is not without its liabilities (Street, 1969). Such techniques as soil tillage, crop rotation and water control can be used to increase the commitment to, and the productivity of, tropical horticulture, but they are also accompanied by increased maintenance costs and lowered efficiency within the agricultural system. They can also result in environmental degradation and general ecosystem simplification. These developments may increase ecosystem instability, a situation which results in lower long-term survival prospects for the group. For example steady state rainforest ecosystems, in which people have a more diversified exploitation strategy with a low environmental impact, have a much

---

* This statement implies that the common anthropological assertion that it is the requirements of hunting which are responsible for settlement dispersion, needs to be qualified (e.g. Carneiro, 1964, 1970; Morren, 1974; Siskind, 1973, p. 39). There is no doubt that hunting, fishing, as well as other animal food-getting strategies are importantly related to settlement and mobility patterns, but one must also consider the fact that there are important differences in the agricultural potential of different tropical environments.

longer life span (see Dornstreich, 1973, pp. 69–72, 79–83, 450–458).*

In this essay I initially described the Gadio Enga subsistence pattern. I hope that the format used here lends itself to a comparison between the Gadio example and the systems of other small-scale societies. I believe that enough information has been presented to show that looking at subsistence organization and operation in this way indicates some of the reasons why these societies differ from one another. But if this is to be done, we must have much better descriptions of small-scale subsistence patterns, and all comparisons between them must be based on a consideration of whole subsistence-dietary systems. Vague classifications and incomplete descriptions of subsistence will only limit our possibilities for explaining the similarities and differences in the adaptation of small-scale tropical societies.

VI. REFERENCES

Armillas, P. (1971). Gardens on swamps. *Science* **174**, 653–661.

Beals, A. R. (1964). Food is to eat: The nature of subsistence activity. *Am. Anthrop.* **66**, 134–136.

Beals, R. L. and Hester, J. A. (1956). A new ecological typology of California Indians. *In* "Men and Cultures" (Ed. A. F. C. Wallace). Philadelphia, pp. 411–420.

Bennett, C. F., Jr (1962). The Bayano Cuna Indians, Panama: An ecological study of livelihood and diet. *Ann. Ass. Am. Geogr.* **52**, 32–50.

Brookfield, H. C. (1962). Local study and the comparative method: An example from central New Guinea. *Ann. Ass. Am. Geogr.* **52**, 242–254.

Brown, J. K. (1970). A note on the division of labor by sex. *Am. Anthrop.* **72**, 1073–1078.

Carneiro, R. L. (1964). Social concomitants of ecological differences among two Amazonian tribes. Paper delivered at the annual meeting of the American Anthropological Association. Detroit.

Carneiro, R. L. (1970). The transition from hunting to horticulture in the Amazon basin. *Proc. Int. Congr. anthropol. ethnol. Sci.* **8**, 244–248.

Chagnon, N. A. (1968). "Yanomamo. The Fierce People". Holt, Rinehart and Winston, New York.

Chagnon, N. A. (1973). The culture ecology of shifting (pioneering) cultivation among Yanomamo Indians. *In* "Peoples and Cultures of Native South America" (Ed. D. R. Gross). Natural History Press, New York, pp. 126–142.

Clarke, W. C. (1966). From extensive to intensive shifting cultivation: A succession from New Guinea. *Ethnology* **5**, 347–359.

---

* This reasoning is purely theoretical and does not refer to any particular historical situation. It also considers only ecological systems of a comparable sort and does not refer to interactions between, for example, small-scale societies and societies possessing mechanized technologies.

Clarke, W. C. (1971). "Place and People. An Ecology of a New Guinean Community". University of California Press, Berkeley and Los Angeles.

Deevey, E. S. (1968). Measuring resources and subsistence strategies. In "Man the Hunter" (Eds R. B. Lee and I. DeVore). Aldine Publishing Co., Chicago, pp. 94–95.

Denevan, W. M. (1966). A cultural–ecological view of the former aboriginal settlement in the Amazon basin. Prof. Geogr. **18**, 346–351.

Denevan, W. M. (1970a). Aboriginal drained field cultivation in the Americas. Science **169**, 647–654.

Denevan, W. M. (1970b). The aboriginal population of western Amazonia in relation to habitat and subsistence. Revta. geogr. am. **72**, 61–86.

Denevan, W. M. (1971). Campa subsistence in the Gran Pajonal, Eastern Peru. Geogrl Rev. **61**, 496–518.

Dentan, R. K. (1965). Senoi Semai Dietary Restrictions: A Study of Food Behavior in a Malayan Hill Tribe. Ph.D. Dissertation, Yale University, New Haven.

Dornstreich, M. D. (1973). An Ecological Study of Gadio Enga (New Guinea) Subsistence. Ph.D. Dissertation, Columbia University, New York.

Dornstreich, M. D. and Buchbinder, G. (1970). Differential female mortality in New Guinea as a factor in population regulation. Paper delivered at the annual meeting of the American Anthropological Association.

Forge, A. (1972). Normative factors in the settlement size of neolithic cultivators (New Guinea). In "Man, Settlement and Urbanism" (Eds P. J. Ucko, R. Tringham, and G. W. Dimbleby). Schenkman Publishing Co., Cambridge, pp. 363–376.

Golson, J. (1970). A hydraulic civilization in the Waghi Valley? Seminar paper, Research School of Pacific Studies, Australian National University, Canberra.

Harner, M. J. (1972). "The Jivaro. People of the Sacred Waterfalls". Natural History Press, New York.

Harris, D. R. (1971). The ecology of swidden cultivation in the Upper Orinoco rainforest, Venezuela. Geogrl Rev. **61**, 475–495.

Heizer, R. F. (1958). Prehistoric central California: A problem in historical–developmental classification. Univ. Calif. Archaeol. Survey Rep. **41**, 19–26.

Holdridge, L. R. (1959). Ecological indications of the need for a new approach to tropical land use. Econ. Bot. **13**, 271–280.

Holmberg, A. R. (1969). "Nomads of the Long Bow. The Siriono of Eastern Bolivia". Natural History Press, New York.

Hughes, I. (1970). Pigs, sago and limestone. Paper delivered to ANZAAS congress, Port Moresby.

Hyndman, D. C. (1973). Using literary sources to investigate various New Guinea ecosystems. Occasional Paper Anthropological Museum, University of Queensland, **1**, 68–94.

Hyndman, D. C. (n.d.) The ecology of subsistence of the Wopkaimin Mountain Ok people of the Western District, Papua New Guinea. mimeo.

Jen Hu Chang (1968). The agricultural potential of the humid tropics. Geogrl Rev. **58**, 333–361.

Lathrap, D. (1968). The "hunting" economies of the tropical forest zone of South America: An attempt at historical perspective. In "Man the Hunter" (Eds R. B. Lee and I. DeVore). Aldine Publishing Co., Chicago, pp. 23–29.

Lathrap, D. (1970). "The Upper Amazon". Praeger, New York.

Linton, S. (1971). Woman the gatherer: Male bias in anthropology. In "Women in Cross-Cultural Perspective: A Preliminary Sourcebook" (Ed. S. E. Jacobs). Illinois Department of Urban and Rural Planning, pp. 9–21.

McArthur, M. (1974). Pigs for the ancestors: A review article. *Oceania* **45**, 87–123.

McIntosh, R. P. (1967). An index of diversity and the relation of certain concepts to diversity. *Ecology* **48**, 392–404.

Meggers, B. J. (1971). "Amazonia, Man and Culture in a Counterfeit Paradise". Aldine Publishing Co., Chicago.

Miracle, M. P. (1973). The Congo basin as a habitat for man. *In* "Tropical Forest Ecosystems in Africa and South America: A Comparative Review" (Eds B. J. Meggers, E. S. Ayensu and W. D. Duckworth). Smithsonian Institution Press, Washington, pp. 335–344.

Morren, G. E. B. (1974). Settlement Strategies and Hunting in a New Guinea Society. Ph.D. Dissertation, Columbia University, New York.

Netting, R. M. (1968). "Hill Farmers of Nigeria. Cultural Ecology of the Kofyar of the Jos Plateau". University of Washington Press, Seattle.

Nietschmann, B. (1972). Hunting and fishing focus among the Miskito Indians, Eastern Nicaragua. *Hum. Ecol.* **1**, 41–68.

Oomen, H. A. P. C. (1971). Ecology of human nutrition in New Guinea. Evaluation of subsistence patterns. *Ecol. Fd Nutr.* **1**, 3–18.

Pospisil, L. (1963). Kapauku Papuan Economy. *Yale Univ. Publs Anthrop.* **67**.

Rappaport, R. A. (1968). "Pigs for the Ancestors. Ritual in the Ecology of a New Guinea People". Yale University Press, New Haven.

Rappaport, R. A. (1971). The flow of energy in an agricultural society. *Scient. Am.* **224**, 116–133.

Robbins, R. G. (1961). The vegetation of New Guinea. *Aust. Territ.* **1**, 1–12.

Sauer, C. O. (1958). Man in the ecology of tropical America. *Proc. Pacif. Sci. Congr.* **9**, 105–110.

Schieffelin, E. L. (1975). Felling the trees on top of the crop: European contact and the subsistence ecology of the Great Papuan Plateau. *Oceania* **46**, 25–39.

Sebrell, W. H. and Hand, D. B. (1957). Protein malnutrition as a world problem. *In* "Amino Acid Malnutrition" (Ed. W. H. Cole). Rutgers University Press, New Brunswick, pp. 47–59.

Siskind, J. (1973). Tropical forest hunters and the economy of sex. *In* "Peoples and Cultures of Native South America" (Ed. D. R. Gross). Natural History Press, New York, pp. 226–240.

Sorenson, E. R., Gajdusek, D. C. and Reid, L. H. (1969). Nutrition in the Kuru region. I. Gardening, food handling and diet of the Fore people. II. A nutritional evaluation of traditional Fore diet in Moke Village in 1957. *Acta trop.* **26**, 281–345.

Spath, C. D. (1971). The toxicity of manioc as a determinant of settlement patterns. Paper delivered at the annual meeting of the American Anthropological Association. New York.

Street, J. M. (1969). An evaluation of the concept of carrying capacity. *Prof. Geogr.* **21**, 104–107.

Townsend, P. K. (1971). New Guinea sago gatherers. A study of demography in relation to subsistence. *Ecol. Fd Nutr.* **1**, 19–24.

Townsend, P. K. (1974). Sago production in a New Guinea economy. *Hum. Ecol.* **2**, 217–236.

Turnbull, C. M. (1972). Demography of small-scale societies. *In* "The Structure of Human Populations" (Eds G. A. Harrison and A. J. Boyce). Oxford University Press, London and Oxford, pp. 283–312.

Vayda, A. P., Leeds, A., and Smith, D. B. (1961). The place of pigs in Melanesian subsistence. *In* "Patterns of Land Utilization and Other Papers" (Ed. V. E. Garfield). Proceedings of the American Ethnological Society, Seattle, pp. 69–77.

Waddell, E. (1972). "The Mound Builders. Agricultural Practices, Environment and Society in the Central Highlands of New Guinea". University of Washington Press, Seattle and London.

Weiner, J. S. (1972). Tropical ecology and population structure. *In* "The Structure of Human Populations" (Eds G. A. Harrison and A. J. Boyce). Oxford University Press, London and Oxford, pp. 393–410.

Zeigler, A. C. (1968). Quasi-agriculture in north-central California and its effect on aboriginal social structure. *Pap. Kroeber anthrop. Soc.* **38**, 52–67.

CHAPTER X

From Hunting to Herding: Pigs and the Control of Energy in Montane New Guinea

GEORGE E. B. MORREN

Cook College, Rutgers University, U.S.A.

I. INTRODUCTION

In this essay I use energetic concepts to describe aspects of the behavioural and biological adaptation of the Miyanmin people of the West Sepik Province, and to compare these with similar features of other montane New Guinea populations. This is with three main objectives in mind: one, to affirm the utility of an energetic approach in the light of criticisms to which it has been subjected, two, to widen the class of human activities and movements which may be usefully viewed as directly influencing the flow of energy and three, to redefine the spectrum of montane New Guinea subsistence patterns by focusing on the food chain(s) relating pigs to man in a number of locations.

A. HUMAN ECOLOGY AND ENERGETICS

By some accounts, ecology is the study of the interactions (or inter-connections) between the living components and non-living elements in a given place. In seeking to understand some of these interactions, energy is a primary common denominator, a characteristic of all exchanges in the biosphere including those not involving elemental flows. Moreover, when so used, energy values are absolute and behave in accordance with the physical energy laws governing all energy transformations in the universe.

The ecologist Howard T. Odum (1971) has developed an "energy language", including a graphical shorthand, which permits the isolation and representation of energy flows and/or transformations along with the internal (to the system) mechanisms and environmental factors controlling the process. It is the latter feature, the ability to deal with control, which is innovative, and makes Odum's approach particularly useful for human ecological studies.

For obvious reasons, Odum's method and procedures cannot be described here in detail and the reader is referred to the original exposition cited or to works of others who have employed them (e.g. Little and Morren, 1976; Thomas, 1973). Nevertheless, a number of important features of the approach can be specified.

a. Odum's "macroscope" or "detail eliminator" involves a systems approach that attempts "to discern broad features and mechanisms of a system of parts" (Odum, 1971, p. 10) and avoids the bog of particularistic detail. The detail eliminator is built into the energy language which, in turn, is premised in physical energy theory.

b. The "language" itself is a working list of, and set of graphical symbols for, the physical sources and transforming components of ecosystems. A modified guide to Odum's energy language is presented in Figure 1. For our purposes, the most important of these is Odum's concept of the work gate which, analogous to a valve in a network of pipes, represents the action of work performed by a living part of the system (e.g. a human population, a herd of grazing animals) and limiting or tolerance factors (e.g. rainfall, temperature, protein) in controlling the flow of energy in the system. The flow of energy through the work gate is proportional to the magnitude of the factor applied to it, and this factor, be it work performed by living things, or perturbations of physical elements, represents the energetic or elemental cost of the process or the necessary degradation of energy or resources at the specified point in the system. Later in this paper, an attempt will be made to classify the kinds of human activities which may be associated with particular work gates in ecosystems involving human populations.

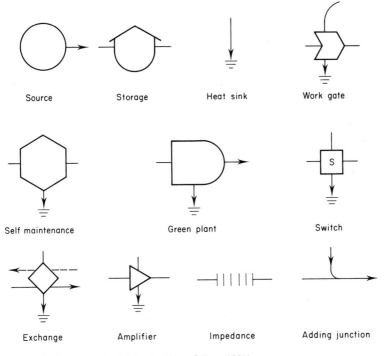

Source   Storage   Heat sink   Work gate

Self maintenance   Green plant   Switch

Exchange   Amplifier   Impedance   Adding junction

FIGURE 1. Energy symbols (adapted from Odum, 1971).

c. The amount of detail "eliminated", that is, the choice of broad features focused upon with Odum's macroscope, depends upon the objective of the study. A human ecological study necessarily focuses on the interaction between the members of a particular population and environmental components. Of course, not all components of the environment are important nor are all human activities and movements in relation to the environment important, or at least important enough to demand attention. Hence, it is valuable to focus on those components of the environment which constitute a past, present or potential problem for a human population and also on how members of that population respond both behaviourally and biologically to those problems.

This latter approach in human ecology has recently been propounded by Vayda and McCay (1975). They have identified as one type of problem those factors, either environmental or man-made, "that carry the risk of morbidity or mortality" (Vayda and McCay, 1975, p. 293). However, in the same paper Vayda and McCay also

take to task anthropologists (and biologists) who have laboured under
what they, following Brookfield (1972, p. 46), call the "calorific
obsession". These critics question the basic assumption of most energy
flow studies that have been conducted to date, that adaptation is a
matter of energetic efficiency. For them energy flow studies may only
be somewhat useful in relation to those particular cases in which energy
itself is a significant problem. However, such valid criticisms must be
interpreted strictly. In the broader context of the general utility of an
energetic approach, their attack is aimed at a "straw-person" called
"studies of the efficiency of energy capture and use" (Vayda and
McCay, 1975, p. 296). As I will argue later in this essay, studies of
human labour input: energy output efficiencies (or what might be
called work gate efficiencies in Odumese) do have only narrow usefulness. However, studies of the flow and control of energy, including the
quantitative aspects, are also studies of "environmental problems"
and of "how people respond to them" (Vayda and McCay, 1975, p.
293).

Vayda and McCay have also implicitly questioned the usefulness
of an energetic assessment of the "cost" of a response. For Vayda and
McCay, as for Slobodkin (1968), the most significant cost of a response
is in terms of reduced flexibility or reduced ability to respond to future
problems. This view is based on the assumption, described above, that
energy is not always limiting to a human population. The objection of
Vayda and McCay can be satisfied, or at least countered, if the unit
of cost is not trophic energy *per se* (i.e., energy available to a human
population in a food chain), but human somatic energy (i.e. labour).
This is a measurement of an organism's behaviour and has little
relationship to the kind of energetic measures which Vayda and McCay
say are being criticized by ecologists. As such, those human responses
which influence energy flows are subject to the same test of effectiveness
which Vayda and McCay advocate. In other words, the kinds of
question which they proposed about how people respond to environmental problems can be stated in energetic terms, with the test of the
operation of a pattern of responses involving not a certain level of
energetic efficiency but, rather, a. the ability of a response to reduce
or mitigate the intensity of a particular problem and b. the biological
state of the population with respect to the problem in question.

Thus, something is a problem for the members of a population if it
interferes with their ability to capture and utilize energy. More
specifically we are interested in how members of a population respond
to any property that has a measurable direct influence on their
fecundity, longevity, speed of development, or spatial location (see
Maelzor, 1965, p. 160), the dimensions of life and the dimensions of

the ability to capture and utilize energy. This is my working definition of "environmental problem". An energetic approach to environmental problems and human responses to them is advantageous because it makes possible a high degree of intersubjectivity and quantification (Jamison and Friedman, 1975, p. 127 *et seq.*). Vayda and McCay make no recommendations in this area. Hence this paper may also be taken as a serious, if preliminary, attempt to apply their methodological conclusions in a practical way to admittedly incomplete case material.

B. HUMAN CONTROL OF ENERGY FLOWS

Since the time of Steward ecological studies of human populations have been equated, in practice if not in theory, with studies of subsistence. In particular, investigations focusing on energetics and work, have tended to define narrowly the spectrum of human activities and movements to be accounted for in quantifying the operation of a pattern of energy transformations leading to man. The concern has been with subsistence activities, with activities directly influencing so-called production. Investigators thus measure such energy input variables as "hunting effort" (Lee, 1969), cultivation work, weeding, herding, harvesting, and occasionally garden to village transportation (Waddell, 1972), dung for fertilizer (Thomas, 1973; Winterhalder *et al.*, 1974) and fossil fuel (Kemp, 1971).

Contrary to the view expressed by Vayda and McCay (1975, p. 296), it is this narrow, unrealistic view of how human life is actually sustained, rather than their emphasis on energetic efficiency *per se*, which is probably the major fallacy in energy studies in human ecology. A good example of the expressions of this problem is Marvin Harris' use of the labour input–food output ratio, or what he calls the Index of Technoenvironmental Efficiency. Harris (1971) illustrates this point, not because he is a proponent of the fallacy *per se*, but rather as a consequence of his advocacy of a materialist research strategy which forced him to base conclusions on poor or partial data or on intuition. Harris assembled quantitative data on five cases. The selection of these cases was partly determined by a paucity of useful data, but they were intended to be broadly representative of different levels of social and technological complexity. His material cannot be reproduced here (and the reader is referred to it) but it is of interest for several reasons. First, a New Guinea Highlands case, the Tsembaga Maring, is included in the sample, and this case will be reviewed later in this paper. Second, a very narrow range of subsistence activities figured in the calculation of labour inputs. Third, an attempt was made to

generalize about the evolution of food production systems as an adjunct
to the presentations of these sample data. We can briefly turn to these
generalizations* inasmuch as they exemplify methodological problems
which are very common.

As the factor of technoenvironmental efficiency has improved, both
the average size of the food-producing work force and the total
number of hours spent on food production has gone up (Harris, 1971,
p. 216).

> labour saving food producing technologies have been employed primarily
> to increase total production rather than to cut back on the work effort per
> food producer. Up till the introduction of industrial agriculture, this meant
> not only a continuous increase in work input per food producer but an
> even greater increase in the total number of food producers per square mile
> of arable land. Thus, in the long run, the increment in the techno-
> environmental efficiency has led to an increment in population density.
> (Harris, 1971, p. 217)

As suggested earlier in the argument, these conclusions have no
meaning if the calculations of technoenvironmental efficiencies are
based on erroneous assumptions; for instance, if only labour inputs to
food production are employed. Technoenvironmental efficiency will
clearly appear to increase if more and more life-supporting work
occurs outside of the food production sector; for example in manu-
facturing tractors, in preserving food, in transportation and so forth.†
In other words, the technoenvironmental efficiency described by
Harris should be interpreted merely as an approximation of the proportion of labour devoted to food production in a larger complex pattern
of life support. Recent assessments of the energetics of modern life
support systems have benefitted from such a perspective (Pimentel
et al., 1974; Steinhart and Steinhart, 1974), affirming that there is
more to making food and other important substances available to
people than merely growing and harvesting them. Similarly, Freeman
(1955, p. 90) argues that in Sarawak there is no difference in efficiency
between a dry rice swidden and a wet rice paddy if the labour expenditure in guarding the former is included. If these considerations are
assumed then the notion that cultural development is accompanied by
an increase in energetic efficiency is likely to be erroneous. Hence, I
further assume that most work activities in all populations are life
supporting. This is consistent with a commitment to study how a

---

* In a later edition of his text book, Harris (1975) modifies somewhat the conclusions in question.
† While the foregoing argument may appear to the reader to be strongly critical of Harris' work,
it should be pointed out that it is Harris who deserves the credit for asking such questions in the
first place. His usual critics deny the relevance of the questions.

TABLE I

Energy flow to man by food chain for three montane New Guinea populations; magnitude and proportion of human controlled energy production

Food chain type	Miyanmin		Tsembaga Maring		Raiapu Enga	
	10^6 kcal	%	10^6 kcal	%	10^6 kcal	%
Root crop	12·1	50·2	46·7	75·7	100·1	91·6
Other crop	0·7	2·9	11·3	18·3	8·5	7·8
Pig	8·5	35·2	3·7	6·0	0·6	0·5
Wild (native) fauna	1·8	7·4	a	—	a	—
Wild vegetable	0·3	1·2	a	—	a	—
Exchange (+)	0·7	2·9	a	—	0·1	0·1
Sub-total	24·1	100·0	61·7	100·0	109·3	100·1
Exchange (−)	0·6	2·5	a	—	1·0	0·9
Pig fodder (−)	3·9	16·2	16·6	27·0	70·8	64·7
Total energy to man	19·6	81·3	45·1	73·0	37·5	34·3

^{a} No quantitative data available in original sources.

particular system—a pattern of energy flow and control—actually works.* From an operational standpoint the objectives I have set out will not be served in any way by calculations of work gate efficiencies. Instead, calculations of the relative proportions of a group's energy expenditure at the various kinds of work dates to be specified below will constitute measurement of response effort.†

Accordingly, from the standpoint of employing an energy language it is apparent that Harris and his original sources were guilty of eliminating the wrong detail; that the categories food production and subsistence activity are unrealistic and arbitrary, and that "they do not work". Inasmuch as our overriding concern is with how people respond to environmental problems, what is required is the identification, in the food chains leading to a particular human population, of all those points or work gates at which human activity affects the magnitude of the energy flows involved.

* For those who may be concerned with the philosophical–political implications of these statements (as I am), I must also maintain that I am not saying that, with respect to any system, this is the way it must be. Asserting that MacDonald's and similar "fast food" institutions are part of the U.S. life support system is not the same thing as saying that it is the "best of all possible worlds" solution to some kind of problem. On the other hand, "fast food" patterns of food distribution are a common feature of the urban scene worldwide.

† The basic data are presented in Tables I and II in such a way as to permit those readers who are committed to the utility of efficiency measurements to calculate them for themselves. Alternatively, I have presented various efficiency measures based on these data elsewhere (Little and Morren, 1976).

II. KINDS OF RESPONSE

The treatment of the Miyanmin data, and also the several cases for comparison, below, reflects these considerations, in that an attempt has been made to include all life supporting human activities, or at least those which can be shown to influence directly energy flows. As presented in Figure 2, the flow of energy to man in montane New

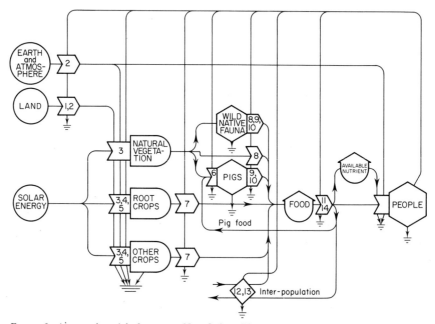

FIGURE 2. A general model of montane New Guinea life support systems. Numerals within work gate symbols refer to the rows in Table II where the magnitude of response in connection with the designated controlling activities and movements is reported for three different populations.

Guinea can be usefully (and arbitrarily) viewed as passing through three or four basic kinds of food chains, including the root crop chain, the pig chain, the other crop chain and the wild fauna chain. To the various manifestation of these in various locations should be added subsidiary chains relating local human populations to each other, including the non-trophic transactions involving traditional or modern exchange, as well as the trophic exchange involved in cannibalism. Such subsidiary chains are particularly important for providing high quality protein and fat. Another subsidiary chain involves the exploitation of wild vegetable products.

The pig chain deserves particular attention as it is related to some of the most pressing environmental problems, and dominates the structure of the larger systems by drawing off a disproportionate amount of human response effort and resources for control purposes. All of these chains are subject to the controlling influence of physical and climatic factors. Of greater interest to us are the internal loops controlling the flow of energy in these food chains. Particularly dominant are the controlling activities of man, which represent his responses to environmental problems, and which include (but are hardly limited to) the so-called subsistence practices such as agricultural techniques, hunting tactics and the like. A wider spectrum of man-influenced work gates can be identified including those which affect 1. territorial integrity and acquisition; 2. the location of population clusters; 3. environmental modification; 4. the management of induced communities; 5. control of the primary production of certain plant species; 6. the degradation of natural communities; 7. the management of domesticate reproduction; 8. the movement of people; 9. the harvesting of plant and animal products; 10. transportation; 11. the political, ritual and economic control of interpopulation economic chains; 12. the conversion of plant and animal products to digestible forms; 13. the direct control of limiting and tolerance factors (e.g. temperature, human pathogens etc) and 14. the direct control of human biology (i.e. health, fertility, rate of growth and mortality). This list should be taken as a tentative catalogue of the ways in which people (in montane New Guinea) respond to environmental problems.

Energy units provide the only extant means of directly measuring and comparing the magnitude and duration of modes of response for a given time period. In practice the proportion of the total labour budget allocated to any controlling activity may be a more useful measurement of the ways in which members of pre-industrial populations respond to environmental problems. This is because labour is, itself, a limited quantity. Thus, in relation to the framework proposed by Vayda and McCay (1976), I argue that human labour devoted to one pattern of activity or response reduces the amount of labour available for other or further responses, thereby reducing flexibility.

A. ENVIRONMENTAL PROBLEMS

The primary environmental problems need also to be identified. For human populations living in montane Papua New Guinea, the significant environmental problems are basically a set of limiting or tolerance factors and infectious disease causing parasites. The actual problems may have included at various times the availability of essential amino acids in protein, the availability of fats, the prevalence of malaria and various respiratory and gastrointestinal infections, the availability of dietary iodine and low night-time temperature.* The distribution of the various infectious diseases, both in New Guinea generally and within particular populations, may also be usefully viewed as a secondary problem in many instances. For example, many infectious diseases are influenced by settlement pattern, crowding and time spent indoors, individual mobility, man–animal interactions, human alteration of habitat and variability in nutritional status related to distributional patterns (including ritual cycles).

Population is also a problem in many localities, and amplifies the effects of other primary problems (see below). It would appear that trophic energy itself is not limiting. A range of secondary problems (e.g. those problems arising from responses to primary problems) might also be identified. Many of these (secondary) problems have a distinctive political character, involving the use of force, the erosion of group sovereignty and the elaboration of local political roles. In the short run the most acute of these has been warfare, itself a universal though variable response to the fundamental problem of maintaining a sufficient territorial base for the operation of a life support system. Military alliances, intergardening and patterns of refuging for the purpose of coping with extreme environmental hazards (Waddell, 1975), along with the operation of areally integrating patterns of exchange (involving the movement of pigs) act to compromise local political sovereignty and thereby reduce the flexibility of responses for individuals and other lower level units of population. The rise of local "bigmen" in connection with control of areally integrating chains results in the loss of resources by some populations (and gains for others) and establishes an emergent pattern of stratified access to resources which is reflected in the maldistribution of dietary resources and apparent inefficiency. However, this kind of inefficiency is a characteristic of all complex (stratified) life support systems and has no bearing on questions concerning the nutritional significance of subsistence practices (see below). In the long run the most acute secondary problem has been population growth, a contingency which increases the intensity of other primary and secondary problems. This is because, all else being equal, many factors which are problems for a

---

* I have purposely limited my discussion of environmental problems to those conditions which numerous authorities have identified as major mortality risks, and have avoided discussion of many other conditions, including infectious diseases such as yaws, tuberculosis, leprosy and tinea. These diseases are or were widespread, but they appear to be less significant.

large population will not be problems for a smaller population, or at least will not be so acute.

Evidence concerned with the prevalence of the problems described above will appear in the case material later in the paper.

B. RESPONSE EFFECTIVENESS

Two related tests of response process effectiveness were proposed earlier in this essay. The first would measure the extent to which a response or set of responses reduces or buffers the intensity of an environmental problem. In the examples which follow the accumulation of essential amino acids by particular life support systems is taken as a measurement of the effectiveness of behavioural responses in capturing meat in relation to the present or potential problem of the availability of high quality protein. If data were available this kind of measurement might also serve as a rough index of effectiveness in relation to the fat and iodine problems insofar as meat constitutes a concentrated source of lipids, and iodine may be concentrated in producer–consumer food chains. A comparable measurement of the response effectiveness for infectious disease is not as clearcut. For example, the distribution of malaria is inversely related to altitude (Stanhope, 1970), and takes its greatest toll among infants and children. Thus, one possible measurement of response effectiveness would focus on the balance of migration between low and high altitudes. The data required for this measurement are sparse. Another possibility is the altitudinal distribution of population, or the distribution of population in relation to altitude and rainfall (Brookfield, 1963), concerning which there is rather more information.

The second general test of the effectiveness of responses to environmental problems involves the measurement of the biological attributes already noted; particularly, fecundity, longevity, mortality, and speed of development or variants of these. In addition to standard demographic measurements, biomedical researchers in New Guinea have devoted much attention to infant and toddler mortality, as well as growth and development, these seen as particularly good indices of the health and nutritional status of the general population (Malcolm, 1970).

III THREE MONTANE LIFE SUPPORT SYSTEMS COMPARED

The presentation that follows is not a study of dietary intake and energy expenditure. This qualification applies equally to the analysis of the original data on the Miyanmin and to the estimates of food production and work derived principally from the work of Rappaport (1968, 1971a) and Waddell (1972). Instead, this analysis focuses on the structure of the energy flow pathways and control mechanisms in general and in the three cases, and uses estimates of inputs and outputs based on indirect or crude field measurements in combination with what I hope are reasonable assumptions.

I can outline my assumptions and procedures briefly here. The Miyanmin estimates, drawn from original field data, are based primarily on measurements of production for sample periods, and work diaries maintained during the same period. For production, I weighed all food entering a residential hamlet during two two-week periods and also measured the distribution of food including that allocated to pig feeding, that shared between households, and that sent (in prepared form) to other residential hamlets. I used the food tables compiled by Dornstreich (1973, p. 422) to compute edible portions and nutritional value. For work, I made daily entries in a diary for every adult sleeping in the hamlet on every day during the sample periods. I also conducted sample time and motion studies for stereotyped work and leisure activities. I then used the energy expenditure values published by Norgan *et al.* (1974) in connection with the New Guinea International Biological Programme (IBP) project, to estimate daily energy expenditure for the population of the hamlet during sample periods. All of these calculations were then converted to an annual time frame.

For the Maring, Rappaport's (1971a) estimates were employed with modifications required to correct miscalculations which cropped up in the editing of his paper (Rappaport, pers. comm.), and to correctly reflect the proportions of land devoted to two different kinds of gardens. All of these estimates were converted then to the scale of one square mile in order to conform more closely to the units of human population involved in the other two cases.

For Raiapu Enga, Waddell's consumption estimates have been converted using Dornstreich's (1973) Food Tables, and his work data have been converted to energy expenditure values using the IBP values cited above.

There are several bases for justifying the obvious lack of precision in these procedures, to note only one kind of shortcoming in the present effort.

a. These are all the data there are!

b. As McArthur (1974 and Chapter V) has noted in connection with a critique of Rappaport's work, it is impossible for a single researcher to do all that "must" be done to satisfy the conflicting requirements of, say, generality and precision. I know of only one field investigation of the energetics of a human population in its environment that has combined precise measurements of dietary intake and energy expenditure with a reasonably realistic model of energy flow and control. This is Brooke Thomas' (1973) study of Peruvian Altiplano Indians. I doubt if there will be too many replications of it, especially given the fact that Thomas' study benefited from its link-up with a large-scale project with good on-site laboratory and technical support, and spare data gatherers when needed.

c. For some purposes, including those outlined at the beginning of this essay, it is probably more important to focus on a realistic and general model, than to be precise. As Norgan and associates (1974, p. 343) have pointed out, for studies of populations or groups, "it is often perhaps of more importance to obtain a detailed record of the pattern of the daily life than to undertake . . . laborious and expensive measurement. . . ." Their tabulated data were presented explicitly to facilitate further studies of New Guineans on a less rigorous basis than they themselves had accomplished. It is noteworthy that, because of the narrowness of the New Guinea IBP project objectives, and lack of general ethnographic and ecological back-up, it was not possible for me to use the Lufa population in the present comparative effort.

Similarly, this is not a study of epidemiology, nor of health problems generally. An attempt is made to describe a range of environmental problems, including health problems, faced by members of particular New Guinea populations, and some information on the health status of these people is a necessary part of any assessment of response effectiveness. The discussion of health problems is otherwise selective and designed to illustrate the application of the methodology proposed in this paper.

For the Miyanmin, quantitative data bearing on such questions as infant and toddler mortality, growth and development, fertility and mortality are incomplete and partially analysed. For the other cases, there are survey data touching on at least some of these measurements (see Buchbinder, 1973; Sinnett and Whyte, 1973; Vines, 1970). In most cases qualitative assessments may be sufficient to illustrate the general points raised.

Estimates of energy flow and energy expended by people in controlling the flow of energy in the three cases are presented in Tables I and II respectively. In Table I, rows refer to the major food chain types and summations, with columns representing the net flows expressed in millions of kilocalories and as a percentage of total energy production for each population. In Table II, rows refer to the various work gates, grouped in broad types as was discussed earlier, and the columns represent net energy expenditures for each expressed in millions of kilocalories and as a proportion of total (estimated) response effort expended in control activities for each of the three cases.

Then, in the sections which follow, I undertake to elaborate the outline presented in the tables, in some detail for the Miyanmin and with a summary discussion for the Tsembaga Maring and the Raiapu Enga. In each case an attempt will be made to assess the effectiveness of the respective life support systems according to the criteria described in the preceding section.

A. THE MIYANMIN AND ENERGY FLOW

The Miyanmin life support system exemplifies a land-extensive swidden and hunting pattern supporting a dispersed population with a crude density of less than three people per square mile. This system manages or controls the flow of energy through three major trophic levels in an ecosystem which is affected by human activity only on a temporary and local scale. The producer level includes the natural vegetation characteristic of what may be designated "lower montane rainforest" and the induced floral associations of cultivated plants and tree crops. The next trophic level of primary consumers consists of an extremely diverse assemblage of wild native fauna, wild pigs, and a relatively small number of domesticated pigs and tamed fauna. The third level of higher order consumers consists principally of the omnivorous human population, but also includes domesticated dogs.

For the purpose of viewing the operations of a life support system, the most significant human unit is the local population. Among the Miyanmin this is a regional cluster of corporate groups or subgroups, ranging in size from 50 to 200 people, which jointly "operate" the life support system. Local populations occupy watersheds and valleys, are named after such features, and are economically self-sufficient with a high degree of co-operation, co-ordination, sharing, and population movement between subunits in connection with the operation of the system. The system is effective and sufficient in the sense that there is a reasonable balance between human labour outputs and food production. Levels of health and nutrition are high by New Guinea standards, and there is no evidence of long-term environmental degradation.

An energy flow model of this situation is presented in Figure 3, and the energy magnitudes presented for comparison with other cases in Tables I and II. The data and observations on which it is based derive from only one subunit of the local populations,* a residential hamlet,

* Ukdabip hamlet of Kome parish in the Hak-Uk valley, in the approximate altitudinal range 870–1220 m (see Map 1).

TABLE II

Magnitude and proportion of response effort in three montane New Guinea populations

Type of control	Miyanmin		Tsembaga Maring		Raiapu Enga	
Work gate	10⁶ kcal	%	10⁶ kcal	%	10⁶ kcal	%
Territorial						
1 War and politics	a	—	a	—	1·1	10·1
2 Settlement	0·7	13·0	c	—	0·5	4·6
Environmental						
3 Clear	0·9	16·7	0·6	13·6	1·0	9·2
4 Control	0·0	0·0	0·3	6·8	2·1	19·2
5 Plant and cultivate	0·6	11·1	1·1	25·0	1·2	11·0
6 Herd	0·0	0·0	1·3	27·3	0·2	1·8
Cropping and location						
7 Harvest and transport	0·5	9·3	1·2	27·3	2·4	22·0
8 Collect	0·1	1·8	e	—	c	—
9 Hunt and slaughter	0·7.	13·0	e	—	c	—
10 Mobility	1·2	22·2	c	—	0·3	2·6
Exchange and preparation						
11 Firewood collection	d	—	c	—	0·6	5·5
12 Purchase	b	—	c	—	0·1	1·0
13 Ritual and exchange	0·1	1·8	c	—	1·1	10·1
14 Cook	0·6	11·1	c	—	0·3	2·8
Total response effort	5·4	100·0	4·4	100·0	10·9	100·0

[a] Warfare had been suppressed in all areas by the time the cited research was conducted among the three populations, but other forms of traditional and introduced political activity have continued. For the Miyanmin, effort involved in intergroup political activity is aggregated in 10. No quantitative data are available for the Maring.
[b] Not measured by the author, but observed to be of small scale.
[c] No quantitative data available in original sources.
[d] Aggregated in 7 and 14.
[e] Rappaport (1968, p. 282) notes that his estimates of energy expenditure should include data on "some casual hunting". Significant kills of wild pigs are reported (included in Table I) and elsewhere Rappaport recognizes the small dietary contribution from the collecting of small fauna and wild vegetable foods by women and children.

for two separate periods of two weeks, but the model does reasonably reflect the main features of Miyanmin life support. Annual estimates of flows and human labour have been projected and are comparable to the two other systems presented later in this study. The main components of the system and their connecting trophic relations can be briefly described. Natural vegetation is important to the human

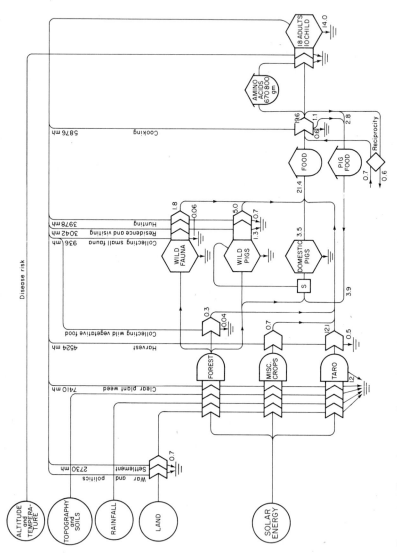

FIGURE 3. Miyanmin energy flow and control. mh represents man-hours.

population in several respects. In season it contributes directly to the human diet a variety of leaves, nuts and fruits. In the form of dead timber left in gardens (a by-product of agriculture) it also provides firewood (not represented in the diagram). Forest vegetation also supports a diverse assemblage of primary consumers of great dietary importance to man including insects and their larvae, various reptiles and amphibians, small to medium sized terrestrial mammals such as small kangaroos, possums and rats, and also birds, including the terrestrial cassowary. Aquatic fauna including turtles, fish, eels and even crocodiles have trophic importance to Miyanmin living at lower altitudes. Treated separately in the model are wild pigs, which on an annual basis are probably the single most important source of high quality protein. Wild vegetation provides the principal support for the wild pig population, but in the rainier season wild pigs often invade gardens and compete directly with man for the crops growing there. Domestic pigs also depend on wild forage during the drier part of the year although a proportion of garden produce, mainly in the form of substandard taros and scraps, are cooked and fed to them on a daily basis. Domestic pigs are most frequently slaughtered at times when their food value will fill gaps arising from the periodic unavailability of other sources of high quality protein, such as wild pigs, which are difficult to hunt in the rainier season in the higher altitude habitats occupied by some Miyanmin local populations. Historically the Miyanmin also resorted to intensive exo-cannibalism during times of extreme protein stress (Morren, 1974a; Dornstreich and Morren, 1974).

Taro is grown in roughly cleared swiddens and is the predominant staple for the Miyanmin both by weight and by proportion of energy contributed to the group's diet (Fig. 4). Other cultivated plants, including leafy vegetables, squash, beans, and some sweet potato, and such tree crops as breadfruit and *Pandanus* are of particular importance as sources of protein, fat, and other nutrients in the diet.

The flow of energy in this system is controlled by environmental factors, and by the operation of internal control loops operated through the activities and movements of the population at the primary and higher-order consumer trophic levels. Both kinds of control factors operate through work gates and switches to increase, decrease or redirect the flow of energy between levels and components.

Altitude and seasonal rainfall have an important general influence on the character of life in montane zones. In the Miyanmin area the rainfall averages 4000–5000 mm per year and is seasonal (Morren, 1974a). The heaviest rainfall occurs between January and May, with somewhat lighter rainfall during the rest of the year. Seasonal varia-

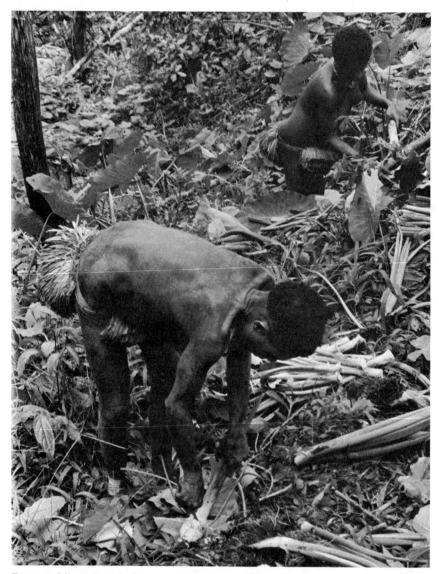

Figure 4. Miyanmin agriculture: a mother and daughter work in a producing garden, harvesting and processing their crop of *Colocasia* taro in a patch of shade. The taro plants are scraped clean of their roots and clinging soil, and the edible corm is then split from the leaf stalk with a bamboo spatula. The leaf stalk will be replanted in a newly cleared site within five days.

tions in rainfall affect vegetation, fauna and man, and also represents a significant environmental problem. The effects of seasonal perturbations on vegetation and animal life have been described elsewhere (Morren, 1974b). Effects in the Miyanmin agricultural sector are also apparent: the cultivation of taro is clearly favoured by the high rainfall and the resulting water-saturated soils; small amounts of white sweet potato, on the other hand, must be grown in extremely well-drained sites, since no form of drainage is provided in the gardens. Seasonal rainfall and cloud also control to a certain extent the growing period of some plantings, so that those made in the rainier season grow through the sunnier days of the drier season later in the year, and may be more productive. However, planting and harvesting are continuous throughout the year.

The temperature gradient associated with altitude operates on the Miyanmin life support system as a determinant of ecological zonation which in turn controls the distribution of certain plant and animal resources. Thus, over the wider Miyanmin area, altitude is associated with the variability displayed by human life support systems. The 500–1200 m range is particularly rich in resources with the most extensive variants of the Miyanmin life support system occurring below this range, where the smallest human population and lowest population densities also occur. The relationship of this temperature gradient to the prevalence of malaria is also visible over the wider Miyanmin area. Malaria is endemic throughout the area but the highest rate of infection occurs amongst the populations at the lowest altitudes and it appears to have an epidemic character among higher altitude populations. It is a major cause of infant mortality with most adults having a partial acquired immunity which somewhat mitigates the symptoms. Epidemics involving respiratory diseases have been a major problem for all Miyanmin groups since at least the early nineteen-fifties. Adults are more at risk than children (Figure 5).

Internal control loops, particularly those consisting of human labour inputs at critical points in the energy flow system, can be described with greater precision. The most basic of all of these are the human inputs which control access to territory and to specialized habitats, which can be labelled warfare, settlement pattern and residence visiting. Warfare belongs to a class of work gates which might well be labelled political. This is because they depend on force or the threat of the use of force for their operation. In the Miyanmin case warfare in connection with territorial defence and acquisition was endemic until the early nineteen-sixties in some areas. During the period of field research local sovereignty was more or less guaranteed by the *Pax Australiana*.

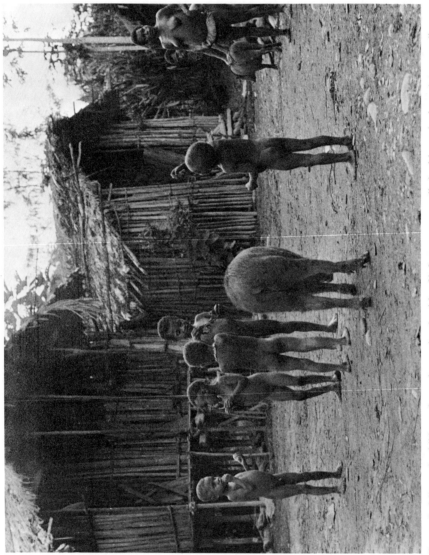

FIGURE 5. Miyanmin children: those who survive the risks of infancy are generally healthy and robust. A very small proportion are defective, possibly as a consequence of iodine deficiency. Children have ready access to most available foods, learn to share before talking, and gather a significant harvest of small vertebrate and invertebrate fauna.

The work gate input labelled settlement pattern has to do with a complex settlement cycle, analysed in detail elsewhere as a process of response to the problem of the availability of meat (Morren, 1974a). A cycle starts when a local population invades a pristine or recovered area that is topographically distinct such as a divide between two rivers. During the initial period of occupation the settlement pattern is nucleated, but over time there is a progressive expansion of the distances between hamlets until a variable limit on expansions is attained. Then there occurs an unidirectional movement of the entire settlement at an average rate of about 1·5 km per year. This continues until a geographic or political boundary is approached, at which time a new occupation area is invaded. The duration of such cycles is approximately eight to twelve years. Settlement pattern "work", consisting largely of house building, is sporadic, although none occurred in the hamlet to which the model pertains during the sample period reported on here. Settlement work (maintenance and repair) amounted to 2730 man-hours (mh) or about 700 000 kilocalories of expended energy. The residence-visiting work gate input has to do with seasonal movements of men and families which have the effect of spatially distributing hunters in relation to harvestable faunal resources. The 3042 man-hours and about 1 200 000 kilocalories of energy expenditure reported here in connection with residence and visiting is an estimate of "travel", specifically the last day of travel resulting in the arrival of a visitor or the return of a household member at the hamlet in question. This amounts to approximately 19% of all energy expended by people in connection with operating the life support system and is the second most costly of all responses.

In the category of inputs to the work gates concerned with the harvesting of wild plants and animals, the collecting by women of wild vegetable foods and small animals (insects, crabs, frogs, rats, bandicoots) expended 937 woman-hours or approximately 100 000 kilocalories, while 3978 man-hours (700 000 kcal) were invested in hunting. This group of inputs accounts for 37% (2 000 000 kcal) of all energy expenditure and produced 29% (7 100 000 kcal) of the total raw food and virtually half of all protein.

The largest inputs are associated with agricultural production. During the period of observation, 7410 man-hours and 1 200 000 kilocalories were expended in clearing, planting and weeding the taro-dominated swiddens and 4524 man-hours and 500 000 kilocalories were expended in harvesting taro and a variety of subsidiary garden and tree crops. This adds up to 37% (2 000 000 kcal) of the total energy expended in life support. Agriculture produced about 53·1% (12 800 000 kcal) of all energy and 31% (207 980 g) of all protein.

Extremely small (and unmeasurable) inputs of human labour are directly expended on pig herding. However, approximately 16·2% (3 900 000 kcal) of human food production is voluntarily surrendered to domesticated pigs in the form of undersized corms and scraps. On this basis one could assign a proportionate amount of 16·2% (324 000 kcal) of human agricultural labour to pig support. On a population basis, this determination has little meaning since it does not represent a significant amount of work that would not be done in any case (but it does have meaning for individuals such as widowers with children, who cannot support a pig and children too!). For comparative purposes (see below) what is important is that no extra land is put under production, and the pig–human ratio is approximately 0·1 : 1.

The final significant human labour input to the system is in connection with food preparation (Figure 6). The input for this work gate involved 11·1% (5876 man-hours; 600 000 kcal) of the total energy expenditure on life support. The data includes routine women's-house and men's-house cooking as well as the more elaborate earth oven "feasts" which involve many guests. The guests participated in the work involved and also contributed 699 300 kilocalories from vegetable foods to the "dinners", and they carried off approximately 590 000 kilocalories from food in the form of prepared vegetables and small portions of meat for people not attending.

It is possible to partially indicate the effectiveness of behavioural responses in reducing the intensity of the varied environmental problems to which the Miyanmin are subject. The success of the Miyanmin life support system in responding to the limited availability of essential amino acids (in protein) is indicated by the ability of the system to deliver an estimated average of 65 g protein per capita per day, a figure that compares very favourably with international standards. Approximately 69% of this is from animal sources most of which is the output of male and female hunting and gathering activities. In addition, the system makes available an estimated 97·5 g of fat, 95% is derived from animal sources. Comparable estimates of iodine availability are not feasible, but a supply of this element is likely to be associated with meat (and accumulated in food chains).

Comparable indications of effectiveness can also be described in relation to responses which may act to reduce the intensity of malaria (although energetic data bearing on this question are not complete). If we can assume that responses which either concentrate population, or particularly vulnerable fractions of the population, in low risk zones are effective in reducing the incidence of malaria, then the effects of a number of such responses can be measured. For example, although the long-term trend (over four or five generations) of Miyanmin expansion

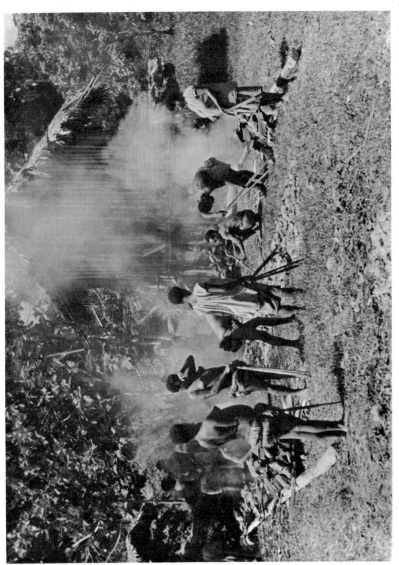

FIGURE 6. Miyanmin food preparation: approximately 11% of Miyanmin labour is devoted to the careful preparation of food. Large leaf ovens are prepared by the residents of a small hamlet whenever a large quantity of some highly valued food—a wild pig, two or three *marita*—is available. The ovens may contain several hundred pounds of taro dough in a huge flat cake, as well as pork, pandanus, leafy vegetables and smaller vertebrates.

has been northwards toward lower altitudes, highest crude population densities occur at higher altitudes in the south (Morren, 1974a, p. 150). More significantly, in the present (living) generation there has been a net migration of women—and their fertility—southwards (Morren, 1974a, p. 248). Hence, to the extent that a larger proportion of total Miyanmin fecundity will be concentrated in higher altitudes, the survival of Miyanmin children, the most vulnerable cohort, will be enhanced.

With the possible exception of infantile diarrhoea (which may be related to malaria or to weaning), dysentery and other gastrointestinal infections are not a problem for the Miyanmin. People spend most of their time in dispersed settlements living in well-constructed and uncrowded individual family houses and men's houses, avoid water sources originating near settlements to avoid female pollution, defecate in a restricted area distant from houses, and wash frequently. House floors are raised off the ground and are easily cleaned. Houses are unoccupied for more than half of the year. Animal foods that are not consumed immediately are preserved by smoking in racks over house hearths or by "canning" in bamboo tubes which hang near the fire. Gastrointestinal disorders introduced by various kinds of external contact do not appear to spread.

When an epidemic involving (typically) an upper respiratory infection strikes a local population, people respond by barring entry to the group territory because of sorcery fears. Although this may have only a small effect on the subsequent contagion within the group, it may act to restrict the spread to other neighbouring groups. The favourable nutritional pattern that I have described and the large proportion of effort that is devoted to food preparation, undoubtedly tends to buffer disease responses. In addition the ingestion of nutritious foods by disease victims is a regular feature of Miyanmin-curing rituals (Morren, 1974a, p. 168).

In general, Miyanmin response processes, especially those concerned with the harvesting and distribution of nutritional resources, evince a high degree of individual and family level flexibility and local population self-sufficiency. However, individual and family level movement is subordinate to local population movement responses (Morren, 1974a).

The effectiveness of Miyanmin responses can also be indicated by assessing the biological state of the population with particular reference to the range of environmental problems already identified. Logically, this assessment involves the determination of the presence of certain physiological responses which can be taken as an index of the success or failure of the buffering effect of behavioural responses (Slobodkin,

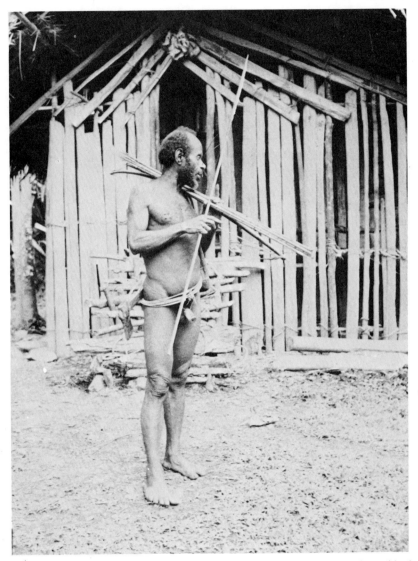

FIGURE 7. Miyanmin male physique: adults are mesomorphic rather than wiry, with the musculature of the thighs and chest particularly well developed. There is a great variability in stature among both men and women. This man, aged approximately 50 years, is 1·68 m (5 ft 6 in) tall.

1968). In practice, it is the presence or absence of the physiological and demographic manifestations of the environmental problems cited. These can be discussed, but with an unfortunate lack of precision.

The clinical signs of protein malnutrition appear to be virtually absent among Miyanmin children, and adults in this group are as tall and robust as any people still living according to an indigenous life-style (Figure 7). In addition, the Miyanmin appear to have achieved a marked recovery from the condition of low fertility and/or high infant mortality that occurred in connection with contact in the nineteen-fifties. The population is expanding, although malaria and iodine deficiency continue to be a problem, especially for children, but apparently mitigated by the availability of nutrients in a relatively large supply of meat.

B. TSEMBAGA MARING

The Maring speaking peoples of the Jimi and Simbai valleys have probably been the objects of more ecologically oriented research than any other ethnolinguistic group in montane New Guinea (see Map 1). They have been the subject of three human ecological monographs based on doctoral dissertation research (Rappaport, 1968; Clarke, 1971; Buchbinder, 1973) as well as numerous scientific articles and reports, the multi-disciplinary research having been initiated by A. P. Vayda. This long-term investigation has resulted in a number of important original contributions to our general understanding of the nature of human ecological adaptations. To be noted in this connection are Rappaport's exposition of the ecological functions of ritual, his rigorous investigation of the agricultural system, and his focus on the influence of the limited availability of protein on a complex adaptive system (1968, 1971a, 1971b), Street's (1969) critique of the carrying capacity concept, and Clarke's (1966) analysis of the contingent nature of agricultural intensification. Undoubtedly, some of these contributions arose from the special characteristics and problems of the Maring that were evinced during the extended period of investigations, though the points cited appear to possess a high degree of general applicability.*

Hence, no comparative study of human ecology in montane New Guinea could fail to exploit the range of material on the Maring. The

* I do suspect that Vayda's recent proposal concerning the test of effectiveness of responses, as distinct from notions of equilibration and efficiency (Vayda and McCay, 1975), arises from the need to accommodate that while the Maring possess a system whose operation has been more or less described, the population appears to be in biological trouble (see below).

statements which follow refer primarily to the higher altitude population of the western end of the Simbai valley; particularly Tsembaga
studied by Rappaport (1968) and Tuguma studied by Buchbinder
(1973), rather than low altitude groups like Bomagai-Angoiang
studied by Clarke. The Maring are presented with a qualitatively
similar set of environmental problems to that described for Miyanmin
and other montane New Guinea populations, including the limited
availability of protein and other nutrients, and disease. The magnitude
of these problems, however, is greater, because of higher population
densities, a relative absence of flat or gently sloping land, and perhaps
other environmental characteristics. However, Buchbinder (in press)
believes that the iodine problem post-dates the contact period. Particularly as manifested at the physiological level, population is clearly a
problem for the Maring under contemporary conditions.

An energy flow model of the high altitude version of the Maring life
support system based on Rappaport's (1971) work is presented in
Figure 8. An inspection of this diagram should immediately acquaint
the reader with important structural differences from the Miyanmin
system already described. This is notwithstanding the fact that the
agricultural classification of Brookfield and Hart (1971) would place
the two in the same taxon. Even from a strictly agricultural viewpoint
this is a distortion. If, moreover, the wider range of life-supporting
activities is used as a basis for judgment, the Maring system more
nearly resembles the systems possessed by such true Highlands peoples
as the Enga (described below) or the Chimbu.

Maring swidden agriculture is clearly more intensive than Miyanmin
agriculture; gardens are fenced, erosion control measures are taken,
there is greater crop segregation, gardens are cropped for several
years and shorter fallows are controlled with respect to composition.
Although sweet potato is the most productive crop, taro is the human
staple (as it is with Miyanmin). The Maring pattern of pig exploitation
consists of some productive hunting and elaborate husbandry practices,
and with a pig–human ratio ranging from $0.8:1$ to $0.3:1$ it is also
clearly a more intensive system. The bulk of sweet potato production
is linked to the pig chain rather than to the part of the husbandry
pattern identified as the root crop chain, and the bulk of the labour
devoted to this forage crop should be accounted as pig management. If
this is done then 2.12×10^6 kilocalories or 48% of the labour reported
by Rappaport is involved in controlling the pig chain. Food crops
other than the staple taro, such as *Setaria*, sugar cane, banana, pit-pit,
and introduced cultigens, are much more significant than among the
Miyanmin. The Maring do employ settlement pattern mechanisms in
connection with pig management, but by comparison with the

Miyanmin they exist on a very reduced scale. Rappaport (1968, pp. 162–164) reports that among moderate to high density groups, residential dispersal accompanies the expansion of the domestic pig herd and that a return to a nucleated pattern follows a large scale pig slaughter. Possibly of more significance are responses in which individuals move out of the group territory or establish intergardening relations, and the very shape of the local population is altered over time. Lower altitude, low density Maring groups are less permanently settled.

Before the coming of Europeans the Maring local populations competed intensively among themselves for territorial resources and warfare was an acute problem for them. This contrasts strongly with the Miyanmin situation in which competition occurred with non-Miyanmin neighbours (Morren, 1974). Maring responses to the problem of warfare have been examined from the standpoint of equilibration by Rappaport (1968) and from the standpoint of maintenance of flexibility by Vayda (1971, 1974), and need not be detailed here. The influence of warfare on the flow of energy to the Maring, and responses to warfare, are both treated in the diagram as territorial questions. Other details are eliminated from consideration because of the lack of quantified data.

Maring local populations participate in an areally integrating exchange cycle (represented by the "traditional exchange" work gate), which is a less intensive version of the Enga's *Te* (Meggitt, 1972). Its elements include the pig festivals and pork prestations described by Rappaport as well as a pattern of exchange and agistment of live pigs over a wide area (Buchbinder, 1973). The quantitative dimensions of this movement are not reported, and we know neither the numbers of animals involved nor the geographic extent of the network, but Buchbinder (1973) feels that the pig herds of most of the higher altitude Maring groups consist of a high proportion of imported pigs.

Notwithstanding Rappaport's model of the ecological functions of the ritual cycle and associated pig slaughter among the Maring, students of New Guinea societies have continued to regard these phenomena as examples of economic irrationality and ritual extravagance, characterized, as they appear to be, by irregular and uneven distribution of pork as well as by a high degree of under-utilization, waste, and spoilage (see Buchbinder, 1973; MacArthur, 1974 and Chapter V).* While this is true on a local group level, it does not necessarily support a general claim that the pig herds are of little importance nutritionally or that the practices in question produce no

---

* For a very early expression of the anti-swine perspective, see Bunzel (1938).

tangible beneficial effects. There are several reasons for the persistence of such claims (aside from the evidence that is thought to support them). One is the belief, described earlier in this paper, that adaptation is to be equated with efficiency. As I have argued, there is no support for the notion that human life support systems are efficient on a group level or for all individual members of the group. The other basis is the tendency to focus only on the group level, rather than on that plus other relevant levels (e.g. the regional level and the individual level). The necessity for focussing on the individual or some other low level entity as a unit of response is most apparent when trying to make sense out of complex life support systems, of which the Maring and the Enga are nascent, unintensive examples. If the individual or family unit is focused upon, what is immediately apparent is the degree of variability in labour, in adherence to the "rules" (Lowman, 1974) as well as in levels of consumption. Pork is nutritionally important to those individuals who manage to consume it, including those who eat more than others because they "violate the rules" by slaughtering and consuming out of turn or in secret, or because they have levers on the situation by virtue of their rank and authority or power; for instance, the ability of the latter to influence or compel the behaviour of the former. The life support systems of traditional and modern societies need similar assessment; for example, is the product of the peasant to be considered "nutritionally unimportant" because 80% of it is eaten by townsmen? And need we look further than modern life support systems for examples of ritual extravagance, waste, under-utilization, and maldistribution?

From the standpoint of the proposals of Vayda and McCay (1976; following Slobodkin, 1968) the cost of an areally integrating response, such as the exchange cycles in which Maring and Enga local groups participate, is stated below.

   a. The loss of flexibility for families and individuals implied in the necessity to constantly defer pig slaughter and to work harder to support the growing pig herd.
   b. The erosion of local group self-sufficiency.

The gains to be associated with such a response include the ability to cope with problems of greater magnitude, more meat per unit of area, more people per unit of area, and, perhaps, lower levels of intergroup violence. The benefit to some individuals has already been discussed. The nutritional benefit to high status members of higher altitude Maring groups derived largely from imported pigs is the case in point.

It is not possible to represent clearly the magnitude of the Maring responses as a proportion of total response effort owing to the incompleteness of the available data. Thus the proportions presented in

Table II are gross underestimations. As in the Miyanmin case it is possible to indicate the effectiveness of responses in reducing the intensity of some of the problems confronting the Maring. For the Tsembaga Maring, the ability of the system to accumulate essential amino acids in protein from both animal and vegetable sources is reported by Rappaport to approximate 35 g per capita per day, or 43–55 g per adult male per day. This measure is likely to vary for a particular population in time and also between classes of people as well as between the systems of different local populations. Clarke (1971) estimates male protein intake for Maring of the Bomagai–Angoiang local population to be 52 g per capita per day. Based on consumption studies of the Tuguma Maring in the Simbai, Buchbinder (1973) estimates adult protein consumption at 34 g per capita per day based on laboratory analysis of locally grown foods. The comparable value for the low altitude Bomagai–Angoiang Maring (who I would expect to replicate the Miyanmin) is 49 g. As in other parts of montane New Guinea, a large proportion, perhaps as great as 90% of protein intake, is derived from vegetable sources. For example, Clarke (1971, p. 181) estimates that as much as 40% of the Ndwimba Basin Maring protein intake comes from green leaves. Similarly Rappaport affirms the importance of non-starchy vegetables (1968, p. 284), and notes the contrast with the Chimbu diet. These proportions contrast strongly with the Miyanmin situation described above mainly because of the prominence of meat in the diet of the latter.

The effectiveness of the Maring system in making fat available to the population is lower than that of the Miyanmin. Buchbinder estimates per-capita fat consumption at 15·5 g for the Tuguma Maring. Estimates of iodine availability in foods, possibly dependent on laboratory analyses of local foods grown in nutrient depleted soils, are not available.

Maring responses to malaria superficially appear to have the same general structure as Miyanmin responses; that is, population is concentrated in the higher altitude portion of the Maring range. This picture, however, appears to be due to a "long run" differential in fecundity and/or infant survival in the higher altitude zone as well as to a net flow of women toward higher altitudes as in the Miyanmin case (G. Buchbinder, pers. comm.).

Maring preferences for locating residences on high ground may also affect the incidence of malaria because of zonation in mosquito habitats and in the incidence of respiratory diseases, and because the ridges are warmer than valley floors at night (Clarke, 1971, p. 100). There is also a tendency for the population to disperse during epidemics affecting people or pigs (Clarke, 1971, p. 102).

Response effectiveness among the Maring can also be examined from the standpoint of the biological and demographic state of the members of the population. If this is done, the members of the Maring populations under discussion display fairly extreme physiological responses to environmental problems, including protein and other nutritional deficiencies. On the basis of actual biological measurement and assays, Buchbinder (1973) found that they displayed very slow growth with ultimate stunting, anaemia, high goitre rates, low resistence to disease, late sexual maturation, low fertility and high infant mortality. She sees these conditions as the result of the synergistic interaction of protein malnutrition, malaria and iodine deficiency (the latter possibly a recent phenomenon). When viewed as a pattern of responses to environmental problems, the Maring life support system is at present clearly ineffective, as is shown by the long-term population decline of a number of these groups.

C. RAIAPU ENGA

The Enga peoples have been studied in sufficient depth to provide a useful case in the present argument. They also present some distinctive responses to the range of environmental problems already discussed. In fact some of their potential problems are very substantial: high population density, high altitude, low night-time temperatures and a floral community dominated by grassy species rather than forest.

An energy flow model of the Raiapu version of the Enga life support system, based on work by Eric Waddell (1972), is presented in Figure 9. This system, too, contrasts with the other cases described, although its basic structure (with the Miyanmin system providing a perspective) is clearly an extension of many features to be seen in the Maring system.

Enga agriculture is very intensive with continuously cultivated open fields devoted primarily to sweet potato (Figure 10). Less intensively cultivated mixed gardens also produce sweet potato, other root crops such as yams, and important subsidiary crops including bananas, sugar cane, beans, *Setaria* and peanuts, as well as cash crops of various kinds. A notable quantitative feature of the agricultural sphere is the amount of effort involved in the intensification of the environmental control work gate, with elaborate fencing, ditching, mounding, composting and the like. Even if the data base is not strictly comparable, the contrast with the Maring—and in particular with the Miyanmin where labour is not spent on such activities—is striking.

Hunting and gathering has no measurable importance among the

Raiapu Enga, with the possible exception of some casual cropping that accompanies other activities such as garden work by women or the play of children. Most animal food derives from domestic pigs and pig herding is very intensive. Although only a small proportion of total effort (1·8%) is directly applied to the care of the herd, some 66% of garden produce, sweet potato and *Setaria* is fed to pigs. If a proportional amount of agricultural labour is assigned to pig support (about 4 370 000 kcal), approximately 42% of all response effort is involved in control of the pig chain. This is related to the high pig–human ratio (2·3:1 is a maximum figure reported by Waddell), the absence of sources of wild forage, the local extinction of wild pigs (necessitating the maintenance of domestic boars for reproduction) and the participation of the Raiapu in the *Te* exchange cycle.

The *Te* exchange cycle analysed by Meggitt (1972) is particularly notable in the present discussion because it probably has important implications for the flow and control of energy over an extensive area, and involves many thousands of people. It represents a degree of extension of the areally integrating pattern described for the Maring that only just falls short of the development of state-like political institutions. Nevertheless, it does function in the political sphere to restrict conflicts, maintaining local group boundaries in the face of intense competition, and in the nutritional sphere it promotes the movement of protein and fat-rich foods over a wide area. Unfortunately, it has not been possible to quantify the flows involved in this chain, but ceremonial activity as a controlling activity is quantified in the model shown in Figure 9.

In recent times the Enga have become increasingly involved in a non-traditional economy, growing cash crops and buying Western goods including food. It is not a significant source of trophic energy nor does it require a large amount of response effort (Table II). It does, however, have other implications as a response to problems (see below).

Enga settlements are relatively sedentary, but there is significant movement and visiting in connection with life supporting activities, including political work, pig exchange and agistment, and as a response to natural and man-made hazards such as frost (Waddell, 1975) and warfare. The information available permits the partial quantification of these movements, but they appear in the category of ceremonial activity (see Figure 9).

The effectiveness of the Raiapu Enga life support system can be partially indicated. Waddell implies that the overall capacity of the system to provide essential amino acids in protein is probably greater than he was able to observe. He reports an average 32 g of protein per capita per day and notes that during the period of his investigation pig

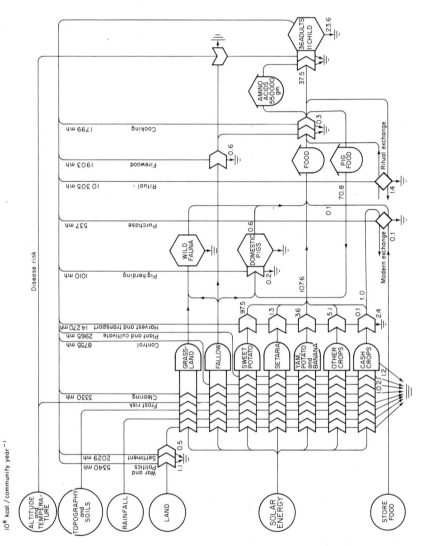

FIGURE 9. Raiapu Enga energy flow and control.

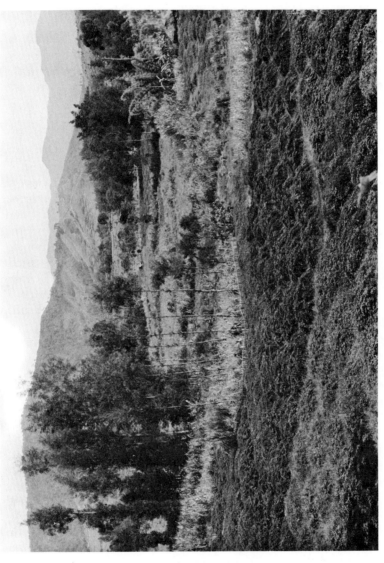

FIGURE 10. Enga agriculture: much of the available land is devoted to the cultivation of sweet potato in the mulched mounds clearly seen in the foreground. Behind these mounds, in the centre of the picture, is a fenced garden in which a variety of vegetables are being grown including the sugar cane and banana which are visible. Behind the fenced garden is a low-lying swampy area where pigs forage. The landscape is dotted with clumps of cultivated casuarina trees. Women's houses can be seen in the middle distance and on the extreme right. The area shown in this photograph is included in Map 4.

slaughter had been deferred due to organizational difficulties accompanying the *Te*. Sinnett and Whyte (1973, p. 261) report somewhat lower levels based on observations among the related Murapin Enga—25 g per capita per day. For the Enga as for the Maring the major environmental problem faced may not be the gross availability of protein or of fat in pork, but rather its distribution or, more properly, its maldistribution. In this connection, the reader should refer to the argument presented in the section of this paper concerned with the exchange cycle of the Tsembaga Maring.

Enga involvement in the cash economy appears to be a particularly effective response in that it provides 35% of the fat and 13% of the protein in the group diet (Waddell, 1972). The response is not, however, without cost, particularly if the results of a future expansion in the cash economy are considered. Such expansion would involve a reduced ability to respond to problems at the local and regional level, as a result of the further erosion of local group self-sufficiency and greater dependency on the national and world economies, and the associated loss of local political sovereignty (a process set in motion by the general pattern of control imposed, initially, by the Australian Administration of Papua New Guinea). The Enga and other peoples of the New Guinea Highlands are well along the road to peasantry.

The Enga have to cope with a somewhat different range of health hazards to that faced by the Miyanmin and the Maring. Malaria is not a problem because they occupy a high and relatively dry intermontane valley. On the other hand, respiratory infections, possibly related to low night-time temperature, as well as to nutrition, smoky house fires, tobacco smoking and other factors, are very common and account for significant mortality (Sinnett and Whyte, 1973, pp. 267–268). Chronic lung disease, clinically resembling chronic bronchitis and emphysema, is common throughout the Highlands (Woodcock *et al.*, 1970; Sinnett and Whyte, 1974) and increases the susceptibility of people to acute infections. Gastrointestinal infections also constitute a significant problem, related to a complex of factors possibly including density of settlement, inaccessibility of water, poor water quality, and poor food preservation and handling. Feachem (1973, 1975) singles out poor personal and domestic hygiene as particularly significant factors in the aetiology of this group of diseases. It is interesting to note that many of the factors cited are what have previously been described as "secondary problems".

The available literature on the Enga does not convey to me a sense of the more intensive long-term ways in which these people respond to disease risks. In the short-term sickness and death triggers a pattern of mourning, the suspension of work, visiting, and feasting which may have biological implications, and which may also trigger different levels of intergroup violence.

From a biological standpoint the effectiveness of the Raiapu Enga system appears to lie somewhere in between the extremes of the Maring and Miyanmin cases. On the one hand the Raiapu population is expanding slowly, the malnutrition does not appear to be as important a factor in Enga mortality as among the Maring. On the other hand, this expansion aggravates the problems associated with pressure on land resources.

IV. HOW MONTANE LIFE SUPPORT SYSTEMS CHANGE

Just as observers have taken too narrow a view of how human life support systems work, so have we tended to use excessively simple criteria for describing the types of life support systems to be found in an area such as the New Guinea Highlands, and on that basis postulating the dimensions of change affecting such systems. In this section I want to look briefly at some of the implications my use of energetic concepts has for an understanding of cultural evolution in montane Papua New Guinea.

Unquestionably, most authoritative writing on such questions has tended to assume that energy is limiting for the human populations of montane New Guinea, and that a description or classification of horticultural methods constitutes a description or classification of a people's solution to their energy problem. The basic fallacy involved in this was discussed in earlier sections of this paper; it should be clear by now that, although New Guineans are faced with many environmental problems, energy is not in a primary sense one of them. Two notable examples can be cited where the expression of this erroneous assumption takes on evolutionary implications. One is Brookfield and Hart's (1971) taxonomy of horticultural systems, and the other is the "Ipomoean Revolution" that Watson (1965a, 1965b, 1967) suggests must have followed the introduction of the sweet potato to the New Guinea Highlands.

The point to focus on here is that in both evolutionary frameworks the "meat question" receives short shrift. In the relevant evolutionary section of Brookfield and Hart, pig herding practices are not coded, dependence on wild animal foods is merely alluded to, and extensive patterns of exchange such as *Te* receive no attention whatsoever. This is despite their claim to "a much closer study of agricultural systems as parts of whole ecosystems than has ever been attempted" (Brookfield and Hart, 1971, pp. 92–93). This produces what I can only call anomalies; for example, when the Brookfield-Hart criteria are applied to the Maring and the Miyanmin, they turn out to have similar scores on the "intensity ranking" scale. More importantly, it distorts the relationship between population pressure and intensification. Watson is guilty of a similar narrowness of vision when, for example, he claims that "nearly all observers of the Central Highlands recognize the sweet potato as the most important single source of subsistence" (Watson, 1965, p. 296). Again, for Watson as for Brookfield and Hart, the criteria of "importance" is implicitly the notion that energy is limiting.

Clearly another approach to the study of the evolution of life support systems in the Highlands of Papua New Guinea is required. For example, it might be fruitful to describe such an evolutionary trajectory as a long-term "response process" (Vayda and McCay, 1975) involving a positive feedback relationship between population and resource management. Hence, it can be argued that the provision of meat and fat are among the most pressing environmental problems for New Guinea Highlanders. It would, therefore, follow that various solutions to these problems, represented by the cases discussed in the preceding section, strongly influence the general character of the various life support systems, including the character of agriculture. All evidence points to the fact that agricultural practices would not be expanded and/or intensified if it were not for the need to support larger and larger pig herds. One needs only to examine the proportion of total response effort directly related to the control of food chains that are capable of accumulating these important nutrients to establish the dominant influence of this problem on the populations themselves, on the character of their responses to it, and on their capacity to respond to other problems. In other words, it is here argued that while the availability of high quality protein and of fats are not the only environmental problems facing New Guinea Highlanders, they are, when amplified by population growth, the most pressing, and provide an additional key to understanding the structure of the various life support systems. It is not only the case that the role of the sweet potato has been exaggerated (Clarke, 1971; Brookfield and White, 1968), but also that the role of agriculture has been exaggerated. Rather it is the expansion and intensification of practices affecting the availability of pork (the most likely source of complete protein and fat) that must command our attention.

This argument regarding the nature of change in life support systems can be translated back into the energy language employed in the main body of this paper. Thus, we conventionally speak of two kinds of change in such systems, expansion and intensification.

a. Expansion involves increasing the territorial base of a particular life supporting activity; a particular chain in which a work gate intervenes becomes more extensive. Thus, a group brings more land under production, or devotes more land to the production of a given commodity, or a group expands its boundaries (often at the expense of another group), or more groups participate in an areally integrating chain.

b. Intensification, as the term is frequently used, has two parts. A particular life support system may be intensified by the establishment of a new chain or the addition of work gates to an existing chain with the concomitant diversion of response effort (labour or resources) to their operation and the elimination of parallel chains and other work gates. The amount of response effort (labour or other resources) applied to a particular work gate may be increased.

c. While both expansion and intensification involve an increase in the capacity of a system to deal with one class of problem, the concomitant diversion of land and the elimination of work gates and food chains entails a loss of flexibility; that is, reduced capacity of some individuals or groups to respond to the problem in question or reduction of the ability of the system as a whole to respond to other problems.

If the essentially synchronic data of the cases presented earlier in the paper are accepted as standing for points in a developmental continuum, the expansion and intensification of controlling activities bearing on the pig chain in montane New Guinea may be described in these terms. The Miyanmin case represents an extensive pattern of pig management.

a. Most pork consumed is wild.

b. Most village pigs are tamed wild piglets.

c. Village boars are castrated.

d. Local human populations denucleate and shift their settlement pattern as local pig abundance falls.

e. Individuals and families shift seasonally with the flux of wild pig activity.

f. No extra land is brought under production to support village pigs and only about 16% of garden production is eaten by pigs in the form of substandard tubers and "kitchen scraps".

g. Parallel food chains such as those involving wild native fauna are affected only by hunting.

h. Live pigs move only within the local population unit (although the Miyanmin may have served as a source of live pigs for the higher altitude Telefolmin people during rare periods of peace in the past).

i. An unmeasurably small amount of effort is involved in herding pigs.

In other words, the Miyanmin evince a great degree of flexibility in this and in other spheres.

Compared to the Miyanmin pattern, the Maring present an intensive pig management pattern.

a. Most pork consumed is domesticated.

b. Most pigs are the issue of domestic sows.

c. Village boars are still castrated.

d. Nucleation and dispersal of settlements is tied to the growth and decline of the pig herds.

e. Seasonal movements of personnel may be tied to gardening.

f. Extra land, especially in the form of higher altitude sweet potato gardens, is brought into production to feed a burgeoning pig herd, with 27% of garden produce fed to pigs primarily in the form of whole sweet potatoes and cassavas.

g. Sufficient amounts of forest remain to support a relict community of wild pigs and native fauna, but hunting returns are small (and, in addition, tracts of anthroprogenic grassland have become established in Maring territory).

h. There is a regional pattern of exchange involving the movement of live pigs, as well as prestations of cooked meat, beyond the boundaries of the local population.

i. 48% of the total measured response effort is devoted to herding and feeding pigs (probably an overestimate).

The Maring loss of flexibility is demonstrated by the destruction of forest and grass-dominated dis-climax, as well as by the erosion of local sovereignty implied by the ritual cycle described by Rappaport (1968), and by the biological state of the population (see the earlier description of this matter). The more intensive forms of agriculture practised by the Maring may be seen as merely a solution to a secondary problem, for instance, a problem arising from the intensification of pig management practices which is, in turn, a solution to the primary problems of the limited availability of protein amplified by human population growth.

The Raiapu Enga pattern of response may thus be seen as an expansion of processes already evident in the Maring pattern.

a. All meat consumed is domesticated pork (or tinned!).
b. All pigs are born by domestic sows.
c. A number of functioning boars are kept.
d. The settlement pattern is sedentary.
e. Some seasonal visiting is conducted in connection with pig exchanges, and with political and ceremonial functions.
f. More than half of all produce from intensively cultivated gardens is fed to pigs.
g. Miniscule amounts of forest remain on ridgetops, with hunting virtually non-existent, and wild forage for pigs also absent.
h. The Raiapu participate in the *Te*, the most extensive exchange cycle reported for New Guinea.
i. Approximately 41% of all response effort is devoted to herding and providing food for pigs.

If the three cases described above fairly represent points on a developmental continuum for the New Guinea Highlands, it is apparent that the very slow "revolution" which has occurred has been Susian rather than Ipomoean; that the most significant feature has been the intensification and expansion of the pig chain at the expense of the elimination or suppression of parallel chains.

V REFERENCES

Bunzel, Ruth (1938). The economic organisation of primitive peoples. *In* "General Anthropology". (Ed. F. Boaz). D. C. Heath, New York.

Brookfield, H. C. (1963). The ecology of highland settlement: some suggestions. *Am. Anthrop.* **66**, 20–39.

Brookfield, H. C. (1972). Intensification and disintensification in Pacific agriculture: a theoretical approach. *Pac. Viewpoint* **13**, 30–48.

Brookfield, H. C. and Hart, D. (1971). "Melanesia: A Geographical Interpretation of an Island World". Methuen, London.

Brookfield, H. C. and White, J. P. (1968). Revolution or evolution in the prehistory of the New Guinea Highlands. *Ethnology* **7**, 43–52.

Buchbinder, Georgeda (1973). "Maring Microadaptation: A Study of Demographic Nutritional, Genetic, and Phenotypic Variation in a Highland New Guinea Population". Ph.D. Dissertation in Anthropology, Columbia University, New York.

Clarke, W. C. (1966). From extensive to intensive shifting cultivation: a succession from New Guinea. *Ethnology* **5**, 347–359.

Clarke, W. C. (1971). "Place and People: An Ecology of a New Guinea Community". University of California Press, Berkeley.

Dornstreich, Mark D. (1973). "An Ecological Study of Gadio Enga (New Guinea) Subsistence". Ph.D. Dissertation in Anthropology, Columbia University, New York.

Feachem, R. G. A. (1973). The pattern of domestic water use in The New Guinea Highlands. *S. Pac. Bull.* **23** (3), 10–14.

Feachem, R. G. A. (1975). Pigs, people and pollution: interactions between man and environment in the highlands of New Guinea. *S. Pac. Bull.* 25 (3), 41–45.

Freeman, J. D. (1955). "Iban Agriculture". Colonial Research Studies 18. HMSO, London.

Harris, Marvin (1971). "Culture, Man and Nature". Thomas Y. Crowell, New York.

Harris, Marvin (1975). "Culture, People, Nature". Thomas Y. Crowell, New York.

Jamison, P. L. and Friedman, S. M. (Eds) (1974). "Energy Flow in Human Communities". Human Adaptability Office of the U.S. International Biological Program, University Park, Pennsylvania.

Kemp, William B. (1971). The flow of energy in a hunting society. *Scient. Am.* **225** (3), 105–115.

Lee, Richard B. (1969). Kung Bushman subsistence: an input–output analysis. *In* "Environment and Cultural Behavior". (Ed. A. P. Vayda). Natural History Press, New York, pp. 47–79.

Little, Michael A. and Morren, George E. B., jun. (1976). "Ecology, Energetics, and Human Variability". Wm. C. Brown, Dubuque, Iowa.

Lowman, Cherry (1974). Unpublished Ms.

Maelzor, D. A. (1965). A discussion of components of environment in ecology. *J. Theor. Biol.* **8**, 141–162.

MacArthur, M. (1974). Pigs for the Ancestors: a review article. *Oceania* **45**, 87–123.

Malcolm, L. A. (1970). Growth, malnutrition and mortality of the infant and toddler in the Asai valley of the New Guinea Highlands. *Am. J. clin. Nutr.* **23**, 1090–1095.

Meggitt, M. J. (1972). System and Subsystem: the *Te* exchange cycle among the Mae Enga. *Hum. Ecol.* **1**, 111–124.

Morren, George E. B., jun. (1974a). "Settlement Strategies and Hunting in a New Guinea Society". Ph.D. Dissertation in Anthropology, Columbia University, New York.

Norgan, N. G., Ferro-Luzzi, A. and Durnin, J. V. G. A. (1974). The energy and nutrient intake and energy expenditure of 204 New Guinean adults. *Phil. Trans. R. Soc.* Ser. B **268**, 309–348.

Odum, Howard T. (1971). "Environment, Power and Society". John Wiley and Sons, New York and London.

Pimentel, David *et al.* (1973). Food production and the energy crisis. *Science* **182**, 443–449.

Rappaport, Roy A. (1968). "Pigs for the Ancestors". Yale University Press, New Haven.

Rappaport, Roy A. (1971a). The flow of energy in an agricultural society. *Scient. Am.* **225** (3), 116–132.

Rappaport, Roy A. (1971b). Ritual, sanctity and cybernetics. *Am. Anthrop.* **73**, 59–76.

Sinnett, P. F. and Whyte, H. M. (1973). Epidemiological studies of a highland population of New Guinea: environment, culture and health status. *Hum. Ecol.* **1**, 245–277.

Slobodkin, L. B. (1968). Towards a predictive theory of evolution. *In* "Population Biology and Evolution". (Ed. R. C. Lewonten). Syracuse University Press, Syracuse, New York, pp. 187–205.

Stanhope, J. (1970). Patterns of fertility and mortality in rural New Guinea. *New Guinea Res. Bull.* **34**, 24–41.

Steinhart, Carol and John (1974). "Energy, Sources, Use and Role in Human Affairs". Duxbury Press, North Scituate, Massachusetts.

Street, John (1969). An evaluation of the concept of carrying capacity. *Prof. Geogr.* **21**, 104–107.

Thomas, R. Brooke (1973). "Human Adaptation to a High Andean Energy Flow System". Occasional Papers in Anthropology No. 7, Department of Anthropology, Pennsylvania State University, University Park, Pennsylvania.

Vayda, Andrew P. (1971). Phases in the process of war and peace among the Marings of New Guinea. *Oceania* **42**, 1–24.

Vayda, Andrew P. (1974). Warfare in ecological perspective. *Ann. Rev. Ecol. Systematics* **5**, 183–193.

Vayda, Andrew P. and McCay, Bonnie (1975). New directions in ecology and ecological anthropology. *Ann. Rev. Anthrop.* **4**, 293–306.

Vines, A. P. (1970). "An Epidemiological Sample Survey of the Highlands, Mainland, and Island Regions of the Territory of Papua New Guinea". Department of Public Health, Territory of Papua and New Guinea, Port Moresby.

Waddell, Eric (1972). "The Mound Builders". University of Washington Press, Seattle.

Waddell, Eric (1975). How the Enga cope with frost: responses to climatic perturbation in the Central Highlands of New Guinea. *Hum. Ecol.* **3**, 249–274.

Watson, James B. (1965a). From hunting to horticulture in the New Guinea Highlands. *Ethnology* **4**, 295–309.

Watson, James B. (1965b). The significance of recent ecological change in the Central Highlands of New Guinea. *J. Polynes. Soc.* **74**, 438–450.

Watson, James B. (1967). Horticultural traditions in the eastern New Guinea Highlands. *Oceania* **38**, 81–98.

Winterhalder, B., Larsen, R. and Thomas, R. B. (1974). Dung as an essential resource in a Highland Peruvian community. *Hum. Ecol.* **2**, 89–104.

Woodcock, A. J. *et al.* (1970). Studies of chronic (non-tuberculous) lung disease in New Guinea populations: The nature of the disease. *Am. Rev. Resp. Dis.* **102**, 575–590.

CHAPTER XI

Energy Use and Economic Development in Pacific Communities

TIMOTHY P. BAYLISS-SMITH

Department of Geography, Cambridge University, England

I. INTRODUCTION

Human ecology has been defined as "the study of the interrelationships of man's exchanges of matter, energy and information" (Flannery, 1973, p. 5). A full understanding of man–environment systems must involve a consideration of all three elements, but as Hornabrook warns (see Chapter III), it may be premature or even counterproductive to attempt any such total analysis at this stage. In this chapter I consider one of these three elements, energy exchanges, in the context of agrarian populations in the Pacific region.

Despite the various criticisms of an energy approach (see Chapter II), energy does have the advantage of being a fundamental and value-free measure of quantity. Shawcross (1967, p. 616) has noted that "the application of thermodynamic concepts . . . supply a unifying principle through which previously unrelated information may be drawn together and organised into an interpretable form". A number of writers have exploited these advantages, and some have attempted to construct general models of social and cultural change by examining the interrelation between change and energy use. I outline some of these ideas below, and then test them against empirical evidence from six Pacific populations.

II. MODELS OF CHANGE IN ENERGY USE

A. ENERGY AND TECHNOLOGICAL INVENTION

Changes in man's use of energy and changes in the efficiency of that use were discussed in an implicit way in many early writings about social and cultural change, but all too often a narrow technological interpretation of change was all that was offered. Descartes, for example, in his "Discourse on Method" (1637) described how, through an understanding of the workings of fire, water, air and the other environmental forces, men might become "masters and possessors of nature". By the seventeenth century this dream of mastery over nature had become possible as a result of technological advances that had begun much earlier (Lynn White, 1962). As early as the fourteenth century Europeans had made great progress towards substituting water and wind power for human labour in the basic industries. More fundamentally, from the tenth century onwards the new agricultural systems of northern Europe, based on the heavy plough, horse traction and a three course rotation, enabled more land to be cultivated. These innovations and the accompanying changes in rural society involved a fundamentally new attitude towards nature. They also provided a food surplus which permitted rapid urbanization, and it was in this new urban environment that there emerged one of the dominant features of the modern world—power technology.

It is not surprising that in the nineteenth century, at the height of this transformation, most writers laid great stress on invention as the key to understanding social change, or social evolution as it came to be called. Whereas in biology evolution was seen as operating on the basis of essentially random mutation, in sociological writings the process was interpreted in more purposeful terms. H. L. Morgan, for example, described the technical inventions in man's prehistory which he saw as being necessary preconditions for "cultural evolution", a process involving a progressive improvement in man's mastery of nature and occurring in distinct stages. Inspired by the work of Morgan (1877) and Tylor (1871), an American anthropologist Leslie White (1943) was later encouraged to examine in a more explicit way the relationship between the technology used at each of these stages and the energy that was thereby harnessed.

B. ENERGY IN CULTURAL EVOLUTION: LESLIE WHITE'S HYPOTHESIS

White (1943, 1959) divided "culture" into three subsystems: technological, sociological and ideological. The primary role is played by the technological system, since without the means and tools for subsistence and shelter none of man's other needs can be met.

> Social and philosophic systems are both adjuncts and expressions of this technologic process. The functioning of culture as a whole therefore rests upon and is determined by the amount of energy harnessed and by the ways in which it is put to work. (White, 1949, p. 367).

It therefore follows that the degree of cultural development (C) can be measured according to the amount of human need-serving goods and per-capita services produced. These products will themselves increase with expansion in the amount of per-capita energy harnessed (e), and/or with an improvement in the efficiency of the technological means by which the energy is put to work (T). In other words,

$$e \times T \rightarrow C.$$

In its original form this statement is not so much a "law" as a hypothesis, or as Harris (1969, p. 636) put it, "a statement of research strategy". It was a deductive model lacking detailed empirical support. White necessarily had to assume that "plant cultivation, fertilization and irrigation served to increase the yield per unit of human energy", in the same way that later innovations (animal husbandry, wind and water power, the Fuel Revolution) had clearly done so (White, 1949, p. 371). His attempt to define an energy resource as an entity separate from the technical efficiency with which it is exploited is also unconvincing, since in practice the total energy resources of an environment (E) only becomes a meaningful concept when it is related to the particular environmental perception and level of technological expertise that exists at a given time and place.

Despite these shortcomings, White's model represents a useful working hypothesis. Three generalized principles of "cultural evolution" stem from it (Meggers, 1960).

(1) If there is no increase in energy or improvement in technology the culture will remain stable.

(2) If either energy or culture or both are increased or improved, the culture will increase in complexity.

(3) If either the energy or the technology or both are diminished, the culture will decline in complexity.

If these principles have any validity they ought to explain many aspects of a society's stability, progression or regression, including aspects of contemporary "development".

On the other hand, expecting White's model to apply directly to particular cases may involve a misunderstanding of its purpose. Sahlins (1960) pointed out that because culture was being viewed by White as a closed system, his concern was restricted to principles of "general evolution". In the real world social change occurs in an open system, and so involves the "specific evolution" (or adaptation) of cultures, thus leading to change that may be contrary to general evolutionary trends. Specific evolution is defined as "the production of an organized cultural whole . . . which copes with the dual selective forces of nature on the one hand and the impact of outside cultures on the other" (Harding, 1960, p. 45). It can be observed as a connected, historical sequence of forms, whereas general evolution is a sequence of levels merely exemplified by forms that show a given degree of development, such as amount of energy transformation, complexity of organization, or degree of adaptability (Sahlins, 1960). These levels are what can usually be classified into cultural stages. It is argued by these authors that it is the failure to recognize this distinction between general and specific that has led to the neglect in human ecology of White's model of how cultures change.

Another reason for the neglect of White's law of energy levels was its inadequate empirical support. Sahlins agreed with White that "in culture . . . thermodynamic accomplishment is fundamental to progress [i.e. general evolution], and therefore would appear useful as a criterion of emergent development", but he could provide no evidence in support of this statement since there was "a lack, for the moment, of ready estimations of cultural progress in energy terms", let alone any satisfactory method whereby the thermodynamic achievements of different cultures could be quantified (Sahlins, 1960, pp. 33–35). In Section V I suggest and illustrate a number of ways of approaching this problem.

Other reasons for the lack of interest in evolutionary principles relate to the question of research priorities. Many would agree with Lucy Mair, that the interesting and urgent practical questions are not why particular inventions have been made at particular times and places, nor even why new technologies have been adopted by particular societies; instead "what everyone is asking today concerns the response to the inventions of recent centuries of peoples to whom these inventions are alien" (Mair, 1965, p. 126). One response, of course, is the conservative one of non-adoption, and to understand this response requires the question "why?" as well as "how?" to be answered. Nevertheless, in most societies the existence of cultural change is so all-pervasive in the modern world as to appear to be self-evident in its rationale. Alternatively, its complexity would seem to defy a simplistic energy-based explanation.

In an effort to dispel this attitude and to disprove Steward's view that White's hypothesis "can tell us nothing about the development of the characteristics of individual cultures" (Steward, 1953, p. 318), an attempt was made by Meggers (1960) to test White's model with detailed ethnographic data. She examined what changes occurred in particular cultures as a result of economic innovations, for example the intensification of rice production by the Tanala of Madagascar and the acquisition of the horse by the Cheyenne. The modifications in socioeconomic organization (White's C) in these societies are related to changes in e (per-capita energy use) or T (technology). The case studies do clearly show the close interrelation of social organization with the quality and quantity of the resource base, but Meggers' data on energy gain and efficiency are wholly qualitative. Since she also neglects to consider the possibility of change in population pressure, the simple one-way links that she implies exist between the environment (equated with e) or technology (T) and increasing social complexity, settlement nucleation etc. (C) are too deterministic to be convincing.

It has in fact been clear since Malthus' "First Essay in Population" in 1795 that the energy potential of a particular type of environment bears no direct relation to the cultural level achieved by its inhabitants.[*]

---

[*] In Malthus' words (1798, p. 364), despite the stimulus of population growth "savages will inhabit countries of the greatest natural fertility for a long period, before they partake themselves to pasturage or agriculture".

Megger's "law of environmental limitation on culture" therefore has very little predictive value even in the closed system world of general evolution processes. Just as carrying capacity formulae are nothing but abstract measures of population potential, calculated using the level of environmental productivity that a given labour input and technology would achieve (Bayliss-Smith, 1974b), so any attempt to suggest that the agricultural potential of an environment determines its cultural level is doomed to failure.

C. HOW SOCIETIES RESPOND TO INCREASED ENERGY EFFICIENCY

Meggers used the traditional measure of the efficiency of a given environment, namely its agricultural yield (energy return per unit of land). Both White (1949, 1959) and Sahlins (1960), on the other hand, recognized that the amount of food produced per unit of labour (i.e. energy return per unit of human energy expended) may be a far more relevant measure of efficiency. Improvements in agricultural yields occur as a result of the kinds of technological change that Wrigley (1969, p. 52) termed "intensive". These are innovations which permit one man to produce more from the same area of land, whereas extensive change simply enables the cultivable land to be extended without adding to the productive powers of the individuals working on it. Some intensive changes are, therefore, likely to raise the efficiency of labour, but even if this occurs it may in itself be insufficient to stimulate structural change in a culture.

One behavioural response that can result in this lack of structural change is when increased efficiency simply enables leisure time to be expanded. In the course of modern development there are many examples of peoples adopting technological innovations that theoretically should double their output, but instead they only work half as long (twice as efficiently) as previously (e.g. Salisbury, 1962). This leisure response will be shortlived unless the population is stabilized. Ultimately the improved technology may simply enable greater numbers to be supported at the same living standard. Instead of producing a single cultural system at a higher order of development increased efficiency may therefore simply result in the proliferation of several societies each at a relatively low level of cultural organization (Sahlins, 1960).*

* This process was also foreseen by Malthus, who considered that mankind was inherently "sluggish and averse from labour unless compelled by necessity", so that population increase would inevitably result in the colonization of new areas in preference to any localized intensification in food production (Malthus, 1798, p. 363).

Only if both of these responses, increased leisure and increased numbers, are averted will technological innovation lead to progress in the general evolution sense of "more goods and services, new political systems, or the promulgation of transcendental philosophies, and so forth" (Sahlins, 1960, p. 34). It was because Malthus, in the late eighteenth century, could only envisage a limited amount of intensive technological change (and, in Britain, no extensive changes at all) that he reached his pessimistic conclusion, that every time "the restraints to population are in some way loosened, the same retrograde movements with respect to happiness are repeated" (Malthus, 1798, p. 31). Half a century later circumstances had changed, so that Engels and later Marx were able to view technology in a more optimistic light, and so reject completely the capitalists' law of diminishing returns.

> The area of land is limited . . . but the labour power to be employed on this area increases together with the population; and even if we assume that the increase in output associated with this increase in labour is not always proportionate to the latter, there still remains a third element . . . namely science, the progress of which is just as limitless and at least as rapid as that of population. (Engels, 1844, reprinted in Meek, 1953, p. 63)

In the view of Marx and Engels agricultural technology could be continually advanced by scientific research, and the means of production and distribution could be politically controlled, so that there was no danger of population outstripping resources and so threatening welfare. A new ideology therefore emerged in the late nineteenth century, which in its crudest form saw the per-capita energy yield of a society as being determined in both quantity and social distribution by the prevailing political organization of that society.

Although preferable to the racial determinism that dominated anthropological thought at the same period, this political determinism is no more satisfactory than the demographic determinism of Malthus, the technological determinism of Morgan (and later White), or the environmental determinism of geographers like Ratzel and Huntington (and later Meggers). For pre-industrial societies none of these writers were able to provide any detailed empirical evidence about the relationships between technology, energy yield and cultural change, and so for this reason if for no other their "explanations" were largely untested hypotheses. The collection and evaluation of data concerning these relationships has been one of the tasks of research in human ecology during the twentieth century, and it is to this same object that this chapter addresses itself: how precisely is contemporary social change manifested in changes in energy yield and efficiency? In the next section I review some recent evidence and ideas that relate to this question, before turning in Sections IV and V to empirical data from agrarian societies in the Pacific.

III. DATA ON THE EFFICIENCY OF ENERGY USE

A. PRE-INDUSTRIAL SOCIETIES

Marvin Harris (1971) has attempted to quantify White's terms e (per-capita energy harvested) and T (technoenvironmental efficiency). For Harris,

$$e = \frac{E}{P}$$

where E is the total food energy that a system produces annually, and P is the total population. T is defined (Harris, 1971, p. 203) as the average number of calories produced for each calorie expended in food production, a ratio which clearly must be greater than one if the energy produced by a system is to exceed the energy expended in producing it. In practice, Harris confines energy expenditure to the energy costs of the human labour expended in production, ignoring for calculation purposes energy subsidies of various kinds.

The results of this analysis can be summarized as follows (see also the discussion by Morren in Chapter X).

TABLE I

Energy expenditure of various societies

Society	Per-capita energy harnessed (e, 10^6 kcal)	Techno-environmental efficiency (Harris' T)	White's C ($= e \times T$)
Kung (hunters and gatherers; Kalahari)	0·77	9·6	7·4
Maring (shifting cultivators and pig herders; New Guinea)	0·82	9·8	8·1
Genieri (cereal and peanut cultivators; Gambia)	0·92	11·2	10·3
Luts'un (irrigation rice farmers; Yunnan, China)	5·41	53·5	289
U.S.A. (1964 agriculture)	1·52 million	210	32 million

The White hypothesis equating cultural level to $e \times T$ appears on the basis of these data to differentiate very poorly between the first three societies, despite the fact that they represent important stages in cultural evolution. The Kung Bushmen of the Kalahari are nomadic hunters and gatherers; the Maring of New Guinea practise extensive shifting cultivation with perennial hamlets; the Genieri villagers of Gambia practise semi-permanent cultivation. Harris (1971, p. 207) concludes that "the advantage of rudimentary forms of agriculture over most hunting and food gathering lies in the ability of agricultural routines to sustain nucleated settlements rather than in any immediate 'labour-saving' improvements in the factor of tecno-environmental efficiency".

B. ENERGY SUBSIDIES IN INDUSTRIALIZED SOCIETIES

The great increase in efficiency that Harris' data suggest occur with irrigation and industrialization (Yunnan, China and the U.S.A. respectively) may be more apparent than real. In these systems the cost of energy inputs other than human labour ought to be included, since in both cases farming activities are largely or wholly integrated within the wider market economy. Some data recently produced for British agriculture indicate the magnitude of these energy subsidies.

Food energy output per capita in Britain ($0\cdot59 \ 10^{12}$ kcal) can be seen from these figures to be under half the American output of 1964 ($1\cdot52 \ 10^{12}$ kcal), but British farming in 1973 had a slightly higher efficiency ratio when efficiency is calculated as food energy produced

TABLE II

British agriculture and energy subsidies

	Wheat farming per acre	British agriculture, 1973
Food output, E (10^6 kcal)	5·59	32·7 million
Per-capita energy ($E/P = e$)	not stated	0·59 million[a]
Technoenvironmental efficiency, T	not stated	267[b]
White's C ($= e \times T$)	not stated	15·88 million
Energy subsidies (10^6 kcal)	3·94[c]	81·9 million
Actual efficiency	1·42	0·40
Source	Lawton, 1973	McFarlane, 1974

[a] Calculated assuming U.K. population of 55 millions.
[b] Calculated assuming 408 000 farmworkers at 2000 hours per year and 150 kilocalories per hour.
[c] Calculated assuming fuels and fertilizers represent 80% total energy inputs (McFarlane, 1974).

per unit of labour energy expended. This higher technoenvironmental efficiency in Britain is, however, achieved only at the cost of massive energy inputs other than human effort, including fertilizers, machinery, fuels, and the transport and processing of foodstuffs. When these energy subsidies are compared with the food energy produced, the ratio of output to input ("actual efficiency") is only 0·40 for agriculture as a whole, and 1·42 for wheat farming—considerably less than the efficiency ratios of the three subsistence societies examined by Harris.

It is clear, therefore, that when applied to post-industrial food production systems the index of cultural development outlined by White and made operational by Harris overestimates severely the actual efficiency of the production process. Arguably it does give some abstract idea of the high yields, heavy subsidies, and the resulting organizational complexity that technologically advanced farming involves. But as H. T. Odum has pointed out, the huge post-industrial expansion in per-capita energy use occurred largely through the application of energy subsidies, rather than through any basic improvement in the efficiency of energy use. Modern methods of intensive farming has generated what Odum describes as a "cruel illusion", since the scale of the energy subsidies required to raise yields has not been appreciated.

> A whole generation of citizens thought that the carrying capacity of the earth was proportional to the amount of land under cultivation and that higher efficiencies in using the energy of the sun had arrived. This is a sad hoax, for industrial man no longer eats potatoes made from solar energy; now he eats potatoes partly made of oil. (Odum, 1971, p. 115)

The productive but inefficient systems of food production of industrial man contrast with the more stable and self-sufficient systems of the pre-industrial world (see Clarke, Chapter XII).

Almost as much energy is therefore being poured into the food production systems of industrialized countries as is gained from them, and it is only the low monetary cost of the non-renewable fossil fuels used as energy subsidies that makes intensive farming profitable. When seen from an energy viewpoint, it becomes obvious that most of the world's food supply depends for its maintenance on continuous high-energy inputs into agricultural systems. Yet the illusion persists that as a result of astonishing scientific and technical achievements mankind has solved "the problem of production". As Schumacher (1973, p. 11) pointed out, this illusion is based on the fundamental failure to distinguish between income and capital at the global scale.

Until recent times isolated populations were among the few that were forced to view their finite resources in a more realistic fashion.

On small islands in particular there developed forms of social organization and land use that enabled an ecological balance to be maintained, as in the Lau Islands of Fiji (Thompson, 1970) and the Polynesian outlier atolls (Bayliss-Smith, 1974b). The growing links of such islands with the outside world mean that the traditional practices are no longer perceived as having functional utility, as the political control of island resources passes into external hands, and as the islanders themselves move away from Sahlins' (1972, p. 39) stage of Primitive Affluence ("want not, lack not") and into the modern world of expanding needs but limited means by which to satisfy them. Pacific island communities can thus be viewed as microcosms of the global trend towards a more and more exploitative relationship to resources and, in agriculture, a less and less efficient manipulation of energy. A study of their human ecology can, therefore, suggest principles that might be of more than local relevance.

IV. ENERGY USE ON ONTONG JAVA ATOLL

A. THE ATOLL ECOSYSTEM

From the earliest times Western observers describing atolls have tended to emphasize eclusively their negative characteristics.

> They are small low islands level with the water's edge . . . covered with cocoanut trees and dense underwood and inhabited by a poor set of naked wretches who must be sorely straitened for food, as the islands are not much more spacious than a good sized orchard and the water probably brackish! (Wilson, 1841, describing Takuu atoll)

> Coral reefs with their low sandy islets provide the most limited range of resources for human existence and the most tenuous of habitats for man in the Pacific . . . The soil is relatively infertile, lacking humus, and fresh ground water is very limited . . . Maintaining a livelihood is a considerable task for man. (Thomas, 1963, p. 36)

> Coral islands vividly exemplify how a stringent and marginally productive habitat . . . continually challenge the intellectual and technological abilities of man to cope with limited resources and ecological restrictions on alternative modes of social behaviour. (Lundsgaarde, 1966, p. 3)

These and other accounts stress the limited range of resources, low productivity, and spatial constraints on total output that are regarded as characteristic of the atoll ecosystem. Two important factors are neglected: the balance between resources and population, and the degree of fluctuation in productivity following droughts or hurricanes.

Arid, drought prone, or overpopulated atolls are certainly marginal
habitats, but where these conditions are avoided a rather different
picture emerges.

The richness of the marine resources of atolls has always been
apparent, and biological research has confirmed that coral reefs are
indeed "'islands' of isolated high productivity in the middle of
comparatively barren tropical seas" (Stoddart, 1969, p. 446). The
terrestrial ecology of atolls has also been investigated through a
number of reconnaissance studies (Wiens, 1962), and some more
detailed studies of atoll human ecology have been made (Danielsson,
1956; Wiens, 1956; Catala, 1957; Huntsman, 1969; Pollock, 1974;
Carroll, 1975). Alkire's (1965) work on Lamotrek in the Caroline
Islands was one of the first atoll studies to quantify some of the labour
inputs into economic activities and the related outputs of taro, coconut,
breadfruit, fish, turtles, copra etc. These data were transformed into
energy units by H. T. Odum (1971) to exemplify human use of a stable
solar-energy-based system. Odum claimed that the relatively stable
climatic conditions on Lamotrek provided a quite considerable
diversity of food sources for the human population, although no great
quantity of energy was available from any one.

> The meagreness of man's role within a very stable system is also a protection.
> The energy resources available to man are insufficient for him to do damage
> to his supporting system. Their diversity is a protection against epidemic
> decimations of his food circuits. (Odum, 1971, p. 105)

The continuity of human settlement on atolls would seem to support
Odum's emphasis upon the more positive aspects of the environment.
The Central Polynesian outlier atolls north of the Solomons, for
example, have probably been inhabited by man since the earliest
prehistoric settlement (Ambrose and Green, 1972; Davidson, 1974;
Green, 1975), and there is evidence that through conscious population
control numbers may have been stabilized at 70–80% of maximum
carrying capacity (Bayliss-Smith, 1974b). The atolls in this region
have a substantial and generally reliable rainfall, and are free from
the malaria, hookworm and other diseases endemic to the high islands
of the Solomons. Their size and location rendered them less susceptible
to the recurrent hazards of drought, hurricane and tsunami which are
emphasized by Vayda (1959) as playing an important demographic
and cultural role in Central Polynesian and Micronesian atolls. It is
hard, therefore, to accept without reservation the notion that atolls
necessarily offered "a harsher and more hazardous life" (Howells,
1973, p. 255) than high islands, or that the habitat is as "tenuous" and
"marginally productive" as is suggested by the popular stereotype.

B. ONTONG JAVA ATOLL

The largest atoll in the Central Polynesian outlier group is Ontong Java (Map 6). The atoll's lagoon has a maximum length of 70 km and a width that varies from 11 to 26 km. Around the reef margin of the lagoon are 108 vegetated islands, and within the lagoon a further 14 islands making a total of 122, of which 92 are less than five hectares in area. The thirty largest islands make up over 90% of the total land area of 777 hectares, and the largest two of all, Luangiua and Pelau, provide sites for the atoll's two main villages (Figure 1). The population is of mixed Micronesian and Polynesian origin, and as a result of introduced disease its numbers declined steeply from about 2000 in 1900 to 580 in 1940. Since then there has been a recovery: in 1970 the resident population numbered 860, and there were a further 200 persons of Ontong Java origin living in the Solomon Islands (Bayliss-Smith, 1974b; 1975).

European influence was spasmodic and superficial until 1874, but in the last quarter of the nineteenth century labour recruiters and traders exerted a growing influence. By 1890 a trading station had been established, and the self-sufficient subsistence economy based on taro (*Cyrtosperma* and *Colocasia*), coconut and fish began to be modified as coconuts were planted more extensively for copra production, and as imported goods were incorporated into production and consumption patterns. There was severe mortality at this time from introduced diseases, notably endemic malaria and epidemics of upper respiratory tract infections. Depopulation in itself accelerated the decline of the traditional political and religious systems (Hogbin, 1934), although mission activity was ineffectual until 1936 and the British colonial government did little to reorganize the structure of political authority until the early nineteen-sixties.

The penetration of the cash economy is still restricted to the production of copra and, to a limited extent, the collection of trochus shell. These products were sold to resident traders until 1939 and have been traded with visiting ships since 1952. A balance now seems to have been reached between the cash and subsistence sectors, where involvement in copra production is restricted more by a limited set of needs for imported goods and by a preference for products and activities which only the subsistence sector can provide, rather than by any restriction on copra output. In the mid-nineteen-sixties, when copra prices were high and when several commercial projects on the atoll provided some incentive for the islanders to maximize production, over 600 tonnes of copra were exported from the atoll each year.

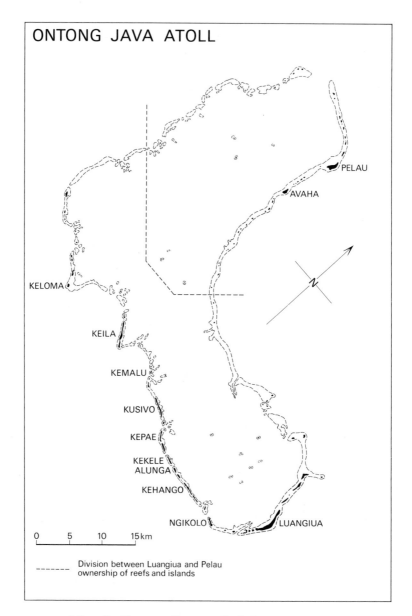

ONTONG JAVA ATOLL

PELAU

AVAHA

KELOMA

KEILA

KEMALU

KUSIVO

KEPAE

KEKELE
ALUNGA

KEHANGO

NGIKOLO   LUANGIUA

0   5   10   15km

- - - - -   Division between Luangiua and Pelau
            ownership of reefs and islands

Map 6. Ontong Java atoll, Solomon Islands.

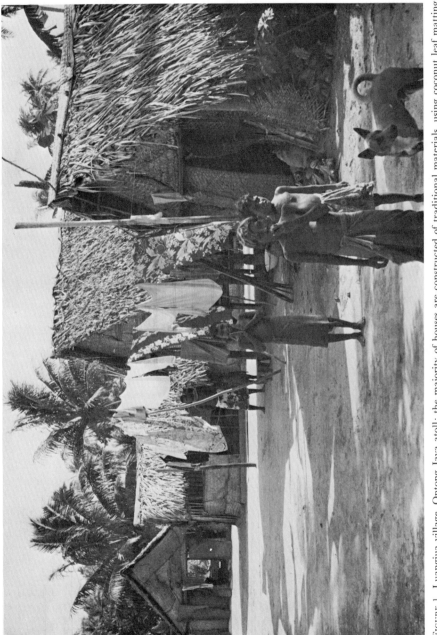

Figure 1. Luangiua village, Ontong Java atoll: the majority of houses are constructed of traditional materials, using coconut leaf matting for the walls and a thatch of pandanus leaves (*Pandanus tectorius*) for the roof.

Output in the year of fieldwork (June 1970 to May 1971) totalled 390 tonnes, and was limited partly by hurricane damage sustained three years previously, but partly also by demand rather than supply. By mid-1971 most islands were back in full production, but many were no longer fully worked, and in 1972 when the price fell to a very low level copra production on Ontong Java was actually abandoned altogether for a while. Ontong Java thus retains some freedom of choice as regards its degree of dependence on the outside world.

C. THE ECONOMIC SYSTEM IN 1970–1971

The approach that I adopted during fieldwork on Ontong Java in 1970–72 was basically threefold: first, surveys were made to determine the structure and distribution of the atoll's population; second, the population's resources were identified and mapped; and third, the relationship between the population and its resources was assessed through sample surveys of activities and production. In combination, these three sets of data enable precise quantitative statements to be made about the aggregate economic system as it was functioning at that time.

An understanding of that system's functioning, as opposed to a mere description of its operation, requires of course other kinds of information. Without such an understanding little can be said about the probable direction of future change. This extra information can sometimes come from a reconstruction of the past, so that one can determine how a society responded to past innovations and in what ways its internal structure was modified in the process. It can also come from a comparative study of the present, to see how other populations occupying similar environments gain their livelihood, and how and why they have responded to change. Third and perhaps most important, an understanding of any society—especially at the micro-scale— requires a knowledge of the needs, motives and aspirations of the individuals that comprise that society. For an outside observer an appreciation of these intangible social catalysts can only be gained from first-hand observation and fieldwork, over as prolonged a period as is feasible (Brookfield, 1973).

In this chapter my main purpose is to describe in energy terms the structure and functioning of the economic system of Ontong Java, and to compare it with other Pacific communities. A degree of explanation may be implicit in the description, but it is not the primary aim. The period to which the data refers is June 1970 to May 1971, and it was during these twelve months that surveys were carried out which recorded: all imports and exports; month by month changes in the population and its location; crop yields and the total output of taro swamps (eight-week sample period); production from fishing (three sample periods totalling 13 weeks); nutritional surveys of sample households; and the work inputs of a sample totalling 86 adults (20% of the adult population) for 4903 mandays in three different locations. Maps were also made of crops, in particular the taro swamps, and other types of atoll vegetation were mapped by air photo interpretation. The methods adopted in these surveys, and the means by which the data were converted into the form shown below, are discussed at length elsewhere (Bayliss-Smith, 1974a).

The way in which the economic system was structured is shown in Figure 2. The atoll environment can be classified into a number of different communities most of which are ecologically distinctive. The majority of islands are wholly planted with coconuts, forming a mixed woodland, but small patches of the original *Pisonia* forest and littoral scrub vegetation remain. The largest islands have freshwater swamps planted with taro (*Cyrtosperma* and *Colocasia*) (Figure 3), and there are also small swampy areas dominated by *Hibiscus*, woodland, by *Cyperus* reed beds, or in brackish sites by mangroves (*Bruguiera gymnorrhiza*). The village areas form another distinct ecological unit, with a largely exotic flora and altered soils planted with gardens of sweet potatoes and bananas.

The work involved in maintaining and exploiting these different ecosystems can be conveniently classified into a subsistence sector and a cash sector. The subsistence activities are either food producing ("subsistence production") or they are concerned with maintaining infrastructure such as houses and canoes. There is also a category of activities somewhat misleadingly termed "non-productive", which include sedentary, home-based activities like food preparation and looking after children.

Relationships between the Ontong Java economic system and the outside world are subsumed in Figure 2 in the category "external human systems", which provide outlets for exported products and migration and which supply imported foods and information. The input of biological production within the various exploited environments of the atoll is represented by "external energy cascades". The other "black box" within the system is the category "socioeconomic organization", which controls the level of inputs into subsistence, cash or other activities through a changing schedule of needs, perceptions and aspirations.

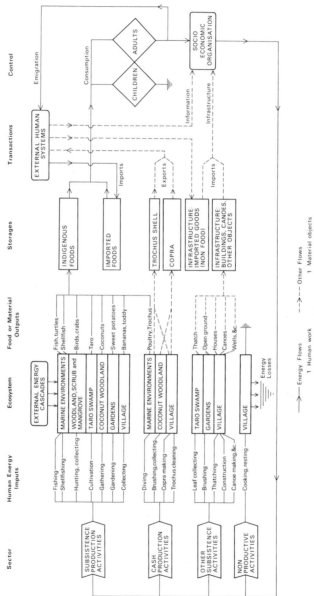

FIGURE 2. The economic system of Ontong Java atoll in 1970–71.

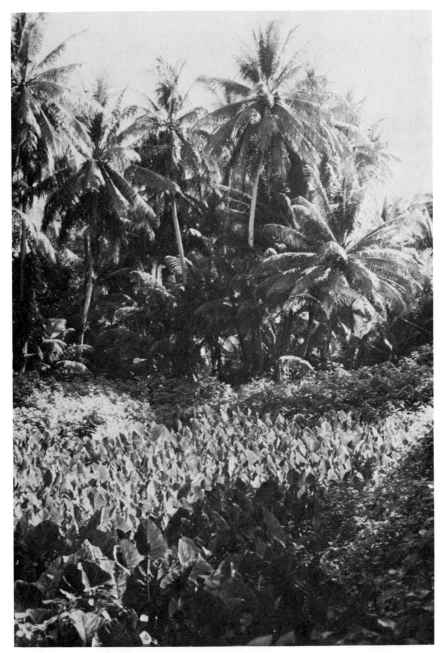

FIGURE 3. Atoll vegetation: this small depression on Pelau island has been excavated to ground water level, and is planted with *Cyrtosperma chamissonis*, a slow growing but non-labour intensive type of taro which will tolerate less favourable soil conditions than *Colocasia*. The coconut woodland surrounding the taro swamp is also easily maintained, as the dense canopy of palms prevents much light from reaching the ground and so suppresses the undergrowth.

D. THE PRODUCTIVITY OF THE LAND

The energy flows shown in Figure 2 consist of labour inputs into different ecosystems and the resulting food production. Money was also generated by the system through the sale of copra and trochus, and in the year 1970/71 it amounted to $A 36 500 or $A 43 per person. Of this income $A 10 200 was spent on imported food and $A 19 900 on non-food imports. Accurate estimates of the total labour inputs and food outputs were obtained through surveys, the results of which are summarized in Table III.

The average productivity of the terrestrial ecosystems ranges between 17·8 million kilocalories per hectare per year for taro grown in the *Colocasia* swamps to only 0·04 million kilocalories for the minor

TABLE III

Main ecosystems of Ontong Java atoll (A), and their productivity
June 1970 to May 1971 (B)

A. Ecosystems

Vegetation unit	Area (hectares)	Main food products	% of total dietary calories
1. *Cyrtosperma* swamp	37·42	*Cyrtosperma* taro	18·2
2. *Colocasia* swamp	3·30	*Colocasia* taro	11·1
3. Village environs	13·33	Sweet potatoes, papayas, toddy, bananas	3·2
4. Woodland, scrub, littoral and strand vegetation	45·83	Birds and eggs, crabs, turtles and their eggs	0·4
5. Coconut woodland	651·11	Coconuts (unripe, ripe and germinating), pandanus and other fruits	21·0
		Imported foods purchased with copra	24·5
6. Mangroves, *Hibiscus* and *Cyperus* swamps, turmeric plots and unplanted taro gardens	26·66	Bananas, sugar cane	0·1
7. Submerged coral reefs, lagoon sand flats, and pelagic waters	n.a.	Fish, molluscs	19·2
8. Reef flats	n.a.	Trochus, and trochus purchased imports	2·4
Ontong Java atoll	777·65 (land)	All foods	100·0

TABLE III—*continued*

B. Productivity

Vegetation unit	Food output		Related work input	
	Energy value (10⁶ kcal)	Productivity (10⁶ kcal/ha)	Energy value (10⁶ kcal)	Productivity (output:input)
1.	96·92	2·59	5·01	19·3
2.	58·82	17·82	9·88	6·0
3.	17·00	1·27	0·38	44·7
4.	2·10	0·04	2·07	1·0
5. a.	111·56	0·17	2·51	44·4
b.	129·91	0·20	48·00	2·7
6.	0·01	—	2·00	—
7.	101·82	n.a.	11·82	8·6
8.	12·35	n.a.	1·51	8·2
Ontong Java	531·12	0·68 (land)	81·18	6·4

n.a.: not available.
Bayliss-Smith (1974a, pp. 319–320).

foods such as birds, turtles and eggs obtained from the woodland and scrub areas. There is a great difference between *Colocasia* and *Cyrtosperma* taro, the latter yielding only 2·6 million kilocalories. *Colocasia* is a labour intensive crop requiring constant weeding and mulching (Figures 4 and 5), so its high yield is only obtained at the cost of a lower return to labour (see Section IV E). Sweet potatoes compare favourably with *Colocasia* taro, yielding 15·0 million kilocalories per hectare, but only restricted areas in and around the main village are suitable for their cultivation.

Coconut productivity is equally variable, owing to differences in soils and in the density of palms, and as a result also of variations in the intensity of cropping (Table IV).

Coconuts have a high de-facto energy value (6312 kcal per kg), but their value to the Ontong Java people is not only as a foodstuff but also as a source of cash income. As such, copra has a perceived energy value that is considerably lower than its de-facto value, and it is one that will change according to the price received for copra, the prices paid for imported goods, and the preferences and priorities among imports. As an approximation, average demand can be represented by the actual food imports of Ontong Java atoll in 1970–71, and this can be used to generate a "perceived" or potential energy value for copra. For the average yield per hectare in 1970–71 (2975 coconuts).

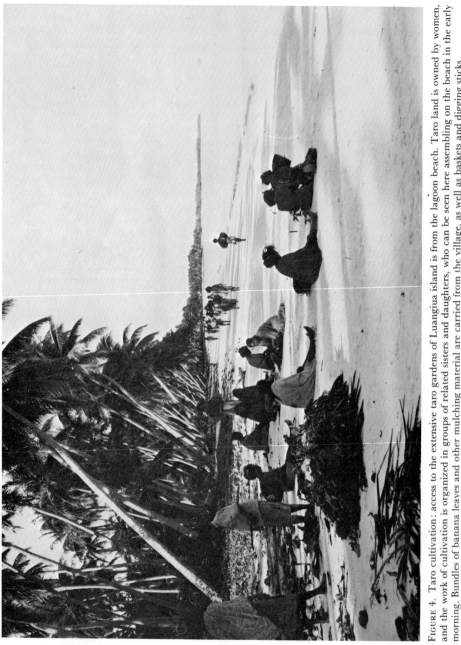

FIGURE 4. Taro cultivation: access to the extensive taro gardens of Luangiua island is from the lagoon beach. Taro land is owned by women, and the work of cultivation is organized in groups of related sisters and daughters, who can be seen here assembling on the beach in the early morning. Bundles of banana leaves and other mulching material are carried from the village, as well as baskets and digging sticks.

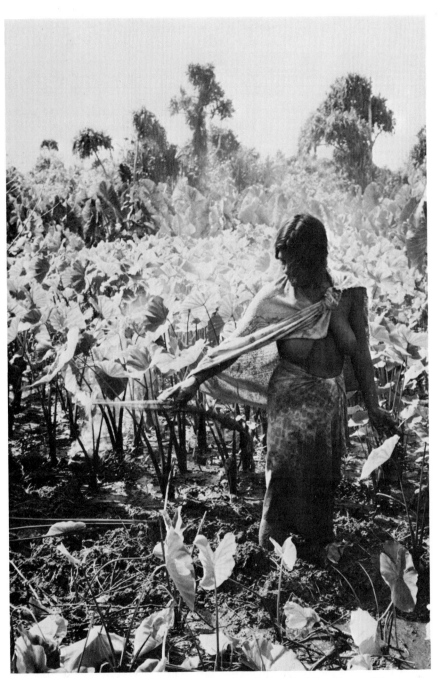

FIGURE 5. Taro cultivation: the planting procedure is described by Morren (Chapter X, Figure 4). The soil has a very high organic content as a result of being almost continually water-logged, and its nutrient level is maintained by continual mulching and weeding around the *Colocasia* plants, which are harvested and replanted every three months. Boundaries between plots are marked with lines of *Cyrtosperma* plants (middle distance). Pandanus palms (background) provide leaves for roof thatch.

TABLE IV

Maximum and average yields in 1970–71

	Yields per hectare per year		De-facto energy value (10^6 kcal)
	Nuts	Copra (kg)	
High yielding plot, Luangiua island	8690	1750	11·05
Ontong Java average	2975	598	3·77

TABLE V

Alternative energy values for coconut

	10^6 kcal per hectare
De-facto energy value	3·77
Food value if consumed as coconut cream	1·62
Perceived value at 1970–71 food and copra prices ($54·7 worth of copra)	0·77
Perceived value at 1972 prices ($32·8 worth of copra)	0·46

TABLE VI

Three estimates of the productivity of Ontong Java
(1970–71 levels of output and price)

	Energy value (10^6 kcal)	
	Total	Yield per hectare
Consumed production (subsistence output and purchased foods actually consumed)	531·1	0·68
Perceived production (subsistence output plus foodstuffs potentially purchasable with cash income)	899·3	1·16
De-facto production (actual calorific value of net biological output of the economy)	2858·6	3·68

Various energy values can therefore be calculated (Table V).

Three different estimates are therefore available of the mean productivity to man of the total atoll ecosystem (Table VI). Unlike estimates of biological production, each is based only on the useful portion of yield, whether in a direct (food) or an indirect form (money and the food that money would buy). Of these three, the consumed production will not alter unless the population's nutritional needs alter through growth or structural change. De-facto production is more volatile, and will alter according to the quantity of surplus output that is traded with the outside world or, in many agrarian societies, fed to domestic animals. In recent years dramatic changes in the terms of trade have also meant that perceived production levels have also been changing, often in an unfavourable way in Third World countries. The 1970–71 output of the Ontong Java system, for example, which had a perceived value of 890 million kilocalories in that year, would have been worth only 700 million kcal in 1972, when the copra price slumped and the price of imports began to undergo a severe inflation.

E. THE PRODUCTIVITY OF LABOUR

As outlined in Section IIIB, between 1900 and 1940 the population of Ontong Java declined at an average rate of 3·3% per year, and despite its subsequent recovery it is still less than half its precontact size. As a result there is no absolute shortage of land, and there is therefore little incentive to maximize production yields.

Gladwin (1970) has argued that on Puluwat atoll in the Caroline Islands the present day population also lives in an environment where survival does not depend on wresting from a hostile environment every scrap of sustenance that it will yield. As a result productive efficiency is not the standard by which all choices on Puluwat must be made, "there are many pathways to plenty, and productive energies need not be guided only by rational economics" (Gladwin, 1970, p. 32).

For Ontong Java the data in Table VII indicate the alternative pathways among which a choice, economically rational or otherwise, must be made by each producer. The activities that provide the most favourable ratio of food output to labour input are the cultivation of sweet potatoes and bananas, the gathering of coconuts for eating, and *Cyrtosperma* cultivation. The village crops and, to a lesser extent, *Cyrtosperma* taro are limited in output by a restricted area of suitable land, while the consumption of coconuts is limited not by supply but by dietary demand. These constraints restrict the actual labour input in these high yielding activities to only 12% of the total hours of work directly concerned with food production. The majority (86%) occurs in activities which provide yields in the range 6·0–10·4, confirming Rappaport's (1968, p. 63) suggestion that very few techniques employed by human groups primarily for the purposes of capturing food energy will have efficiency ratios much below 10. The only two major exceptions on Ontong Java are shellfish gathering (1·2) and

TABLE VII

The allocation of time between various activities, and the productivity of labour
expended in each: Ontong Java, 1970–71

Category and activity	Total work input (10³ hours)			Productivity[a,b] (energy gained per labour energy expended ratio)
	Males (172 adults)	Females (246 adults)	Population (850 persons)	
Environmental—land				
Colocasia cultivation	7·0	44·3	51·3	6·0
Cyrtosperma cultivation	3·6	22·4	26·0	19·3
Turmeric cultivation	0·2	9·0	9·2	—
Village crop cultivation	0·5	1·3	1·8	44·7
Coconut collection	7·6	1·3	8·8	43·6
Copra, plantation work	54·0	46·5	100·5	10·4
Copra, village work	49·0	44·6	93·6	
Birds, eggs, wild fruits	1·1	0·4	1·4	9·3
Environmental—sea				
Fishing	59·2	0·1	59·3	8·6
Shellfish collection	1·4	2·4	3·8	1·2
Trochus diving	4·6	—	4·6	8·2
Trochus cleaning	1·2	3·7	4·9	
Turtles and eggs	9·7	—	9·7	0·5
External transactions				
Storekeeping	2·9	—	2·9	—
Trading with ships	4·7	1·6	6·3	—
Infrastructure				
House construction and maintenance	18·2	26·9	45·1	—
Canoes	11·2	0·1	11·3	—
Village maintenance	6·6	9·4	16·0	—
Weaving mats	—	32·5	32·5	—
Coir manufacture	—	5·3	5·3	—
Clothes	—	3·3	3·3	—
Turmeric, other crafts	—	3·3	3·3	—
Travel				
Inter-island travel	14·2	11·0	25·2	—
Politics, ritual, etc.				
Public meetings	5·7	1·3	7·0	—
Dancing and ritual	6·8	15·7	22·5	—

[a] The energy gained is calculated from de-facto production, except for copra which is perceived potential production.
[b] The energy inputs are calculated from the hours of work using the energy expenditure rates of Hipsley and Kirk (1965).
Bayliss-Smith (1974a, tables 51–59 and 66).

turtle hunting (0·5), and here it is clear that Gladwin's non-rational motives do operate. On the other hand, these two activities which are inefficient in energy terms only account for 2% of the total hours of "productive" work on the atoll (Figure 6).

An average efficiency ratio can be calculated from these data on labour input, which for the food and money gaining activities alone amounts to 80·1 million kilocalories of work per year. Using the same figures given in Table VI for consumed production, perceived production, and de-facto production, this input generates the following efficiency ratios for the Ontong Java economic system as a whole:

Consumed Production Efficiency	6·6
Perceived Production (indigenous) Efficiency	11·2
De-facto (technoenvironmental) Efficiency	35·7

Of the three, the de-facto efficiency is the one which corresponds to Harris' T measure of technoenvironmental efficiency discussed in Section III. By comparison with the societies discussed by Harris (1971), Ontong Java is intermediate in efficiency between the purely subsistence economies of hunters, gatherers and shifting cultivators ($T = 10$–11) and the intensive rice farmers of Yunnan Province in China ($T = 54$). The per-capita energy output on Ontong Java is also midway between the subsistence producers' and the rice farmers' outputs (3·4 10^6 kcal compared with 0·8–0·9 and 5·4 respectively). On the basis, therefore, of White's C index of cultural evolution ($= T \times e$), Ontong Java also stands in an intermediate position.

It is arguable, however, that the de-facto efficiency (T) measure overestimates considerably the productivity of the economic system as viewed from the producers' own point of view. In terms of the goods that they actually receive for their work, the perceived measure of output is the more realistic. The ratio of this quantity to the primary (labour) input provides an "Indigenous Efficiency", which for Ontong Java was 11·2, scarcely different from the comparable T efficiency of subsistence societies not involved in producing a surplus for the market economy (e.g. Kung, Maring and Genieri). If economic development does involve "cultural evolution", then contrary to White's hypothesis change for Ontong Java seems not to have led to any real increase in either technical efficiency or perceived output per capita.

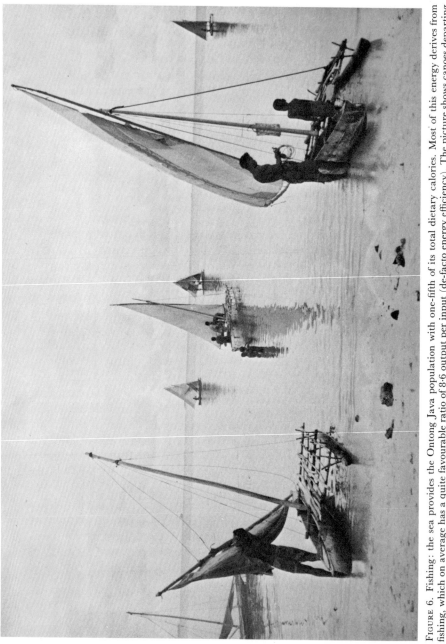

FIGURE 6. Fishing: the sea provides the Ontong Java population with one-fifth of its total dietary calories. Most of this energy derives from fishing, which on average has a quite favourable ratio of 8·6 output per input (de-facto energy efficiency). The picture shows canoes departing from Luangiua for a day's fishing in the lagoon. The use of sailing canoes extends the zone of feasible exploitation to 15–20 km for day trips.

V. ENERGY USE IN SIX PACIFIC COMMUNITIES

A. SIX COMMUNITIES COMPARED

Data on other societies are obviously needed in order to test further the above suggestion, that current economic development in the Pacific is increasing neither the perceived efficiency of work nor the level of perceived per-capita output. Some information is beginning to become available as a result of quantitative, micro-scale studies by anthropologists and geographers, three of which have been reviewed by Morren in Chapter X. To the three New Guinea communities discussed by Morren three others are added for comparative purposes: Ontong Java atoll in 1970–71; the village of Nacamaki on Koro Island in Fiji, for which data are available for two annual periods between 1972 and 1974; and the village of Nasaqalau on Lakeba Island in the Lau group of Fiji, using data for 1974.

For descriptions of the Miyanmin, Tsembaga Maring and Raiapu Enga of New Guinea, the reader is referred to Chapter X, while Ontong Java has been discussed already in the previous section. The two Fijian communities are of particular interest because of their longer exposure to the influence of foreign values and the market economy, so that by any standards of "development" (e.g. monetary income, literacy, welfare services, social and political change) they ought to have experienced more "cultural evolution" in the White–Sahlins sense than have the other societies. The first, Nacamaki, is situated on the wet and fertile volcanic island of Koro. Since about 1910 it has exported copra and kava (*yaqona*) to supplement its subsistence crops, which consist of yams, cassava, dryland *Colocasia* taro and bananas. Of these all except yams are introduced. Purchased foods in Nacamaki comprised 33% of the total diet in 1973–74, compared with 24% on Ontong Java and only 3·5% among the Enga. The second Fijian community is Nasaqalau, on Lakeba island in the Lau group, which has poorer soil resources and less rainfall than Koro but has had an even longer experience of modernization as a missionary centre since 1835 and an exporter of coconut oil since the eighteen-fifties. At Nasaqalau cassava and sweet potatoes supplement the traditional irrigated taro and have largely replaced yam cultivation. Copra and trochus shell are the main sources of a substantial cash income which in 1974 enabled 49% of the diet to be obtained from imported foods.

B. PER-CAPITA ENERGY INCOME

Koro and Lakeba therefore lie further along the development continuum than does Ontong Java, which in turn seems more altered than the Enga and particularly more so than the Miyanmin or Maring of New Guinea. These six societies represent stages along the road which leads from total self-sufficiency towards total involvement with external systems, a trend which the transition from subsistence agriculture to a commercial economy inevitably involves. In Table VIII the annual per-capita cash income of these societies is shown, ranging from nil for the Miyanmin and Maring to $190 for Lakeba. One way of expressing this income in energy terms is to adopt the procedure used to calculate the perceived production of Ontong Java (see Table VI). The surplus cash income (i.e. that portion not spent on imported foods)

TABLE VIII

Annual energy incomes in five Pacific communities, calculated from incomes of consumed subsistence foods and from the potential energy equivalent of cash incomes

	Tsembaga Maring[b]	Raiapu Enga	Ontong Java	Nacamaki, Koro	Nasaqalau, Lakeba
Population	64	47	850	309	265
Year studied	1963	1966–67	1970–71	1973–74	1974
Per-capita income Cash					
Total	0	$A 10	$A 45	$F 140	$F 190
Not spent on food	0	$A 3	$A 21	$F 97	$F 110
Income not spent on food converted to purchased food equivalent (10³ kcal)[a]	0	13	296	578	515
Subsistence Consumed output (10³ kcal)	705	798	625	764	760
Total (10³ kcal)	705	811	921	1342	1275

[a] Conversion factors are as follows (kcal of locally purchased food per $1): Raiapu Enga 4375, Ontong Java 13996, Nacamaki 5960, Nasaqalau 4678.
[b] The Miyanmin are similar to the Maring, having an annual consumed output of 696 000 kcal (see Morren, Chapter X).
The data in Tables VIII, IV and V are computed from the following, Maring: Rappaport (1968, 1971); Enga: Waddell (1972). Estimated cash incomes are derived from Waddell (1972), pp. 119, 199) and Freund (1971, pp. 103–106). Ontong Java: Tables III and VII, and Bayliss-Smith (1974a); Koro: Bayliss-Smith (1976a); Lakeba: Bayliss-Smith (1976b).

is converted into a purchased food equivalent, and this potential energy is then added to that contained in the actual diet. The procedure is the reverse of that now adopted by some economists, in quantifying subsistence output for the purpose of gross domestic production statistics (Dommen, 1974). The conversion uses the mean calorific value of the foods actually purchased, and so incorporates automatically the local pattern of food prices and food preferences.

A comparison of the four societies shows that the transition from complete subsistence (Maring) to a part-commercial economy (Koro and Lakeba) does involve a progressive increase in the total energy income. The per-capita annual income (in 10^3 kcal of perceived food energy) increases from 700 for the Maring to 800 for the Enga, over 900 for Ontong Java, and around 1300 for Koro and Lakeba.

C. DE-FACTO PRODUCTION, AND ENERGY SUBSIDIES TO PRODUCTION

It can be argued that the "energy income" method of analysis severely underestimates the productivity of the two New Guinea populations, whose output of subsistence crops is considerably more than the autoconsumption proportion that is shown in Table VIII. Although the quantity of sweet potatoes and other crops fed to pigs varies markedly in traditional Highlands societies according to the stage reached in the ritual pig cycles, at all times there are substantial pig populations being supported. Among the Maring and Enga, for example, the pigs consumed 27% and 49% respectively of the crops produced, mainly sweet potatoes. The de-facto energy generated by a community should therefore be considered, calculated from the total net primary production. In this case, however, the primary products exported by the other three populations must also be assessed in a similar way. The results of such an analysis, shown in Table IX, do not contradict those obtained by the first method but merely enlarge the differentials between the populations, which are still ranked in the same order. The positions of Koro and Lakeba are, however, reversed, as a result of the smaller copra production of Lakeba. Its primacy in cash income terms resulted purely from the very favourable copra price that prevailed through the twelve months for which data are available.

To achieve an estimate of the total turnover of energy in these communities an attempt must also be made to calculate on what scale energy subsidies are being imported into the economic systems. Not all material imports can be quantified in energy terms, but the second part of Table IX shows two categories of subsidy, imported foods and imported fossil fuels, which are together termed the secondary inputs.

Neither imported foods nor fuels were used by the Maring, who were essentially pre-contact at the time they were studied. The Enga were beginning to import purchased foodstuffs, but on a very small scale. On Ontong Java, however, imported food and fuel were both becoming important. Rice, flour, sugar and biscuit provided Ontong Java with

TABLE IX

De-facto energy production, imported energy subsidies, and perceived energy production in five Pacific communities

	Energy (10^3 kcal per person per year)				
	Tsembaga Maring	Raiapu Enga	Ontong Java	Nacamaki, Koro	Nasaqalau, Lakeba
De-facto output					
Consumed plants[a]	905	2283	336	534	295
Land animals[b]	60	13	2	4	5
Marine foods[c]	—	—	134	52	90
Exports[d]	—	17	2811	7660	4290
Total de-facto output	965	2313	3363	8250	4680
Imported energy inputs					
Foods	—	28	167	260	386
Fuels[e]	—	—	15	156	450
Total secondary input	—	28	182	416	836
Perceived output					
Consumed plants	645	757	336	534	295
Animals[f]	262	1526	136	56	95
Cash income[g]	—	38	586	611	889
Total perceived output	907	2321	1058	1201	1279

[a] Main plant foods for human and animal consumption are as follows; Maring: sweet potato, taro, Xanthosoma, yams, banana; Enga: sweet potato, yams, banana; Ontong Java: coconut, Cyrtosperma, taro; Koro and Lakeba: taro, cassava, yams, coconut.

[b] Non-marine animal foods are, Maring and Enga: pigs; Ontong Java: seabirds, eggs and poultry; Koro and Lakeba: pigs, cattle and poultry.

[c] Marine foods are predominantly fish, but include also molluscs, turtles etc.

[d] The export crops quantified are copra (at 6312 kcal per kg) for Ontong Java, Koro and Lakeba, and mixed vegetables for the Enga. Total quantities of exports not given an energy value are, Enga: 570 kg coffee; Ontong Java: 10 900 kg trochus shell; Koro: 840 kg kava and about 1000 kg shell; Lakeba: 6380 kg shell.

[e] Imported fuels were mainly kerosene and petrol, which totalled as follows, Ontong Java: 300 gallons; Koro: 1025 gallons; Lakeba: 2815 gallons.

[f] This category includes animals obtained by hunting or fishing, together with domesticated animals assessed according to the energy value of the subsistence foods supplied to them.

[g] The environmental incomes (cash crops, sale of pigs etc.) used to calculate these figures are somewhat smaller than the total incomes used in Table VIII. Incomes from non-environmental sources (e.g. remittances, government salaries) contribute the following percentages of the total incomes in each community, Enga: 14; Ontong Java: 4; Koro: 14; Lakeba: 19.

Sources, see Table VIII.

98% of its imported food energy, which in total absorbed about one-third of the total cash income. Of the fuels, kerosene was used extensively for domestic lighting, replacing home produced coconut oil in most houses except in times of shortage. A little petrol was also being used for the outboard engines of canoes. Imported food and fuel contributed 5·1% to the total energy used by the Ontong Java population.

In Nacamaki village on Koro the same two categories of imports provided a similar proportion of the total energy turnover (4·7%), but the fuels were relatively more important than on Ontong Java atoll. The community's per-capita consumption of kerosene and petrol during the year 1973–74 was ten times the Ontong Java level, as a result mainly of domestic cooking as well as lighting demands. Koro's consumption of fuels fluctuates according to the level of cash income. In the previous twelve months (1972–73) when low copra prices depressed incomes at Nacamaki to only 35% of their 1973–74 level, total imports of fuel energy fell to 51% of the 1973–74 level. Despite such fluctuations, and despite the rising price of fuel, the dependence of island populations like Koro on imported fuels seems likely to increase steadily. In 1974 Nasaqalau on Lakeba used much of its higher cash income to increase still further its dependence on imported fuels, the consumption of which was three times as great as on Koro, averaging 450 000 kilocalories per person despite a higher price.

These data show that in total energy production and use there is already almost an order of magnitude between the Miyanmin and Maring ($0·9 \times 10^6$ kcal per person per year) and Nacamaki ($8·6 \times 10^6$ kcal), with the other three populations intermediate. According to a recent estimate a further factor of ten separates rural Fiji from the U.S.A., where about 84 million kilocalories per person are generated each year (Cook, 1971). In that the present direction of cultural change in the Pacific is tending rapidly towards a greater involvement in the market economy, these six populations provide clear evidence that the quantity of de-facto energy harnessed is a valid measure of cultural evolution, as White (1943) suggested.

D. PERCEIVED POTENTIAL PRODUCTION

From the point of view of people inside these communities, de-facto energy production is too abstract a measure of performance to be useful conceptually. As explained in Section V B above, a much closer approximation to indigenous values is the perceived measure of potential output, based on the energy purchasing power of any cash income received together with the food energy that is expended in animal husbandry (Table X).

TABLE X

Three different ways of measuring energy gain

Energy output	Subsistence sector	Cash sector
Consumed	Subsistence foods eaten	Imported foods eaten
Perceived	Crops eaten, traded, or fed to domestic animals, plus animals or plants hunted or gathered	Total cash income, converted into imported food equivalent
De-facto	All subsistence foods eaten including domestic animals, plus the surplus foods traded or fed to domestic animals	Direct energy value of all exported cash crops

Data on the levels of perceived energy production are also given in Table IX, where the Raiapu Enga of New Guinea rank highest on a per-capita basis as a result of the very substantial quantity of crops produced and fed to herds of domestic pigs at the time of Waddell's (1972) research. In the traditional economy of the Enga

> Pigs were the most important medium of exchange . . . They were the means whereby an Enga household could convert resources mobilized in gardening into objects of wealth which could be traded and exchanged in almost any economic or socio-economic transaction. (Freund, 1971, p. 100)

These data therefore suggest that on a perceived energy basis the Enga are richer in pigs than are Ontong Java, Koro or Lakeba in copra production. In other words, the foods that are fed to pigs have two to three times the energy value of the foods that would be bought with the copra incomes being received by the other populations.

The comparison is, perhaps, not strictly accurate, since it is debatable whether the cost of pig keeping can be equated with its perceived value (Rappaport, 1967, p. 64). Moreover, money from copra is a more flexible commodity than pigs, which are seldom sold for cash. In this respect it is interesting that the monetary value that the Enga themselves would place on their herd, which in Waddell's sample community totalled 108 animals, corresponds much more closely to the energy cost of feeding them than does either the labour cost of keeping them, or their direct calorific value as meat, or the monetary value that they would fetch in the outside world.

Of these five alternative ways of assessing the energy value of pigs, only the two energy costs (food supplied and labour expended) would

TABLE XI
Alternative energy values for Enga pigs

Energy value	Method of calculation	10^3 kcal per capita
a. Annual cost of maintenance	Perceived cost (see Table IX)	1526
	Labour cost (Waddell, 1972, pp. 104, 119)	62
b. Value of total herd	De-facto, assuming 30·6 kg meat per animal at 2906 kcal (Rappaport, 1967, p. 62)	203
	Monetary value in external markets, assuming $15 per animal, converted to Enga perceived energy potential at rate 4375 kcal per dollar (see Table VIII)	151
	Enga cash valuation, assuming average sale price of 30 cents per half pound portion of meat (Feachem, pers. comm.), converted as above	407

have any perceived meaning to the Enga. For the Raiapu Enga "the pig is central not only to nearly all ceremonial and religious occasions but also to the whole mechanism by which a male seeks to acquire the status of big man" (Feachem, 1973, p. 26). In this situation any conversion to energy value via some assumed monetary value is meaningless, and the best measure of the perceived cost of keeping pigs would appear to be the energy value of the human foods that are required to maintain them.

Whether or not the Enga data are used for comparative purposes, the three copra producing communities (Ontong Java, Koro and Lakeba) are certainly comparable. They display no significant differences in perceived potential per-capita output, contradicting the trend towards increasing energy capture with economic development that is suggested by the de-facto data.

E. THE EFFICIENCY OF ENERGY USE

In order to generate ratios of output to input, the nature of the inputs into each economic system needs to be defined carefully. The "primary" inputs represent the cost in human effort for each population to supply itself with the goods to maintain it and enrich it. In addition there are the imported or "secondary" energy inputs, which represent the cost to society as a whole of maintaining or enriching any particular enclave within it. It is usually not feasible to measure in energy terms all such subsidies, but fortunately the two which are frequently the most important for Pacific populations, foods and fuels, are also the easiest to quantify (see Table IX).

The primary inputs into food-gaining and cash sector activities in five of the societies are shown in Table XII, which also give the secondary inputs, the per capita outputs (perceived and de facto), and efficiency ratios. The following four types of efficiency are distinguished:

$$\text{Indigenous efficiency} = \frac{\text{perceived output}}{\text{primary input}}.$$

$$\text{Exogenous efficiency} = \frac{\text{exported de-facto output}}{\text{secondary input}}.$$

$$\text{Technoenvironmental efficiency (Harris' } T) = \frac{\text{total de-facto output}}{\text{primary input}}.$$

$$\text{Total efficiency} = \frac{\text{total de-facto output}}{\text{primary + secondary input}}.$$

F. INDIGENOUS EFFICIENCY IN PIG KEEPING SOCIETIES

The "indigenous" measure of efficiency is an attempt to quantify the meaning of economic change from the point of view of those involved in it. If the level of perceived output that a person receives stays unchanged and his work load increases, then this ratio will fall, indicating declining standards of living. If, on the other hand, perceived output itself declines on a per-capita basis despite an unchanged or even slightly reduced workload, then the indigenous efficiency ratio will again fall. The data in Table XII indicate the sensitivity of this index to variations in both perceived output and labour input.

The three New Guinea populations vary in mode of livelihood and population density, and represent three different stages in agricultural intensification. The Miyanmin are hunters, gatherers and extensive shifting cultivators; the Maring are entirely shifting cultivators; and the Enga practise intensive shifting cultivation (see Morren, Chapter X). The three societies also vary in the importance of pig herding, with pig–man ratios of 0·1, 0·8 and 2·3 respectively, and total labour inputs into pig herding and feeding of 12, 19 and 62 thousand kilocalories per person per year respectively. The indigenous efficiency ratios of the total Miyanmin, Maring and Enga economies are 7·1, 12·6 and 15·8 respectively, and it is not surprising that they reflect the

TABLE XII

Summary indices of the efficiency of energy use in six small-scale economic systems

	Miyanmin	Tsembaga Maring	Raiapu Enga	Ontong Java	Nacamaki	
					1973–4	1972–3
Energy inputs (10³ kcal per person per year)						
Primary	100	72	147	94	116	139
Secondary	—	—	28	182	408	176
Total	100	72	175	276	524	315
Energy outputs (10³ kcal per person per year)						
Perceived	708	907	2321	1058	1201	912
De-facto						
total	833	965	2313	3363	8250	10 551
exports only	—	—	17	2891	7660	9806
Output–input ratios						
Indigenous efficiency	7·1	12·6	15·8	11·2	10·4	6·6
Exogenous efficiency	—	—	0·6	15·9	18·8	55·7
Technoenvironmental efficiency (T)	8·3	13·4	15·7	35·7	71·1	75·9
Total efficiency	8·3	13·4	13·2	12·2	15·7	33·5

Sources. Nacamaki, Koro 1972–73: Bayliss-Smith (1976a); Miyanmin: Morren, Chapter X; others: primary inputs: see footnotes to Table VIII, and for Ontong Java Table VII; secondary inputs, perceived outputs, de facto outputs: Table IX and original sources.

differences in the importance of pigs since the surplus crops fed to pigs are a major part of the perceived production of these systems. The high value placed on pigs in New Guinea highland cultures as a way in which wealth can be stored and status achieved means that these ratios provide an interesting measure of the extent to which the raising of pig productivity is a dominant concern in the three communities.

G. INDIGENOUS EFFICIENCY IN COPRA MAKING SOCIETIES

The finding that the indigenous efficiency of the Ontong Java and Koro systems is similar or lower than those in New Guinea is more unexpected. Ontong Java had a ratio of perceived output to primary input of 11·2, whereas Nacamaki on Koro had a ratio of 10·4 in 1973–74 and only 6·6 in 1972–73 (see Table XII). In both economies the ratios are dominated by the copra sector, and by the fact that the return from copra varies substantially according to changes in the terms of trade.

The actual productivity of labour (kg copra per manhour) on Koro is in fact three times the productivity on Ontong Java. The coconut plantations on Koro are much less scattered than those on the atoll, horses are used for transporting the nuts, and the copra is dried on a centralized basis by the Nacamaki Cooperative Society, rather than being sun-dried in small lots by individual family groups, which is the normal practice on Ontong Java. In all these ways the Koro system is more efficient on a de-facto basis.

The prices received for copra and paid for imported goods were, however, much less favourable in Fiji in 1972–74 than in the Solomon Islands in 1970–71. In addition, producers on Ontong Java used their money to obtain the cheapest forms of imported food energy, whereas on Koro tastes were somewhat more varied and prices considerably higher (see Table VIII). As a result, copra on Koro Island generally provided poorer returns to labour than on Ontong Java atoll.*

The commercial sector has the advantage of providing its return in a more flexible form, for instance, money, but apart from this consideration there was no strong incentive for the Koro people to become involved full time in copra production until 1974, and even then the boom in copra prices was short lived. Rather than being represented as a manifestation of blind conservatism, the continued existence of a substantial subsistence sector in economies like that of Koro should be seen as a thoroughly rational, energy-maximizing response.

Even in 1973–74 the indigenous efficiency of the Fijian village economy compared poorly with the returns available from unskilled wage labour. For a 44-hour working week and assuming the same energy expenditure rate as for copra making (200 kcal per hour), the total work input of a full-time labourer can be estimated as 430 000 kilocalories per year. This primary input compares with a perceived output of 6 032 000 kilocalories, using 1973 wage rates and Koro food prices (Fiji PIB, 1975). These figures produce an input–output ratio of 14·0, which is an attractive return for a villager prepared to work longer hours but for a more reliable income. In Fiji the difference

---

* In the copra sector alone the average ratio of perceived output to labour input was: Nacamaki, Koro 1958 about 5·3 (January to December), 1972–73 4·0 (September to August), 1973–74 13·6 (September to August); Ontong Java 1970–71 10·4 (June to May) (Watters, 1969; Bayliss-Smith, 1976a and 1974a). In other words, the perceived efficiency of copra production on Koro was low until the price rose sharply (and temporarily) in 1974. When compared to the efficiency ratio for subsistence crops (yams, taro and cassava), which on Koro is 11·8 or 12·5 when the value of surplus taro is included, then until 1974 the returns to be gained from copra were clearly inferior.

between the returns from wage labour and the returns from village agriculture have widened still further since 1974 as a result of wage increases and a slump in the price of copra. This growing disparity goes a long way towards explaining the drift of population to the towns and the growing poverty and depopulation of some of the outlying islands (Brookfield et al., 1976).

H. EXOGENOUS EFFICIENCY RATIOS

In an interdependent economic system it is inevitable that small, peripheral village communities will be in a highly dependent position, with only limited control over the flows and relationships that link the whole system together. It is clear that if strictly exploitative values were to prevail, then the internal dynamics and welfare of the small, dependent components of the system would be of no concern to the control centre, unless for example price changes meant that the perceived returns to labour dropped so low that the production of export crops ceased altogether, or disruptive population movements began to occur.

On Koro Island both symptoms of distress began to show during the slump in copra prices in 1972–73. The two annual periods that are compared in Table XII, 1972–73 and 1973–74, are contrasting in this respect. Whereas 1974 was a year of comparative affluence, 1972 is remembered as being a time of great stringency. Low copra prices meant harder work, a greater degree of self-sufficiency, and a lower consumption of imports. A number of people emigrated from Koro to find employment in Suva, some of whom returned the following year when the copra price recovered.

It is interesting that during this crisis period of 1972–73, when the perceived efficiency of the economic system was extremely low, its

TABLE XIII

Copra price and efficiency

Economy	Copra price	Indigenous efficiency	Exogenous efficiency
Nacamaki, Koro, 1972–73	Low	6·6	55·7
Nacamaki, Koro, 1973–74	High	10·4	18·8
Ontong Java, 1970–71	Moderate	11·2	15·9

efficiency of energy production from the external point of view was very high. Copra production was maintained but much less imported food and fuel was used, so that the disparity between the indigenous perception of efficiency and the external view became very substantial (Table XIII).

The large discrepancy between the internal and the external view of efficiency in these economies, and the very different responses of the two output–input ratios to price changes, are indications of the high dependency of small islands. On both Koro and Ontong Java the people themselves clearly receive greatly inferior energy returns than do those who control the trading systems of which they are small components. Current trends in the prices of primary products and of imported foods and fuels are not improving the situation. In view of the inequities between indigenous and exogenous energy returns, and in view also of the unpredictable but generally unfavourable movement in prices, then the continued participation of small Pacific communities in so-called subsistence activities is scarcely surprising. On islands like Koro such behaviour is, in fact, the most rational economic response that is feasible.

I. LESLIE WHITE'S HYPOTHESIS RECONSIDERED

Neither of the two indices of energy efficiency discussed above appears to be the one that White had in mind when he suggested that "culture evolves . . . as the efficiency of the instrumental means of putting energy to work is increased" (White, 1949, p. 368). This index could be what Harris (1971) termed technoenvironmental efficiency (see Section III), which is the ratio of total de-facto output to primary input. A comparison of the five populations in Table XII shows that this T ratio does increase in value with development.

On the other hand, it could be argued that White envisaged efficiency as including man's use of energy subsidies, represented by the secondary inputs in Table IX. This ratio, which is termed total efficiency, is remarkably similar for all five populations in Table XII, ranging from 8 to 16 with only one exception. The exception is Nacamaki in 1972–73, which has a ratio of 33·5, at a time when its population was experiencing the kind of crisis which some pessimistic predictions of the future suggest will become more general in the Third World. If the world's culture is indeed evolving in this direction, then the energy efficiency of its dependent primary producers will—of necessity—increase, as Leslie White perhaps unwittingly predicted.

At the same time, the data in Table XII suggest that economic development is definitely a retrograde process when measured as the return of perceived energy per unit of labour input. This ratio of indigenous efficiency seems to be highest in subsistence societies heavily involved in livestock production (Enga), is intermediate when economic development is partial and prices are relatively favourable (Ontong Java), and is lowest when market involvement is the greatest and cash incomes the highest, especially at times when the terms of trade deteriorate (Nacamaki). Although based on a small sample of communities, these findings are sufficiently clearcut to suggest that from an indigenous viewpoint cultural evolution in the modern world will generally involve a less efficient use of energy, and must therefore occur because it provides substantial intangible benefits which are not measurable in energy terms.

VI. REFERENCES

Alkire, W. H. (1965). "Lamotrek Atoll and Inter-Island Socio-Economic Ties". University of Illinois Press, Urbana.

Ambrose, W. R. and Green, R. C. (1972). First millenium B.C. transport of obsidian from New Britain to the Solomon Islands. *Nature* **23**, 31.

Bayliss-Smith, T. P. (1974a). "Ecosystem and Economic System of Ontong Java Atoll". Ph.D. Dissertation, University of Cambridge.

Bayliss-Smith, T. P. (1974b). Constraints on population growth: the case of the Polynesian Outlier atolls in the pre-contact period. *Hum. Ecol.* **2**, 259–295.

Bayliss-Smith, T. P. (1975). Ontong Java: depopulation and repopulation. *In* "Pacific Atoll Populations" (Ed. V. Carroll). University of Hawaii Press, Honolulu, pp. 417–484.

Bayliss-Smith, T. P. (1976a). "Koro in the 1970s: Prosperity through Diversity?". Development Studies Centre, Australian National University, Canberra. Project Working Paper No. 7, UNESCO/UNFPA Population and Environment Project.

Bayliss-Smith, T. P. (1976b). "Hurricane Val in north Lakeba: a multiple crisis of dependence". Development Studies Centre, Australian National University, Canberra. Project Working Paper No. 9, UNESCO/UNFPA Population and Environment Project.

Brookfield, H. C. (1973). Introduction: explaining or understanding? *In* "The Pacific in Transition" (Ed. H. C. Brookfield). Methuen, London, pp. 3–24.

Brookfield, H. C., Bayliss-Smith, T. P., Bedford, R. D., Brookfield, M., Campbell, J. C., Hardaker, J. B. and Latham, M. (1976). "The Eastern Islands of Fiji: Ecology, Population and Development". Development Studies Centre, Australian National University, Canberra. Draft General Report No. 1, UNESCO/UNFPA Population and Environment Project.

Carroll, V. (Ed.) (1975). "Pacific Atoll Populations". University of Hawaii Press, Honolulu.

Catala, R. L. A. (1957). Report on the Gilbert Islands: some aspects of human ecology. *Atoll Res. Bull.* **59**, 1–187.

Cook, E. (1971). The flow of energy in an industrial society. *In* "Energy and Power" (Scientific American pubn). W. H. Freeman, San Francisco, pp. 83–94.

Danielsson, B. (1956). "Work and Life on Raroia". Allen and Unwin, London.

Davidson, J. M. (1974). Cultural replacement on small islands: new evidence from Polynesian Outliers. *Mankind* **9**, 273–277.

Dommen, E. C. (Ed.) (1974). "Estimating Non-Monetary Economic Activities: A Manual for National Accounts Statistics". UN Development Advisory Team for the South Pacific, Suva.

Feachem, R. G. A. (1973). The Raiapu Enga pig herd. *Mankind* **9**, 25–31.

Fiji, Prices and Incomes Board (1975). "Inflation in Fiji". Government Printer, Suva.

Flannery, K. V. (1973). Introduction. *In* "The Use of Land and Water Resources in the Past and Present Valley of Oaxaca, Mexico". Memoirs of the Museum of Anthropology, No. 5, University of Michigan.

Freund, R. P. (1971). "The Enga Economy and Economic Development". Problem Paper, Institute of Extension Personnel, Michigan State University.

Gladwin, T. (1970). "East is a Big Bird: Navigation and Logic on Puluwat Atoll". Harvard University Press, Cambridge, Massachusetts.

Green, R. C. (1975). Comment on Peter Bellwood's "The Prehistory of Oceania". *Curr. Anthrop.* **16**, 20–21.

Harding, T. G. (1960). Adaptation and stability. *In* "Evolution and Culture" (Eds M. D. Sahlins and E. R. Service). University of Michigan Press, Ann Arbor, pp. 45–68.

Harris, M. (1969). "The Rise of Anthropological Theory". Routledge and Kegan Paul, London.

Harris, M. (1971). "Culture, Man and Nature". T. Crowell, New York.

Hipsley, E. H. and Kirk, N. E. (1965). "Studies of Dietary Intake and the Expenditure of Energy by New Guineans". South Pacific Commission, Technical Paper No. 147, Noumea.

Howells, W. (1973). "The Pacific Islanders". Reed, Wellington, N.Z.

Huntsman, J. W. (1969). "Kin and Coconuts on a Polynesian Atoll: Socio-Economic Organisation of Nukunonu Atoll". Ph.D. Dissertation, University of Auckland.

Lawton, J. H. (1973). The energy cost of "food-gathering". *In* "Resources and Population" (Eds B. Benjamin, P. R. Cox, J. Peel). Academic Press, London and New York, pp. 59–76.

Lundsgaarde, H. P. (1966). "Cultural adaptation in the southern Gilbert Islands". Ph.D. Dissertation, University of Wisconsin.

McFarlane, N. R. (1974). Energy in agriculture. *Nature* **252**, 531.

Mair, L. (1965). How small-scale societies change. *Adv. Sci.* **21**, 308–315.

Malthus, T. R. (1798). "First Essay in Population" (repr. 1966). Macmillan, London.

Meek, R. L. (1953). "Marx and Engels on Malthus". Lawrence and Wishart, London.

Meggers, B. J. (1960). The law of cultural evolution as a practical research tool. *In* "Essays in the Science of Culture" (Eds G. E. Dole and R. L. Carneiro). T. Crowell, New York, pp. 302–316.

Morgan, L. H. (1877). "Ancient Society". Macmillan, London.

Odum, H. T. (1971). "Environment, Power and Society". John Wiley and Sons, New York and London.

Pollock, N. J. (1974). Breadfruit or rice: dietary choice on a Micronesian atoll. *Ecol. Fd Nutr.* **3**, 107–115.

Rappaport, R. A. (1968). "Pigs for the Ancestors: Ritual in the Ecology of a New Guinea People". Yale University Press, New Haven.

Rappaport, R. A. (1971). The flow of energy in an agricultural society. *In* "Energy and Power" (Scientific American pubn). W. H. Freeman, San Francisco, pp. 69–82.

Sahlins, M. D. (1960). Evolution: specific and general. *In* "Evolution and Culture"

(Eds M. D. Sahlins and E. R. Service). University of Michigan Press, Ann Arbor, pp. 12–44.

Sahlins, M. D. (1972). "Stone Age Economics". Aldine, Chicago.

Salisbury, R. F. (1962). "From Stone to Steel". Melbourne University Press, Melbourne.

Schumacher, E. F. (1973). "Small is Beautiful". Blond and Briggs, London.

Shawcross, W. (1972). Energy and ecology: thermodynamic models in archaeology. In "Models in Archaeology" (Ed. D. L. Clarke). Methuen, London, pp. 577–622.

Steward, J. H. (1953). Evolution and process. In "Anthropology Today" (Ed. A. L. Kroeber). University of Chicago Press, Chicago, pp. 313–326.

Stoddart, D. R. (1969). Ecology and morphology of recent coral reefs. Biol. Rev. 44, 433–498.

Thomas, W. L. (1963). The variety of physical environments among Pacific islands. In "Man's Place in the Island Ecosystem" (Ed. F. R. Fosberg). Bishop Museum Press, Honolulu, pp. 7–37.

Thompson, L. (1970). A self-regulating system of human population control. Trans. New York Acad. Sci., Ser. 2, 32, 262–270.

Tylor, E. B. (1871). "Primitive Culture". J. Murray, London.

Vayda, A. P. (1959). Polynesian cultural distributions in new perspective. Am. Anthrop. 61, 817–828.

Waddell, E. W. (1972). "The Mound Builders: Agricultural Practices, Environment and Society in the Central Highlands of New Guinea". University of Washington Press, Seattle.

Watters, R. F. (1969). "Koro: Economic Development and Social Change in Fiji". Clarendon Press, Oxford.

Wiens, H. J. (1956). The geography of Kapingamarangi atoll in the eastern Carolines. Atoll Res. Bull. 48, 1–87.

Wiens, H. J. (1962). "Atoll Environment and Ecology". Yale University Press, New Haven.

White, L. A. (1943). Energy and the evolution of culture. Am. Anthrop. 45, 335–356.

White, L. A. (1949). "The Science of Culture". Farrar, Straus, Cudahy, New York.

White, L. A. (1959). "The Evolution of Culture". McGraw-Hill, New York.

White, Lynn (1962). "Medieval Technology and Social Change". Clarendon Press, Oxford.

Wilson, D. P. (1839–43). Log and private journal of Dr D. Parker Wilson. Ms., Royal Geographical Society, London.

Wrigley, E. A. (1969). "Population and History". Weidenfeld and Nicholson, London.

Part 5

Environment and Man: Policy, Perception and Prospect

The Structure of Permanence: The Relevance of Self-subsistence Communities for World Ecosystem Management

WILLIAM C. CLARKE

University of Papua New Guinea

From an economic point of view, the central concept of wisdom is permanence. We must study the economics of permanence. Nothing makes economic sense unless its continuance for a long time can be projected without running into absurdities. . . . The economics of permanence implies a profound reorientation of science and technology, which have to open their doors to wisdom and, in fact, have to incorporate wisdom into their very structure. (E. F. Schumacher, 1974, pp. 26–27)

I. INTRODUCTION

Readers of this essay will be familiar with the accelerating deterioration of the human environment that marks our world today. I will, therefore, not repeat in any detail what is contained in an also accelerating number of books and papers on the ecological crises associated with too many people or too much technology or both. Instead I will shuttle between a small, technologically simple community in Papua New Guinea and the whole endangered ecosphere, looking as I go at the lessons that the whole might learn from a tiny part. My effort is motivated by two tenets. The first is that studies of small communities and micro-regions can reveal something about larger regions and worldwide socio-economic processes. I do not mean by this, as has been argued by some geographers in the past, that combining many studies of micro-regions will somehow produce a synthetic understanding of larger regions; rather, it is my belief that the intimate understanding available from the study of even one small system may make the larger more comprehensible. My second tenet is that geographers and anthropologists, who more than other scientists have studied human ecology at the micro-scale, should try more to apply their findings to the world's ecological crises. This means less of an "objective" role for human ecologists. As Anderson has written with regard to human ecology as practiced by anthropologists

> The myth of 'value-free' social science is now thoroughly dead, and we must take responsibility for our actions. In anthropology, this will mean on the one hand an expansion of applied anthropology from its present rather *ad hoc* shape to a synthesizing discipline at least as powerful as economic development theory, and on the other a concern by human ecologists with applied anthropology and with the wider context of the world crisis. It will mean a broader focus of research. (Anderson, 1974, p. 266)

II. STUDIES OF THE MARING

My introduction to the Pacific region and to a lesser extent my entry into human ecology as a named discipline* came in 1964 when I and another geographer, Dr John M. Street, joined a research project that had been initiated in 1962 by the anthropologist Andrew P. Vayda under the title "Human Ecology of the New Guinea Rainforest". The people under consideration were the Maring, a linguistically united group of about 7000 shifting cultivators who live and garden on the rugged slopes of the Bismarck range in Papua New Guinea (see Map 1). The geographers were invited to join the project in the hope that information they would collect on Maring environment and land use would contribute to the full development of the anthropologists' hypotheses. Later published works by the anthropologists show their particular concern to have been with elements of cultural behaviour

* Scholastic argument has come to be the main result of trying to define or defend "human ecology" or other similar names for what some geographers and anthropologists have been doing. To avoid such argument and because I see no value in a finely honed definition, I used "human ecology" in an encompassing way to mean the study of ecosystems that contain human beings or that are influenced by human activities. I would as soon settle for "cultural ecology" or even "ecological anthropology"; however, cf. Vayda and McCay (1975).

that appeared to have ecologically adaptive functions—for instance, Vayda's (1971) analysis of Maring war and peace as a multi-phase process that could serve to adjust man–resource ratios, and Roy Rappaport's (1967) classic study of the functions of ritual within the ecosystem of the Tsembaga, a Maring speaking group of about 200 persons. Rappaport (1967, p. 224) regarded the Tsembaga ritual cycle as a complex homeostatic mechanism, operating to maintain the values of a number of variables within "goal ranges" (ranges of values that permit the perpetuation of a system as constituted, through indefinite periods of time). Rappaport argued that the regulatory function of ritual among the Tsembaga and other Maring helps to maintain an undegraded environment, limits fighting to frequencies that do not endanger the existence of the regional population, adjusts man–land ratios, facilitates trade, distributes local surpluses of pig in the form of pork throughout the regional population, and assures people of high-quality protein when they most need it.

My research among the Maring, which provided the data for a later publication (Clarke, 1971), was directed more simply towards an investigation of the interactions among the elements of the habitat and the activities of another small Maring group, known as the Bomagai-Angoiang. During my fieldwork and subsequent writing-up I read widely in human or cultural ecology, much of which could now be included under the term "ecological anthropology" (Vayda and McCay, 1975), and on systems theory.* Although I was impressed and undoubtedly influenced by many of these works, I did not feel that they provided me with as startlingly new and revealing an approach as many of them purported to offer. I assume I so responded because I was a product of the "Berkeley School" of Geography, which stressed from its beginnings under Carl Sauer in 1923 the integration and interplay of physical and cultural components within landscapes or, as we might now prefer, within ecosystems.† If "system" is defined as a recognized "set of objects together with relationships between the objects and between their attributes" (Hall and Fagen, 1956, p. 18), then "systems theory" has always permeated human or cultural geography. The main theoretical contribution to geography of the recent emphasis on systems theory and ecosystems has been the explicit stress put on the reciprocity of the relationships among human beings, their activities and their environments. Acceptance of the idea of reciprocal relationships and feedback mechanisms removes the controversy between cultural and environmental determinists that has

---

* Some of the publications then consulted are cited in Appendix A of "Theoretical Considerations and Practical Problems", Clarke (1971).
† See Leighly (1963) for a selection of the writings of Carl Sauer.

occupied too much time in the history of thought of many social sciences. In my study of the Bomagai-Angoiang I, therefore, made explicit the idea of the ecosystem.

> Considered thus as components of an ecosystem, both man and environment are seen as parts of a single unit, the whole of which is worthy of study. Concern shifts from which part most influences the other to the structure of the whole system and how it operates and changes. (Clarke, 1971, p. 200)

My not wholly successful attempt to introduce a description of ecosystemic change into my study was more of a departure from much I had read on systems theory and ecological anthropology, wherein there was a stated or implicit stress on equilibrium. But it was wholly consistent with my background in a human geography that made history its central theme. As Carl Sauer wrote in 1941 in his paper "Foreward to Historical Geography"

> Knowledge of human processes is attainable only if the current situation is comprehended as a moving point, one moment in an action that has beginning and end. This does not constitute commitment as to the form of the line, as to whether it has cyclic qualities or shows no regularity; but it does guard against overemphasizing the importance of the current situation. The only advantage of studying the present scene is that it is most accessible to inspection. Yet out of the contemporary data in themselves it is not possible to find the means of selecting what is diagnostic of important process and what is not. (Leighly, 1963, p. 361)

Influenced as I was by such a view and having been exposed to a historical geography that dealt with the crumblings of successive civilizations over millennia and the severe modifications of the face of the earth by man over a far longer period, I was made uneasy by ahistorical studies of ecosystems, especially where great emphasis was put on homeostasis or what appeared to be static equilibrium. Thus it seemed to me that in his functional analysis of ritual among the Tsembaga Maring, Rappaport (1967) was describing adaptation without evolution. His study was ground-breaking because of his analytical isolation of measured variables within a human ecosystem and his hypothesis that ritual can function to regulate the relationships of a population with components of its environment. Criticism of his study arose because the linkages between variables seemed just too good and the operation of the feedback controls just too smooth to be quite real in a world where failure and waste are essential parts of an ever continuing evolution. Feedback exists, but in a system as complex as a human ecosystem its operation is seldom purely cyclic. The resulting situation is always new and contains new necessities of adaptation.

Since Rappaport's study was published, other researchers have argued that the Tsembaga Maring are not as "well off" nutritionally and environmentally as Rappaport suggested (Buchbinder, 1973) and that several of the Tsembaga behavioural mechanisms described by Rappaport do not function as beneficially or wholly beneficially as he believed them to (McArthur, 1974 and Chapter V). McArthur also argues that Rappaport ignored political and prestige-gaining motives in his analysis of the growth of the Tsembaga pig herd and the instigation of ritual pig-killing ceremonies.* In one way this criticism is unjustified because Rappaport's stated concern (1967, p. 230) was with the role of ritual, not with its origin. However, if we are to look at human ecosystems through time, human motives must be considered, for man's motivated actions habitually involve a greater change in the environment than the behaviour of other animals. What Waddell, a geographer concerned with the evolution of agricultural systems in the New Guinean Highlands, has written of both pre- and post-contact change within a group that he studied applies in greater or lesser degree to all New Guinean communities.

It has been suggested that the Raipu themselves are 'pathological innovators', pragmatists with their eyes constantly on 'the main chance'. The changes themselves are not associated uniquely with the contact situation and certainly not only with the external sector of the economy, although increased mobility has accelerated the rate of change. . . . All these processes demonstrate that any suggestion of immutability of the subsistence system is quite untenable. (Waddell, 1972, pp. 193–194)

On the other hand, the change posited for the New Guineans was obviously limited. Although evolving, their ecosystems also survived and so must have possessed the property of coherence as well as "certain rules of equilibrial activity" (Beer, 1972, p. 167). An effective concept for expressing this ability to survive within a framework of change is "resilience", which can include the rejection of an equilibrium-centred view without the abandonment of the study of the processes

---

* Brookfield (1973) and Hide (1974) also believe that Rappaport may have stressed ecological functions at the expense of sociological explanation with regard to New Guinea Highlands pig cycles. In speaking of the Chimbu, Brookfield (1973, p. 155) wrote

Rappaport indicates that it is the level attained by the pig population, and its burdensome role on the human population, that triggers off the need for a new ceremony. But this is in a small population; such quasi-automatic regulatory mechanism as Rappaport postulates would hardly be conceivable among the numerous Chimbu with their interlocking cycles. Pig herds are rebuilt to an intermediate level fairly swiftly after a ceremony, and the rebuilding can be accelerated by trade. They are then managed about this level until such time as the need for a ceremony arises from other causes, when they are permitted to increase. Ceremonies are not held primarily to dispose of pigs; they have complex objectives in the maintenance and re-inforcement of the whole system of social relationships.

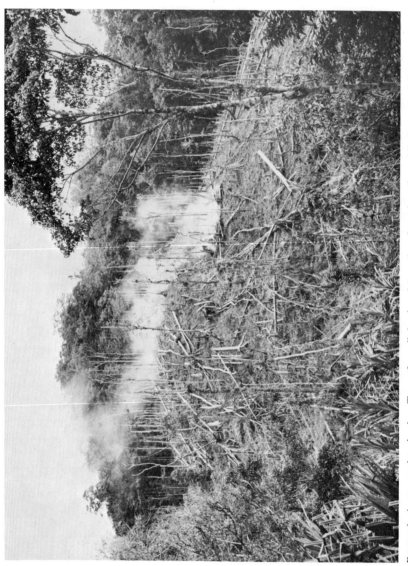

FIGURE 1. A new garden clearing. Trees of a well-developed secondary forest have been felled or pollarded preparatory to establishing a garden. Some of the debris is burned; much of it is left on the ground, adding to the store of organic matter in the top soil horizons. After crops are planted, the garden will be attended to for about a year. After that, weedy regrowth will be allowed to take over the site, beginning the cycle of rejuvenating fallow. Some garden plants—such as bananas, manioc, sugar cane and pawpaw—continue to yield among the regrowth so that production trails off only gradually for another year or more.

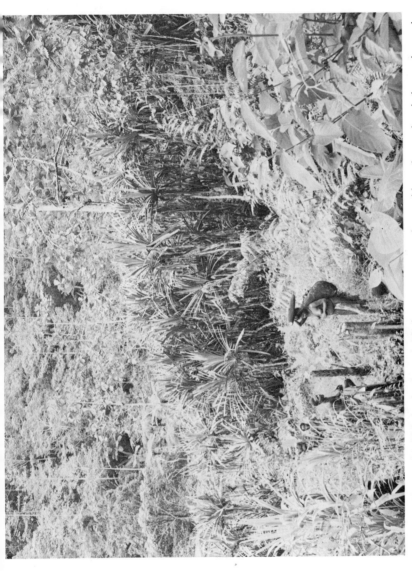

FIGURE 2. The mosaic of Maring land use. A Maring woman returns home with garden produce in her net bag and a *Pandanus* fruit on her head. A short distance behind her is an orchard of *Pandanus*, breadfruit and *Gnetum gnemon* trees. Such orchards produce for decades, yielding edible fruits, seeds and leaves as well as useful fibres. The only maintenance they require is an occasional clearing of the undergrowth. In the left foreground is a garden fence; in the enclosed garden to the left of the fence is a mature mixture of many of the Maring's crops. On the slope in the background is well-developed secondary forest.

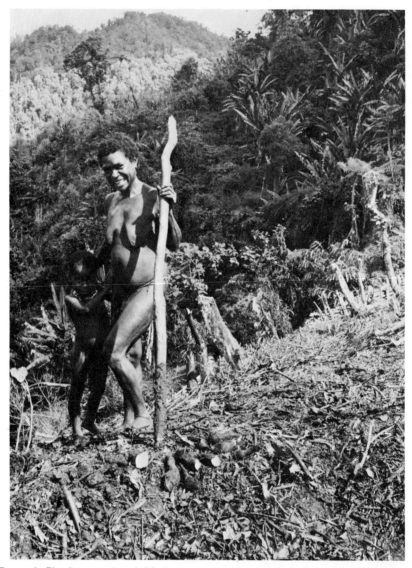

Figure 3. Planting a garden. A Maring woman and her daughter are engaged in planting a section of a newly cleared site. With her heavy dibble, her only tool, the woman pivots out in the litter-covered soil a hole suitable for inserting each of the tuber stocks seen on the ground in front of her. The source of the tubers is a now mature or ageing garden planted previously; thus the stock of crops flows from garden to garden as the gardens themselves move from site to site. In the background is a mosaic of different stages of regrowth vegetation serving to build up soil fertility and as a source of raw materials and a habitat for useful animal life.

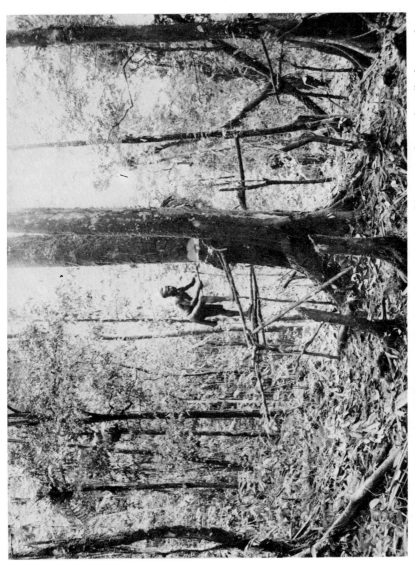

FIGURE 4. Clearing for a garden. A Maring man fells a large forest tree as part of the process of preparing a site for a garden. Given a long fallow period (possible with a low population density), the same sort of forest will again grow on the site after gardening and so sustain conditions favourable for a system of shifting cultivation with a low input of human energy.

by which some properties of systems remain unchanged even as other properties are changing (Vayda and McCay, 1975, p. 298).

Thus it was that though I saw the Bomagai-Angoiang as functioning in a less nicely regulated and balanced way than Rappaport conceived for the nearby Tsembaga, I was impressed by what I took to be the potential of all the Maring groups for continued existence—that is, for permanence. Only recently touched by the influence of the Western, industrial world, the Maring had existed previously for centuries or millennia with stone-age habits and technologies (see Figures 1–4); under the same conditions their survival could be projected far into the future, whereas the habits and technologies of the industrial world pointed to imminent collapse. In the light of this contrast, the Bomagai-Angoiang appeared as a balanced community on the fringe of a madhouse; and as I came near the end of writing my description of their subsistence system, I found rising within me a conclusion that was the reverse of standard ideas about economic development.

> It is an irony that while the Bomagai-Angoiang still live in a relatively stable ecosystem they are becoming so impressed and intrigued by the artifacts of the outside world's plundering economy that they feel that they can only learn from that world, that they have nothing to teach it in return. (Clarke, 1971, p. 196)

III. THE PRINCIPLES OF PERMANENCE

Because the Bomagai-Angoiang have little to offer in the way of explicit statements as to what gives their ecosystem the property of resilient permanence, we must look directly at the system's structure and function in order to derive principles of permanence. Seven such principles are briefly discussed in the following paragraphs.

One, the Bomagai-Angoiang strategy of agriculture is "palaeotechnic" rather than "neotechnic", in the sense that it is not dependent on an energy subsidy or extra-system nutrient sources. As described in detail in Clarke (1971), the Bomagai-Angoiang are classic shifting cultivators who utilize forest to inhibit weeds and erosion, to maintain soil structure and fertility at levels adequate for intermittent crop production, and to provide materials and supplementary sources of food (Figures 1 and 2). Locally captured solar radiation provides the energy for the trophic structure; and all nutrients are internal to the system except for a small, natural input and output associated with rainfall and the outflow of streams. The inherent permanence of such a system contrasts clearly with the precarious security of neotechnic systems with their breached nutrient cycles and their requirement for artificial extra-system inputs from an ever-dwindling reserve. Papers by Manners (1974) and Groth (1975) provide recent details on this as well as other neotechnic dangers discussed below.

Two, Bomagai-Angoiang agricultural behaviour is not self-poisoning. As is now widely acknowledged for the ecosphere, hyper-pollution provides a limit to growth even if energy supply does not. The plant–soil complex is unable to use, hold or recycle fully the massive inputs of fertilizer associated with neotechnic agriculture. The resulting outflow, together with the intentional biotoxins applied to control crop pests, diseases and weeds, is a poisonous or eutrophic component in ecosystems that include neotechnic agricultures. Bomagai-Angoiang agriculture has no comparable toxic flow, and the waste products of their agriculture are promptly assimilated back into the local organic complex.

Three, net energy yields of Bomagai-Angoiang agriculture are strongly positive. For Tsembaga agriculture, Rappaport (1971, p. 127) estimated normal ratios of garden yield to labour input at from 18–20 to one. That is, for every calorie of energy they invested, the Tsembaga received 18–20 calories of food energy—a return similar to that of the Bomagai-Angoiang. Hodder (1973, pp. 97–98) has summarized several other examples of the relatively high energy returns of palaeotechnic shifting cultivation. Steinhart and Steinhart (1974) expand the comparison from shifting cultivation through more intensive palaeotechnic agricultures to the most intensive neotechnic food-supply systems of the U.S.A., which require 5–10 calories of fuel-supplied energy to obtain one food calorie; that is, a negative energy yield. It is further reported (Pimentel et al., 1973) that food-related energy use is continuing to increase in the U.S.A., whose style of "productive" agriculture is presented as a model for regions that have a lower yield per hectare or per farmer hour but still have a positive yield of energy. Making the situation even more threatening in both energetic and environmental terms is the diminishing return associated with increasing neotechnic inputs. Doubling yields often requires many times as great an increase in inputs of fertilizer, energy, pesticides and other technological inputs (Groth, 1975; Hewitt and Hare, 1973, p. 30). Such a relationship is only one facet of the general decline in efficiency levels that comes with economic development and increasing energy consumption per capita (Jackson, 1975). Although they now have a high value productivity, the high input systems cannot be permanently maintained because of Odum's law (Odum, 1973) that net energy is the only energy with true value to society. Until recently, of course, the Bomagai-Angoiang thought of their agricultural system only in terms of an energy budget, not a cash-return budget, and had no choice but to accept Odum's law if they were to survive into the following year.

Four, Bomagai-Angoiang agriculture utilizes the products of bound time but only within the scale of a human life and only within the absorptive capacity of the existing ecosystem. All ecologists know that a mature natural ecosystem such as a tropical forest uses its photosynthetic product largely for maintenance (e.g. Golley, 1972, p. 79). But the complex organization and sizeable biomass of the forest are the result of an accumulation of negentropy through time, the time required for plant succession to move toward maturity. The Bomagai-Angoiang make use of this time-binding process when they fell the forest (Figure 4) and incorporate the effects of plant succession into their gardens (Figure 3). It is this process that makes their agriculture less labour demanding then an intensive palaeotechnic system such as wet rice cultivation, which lacks fossil-fuel technology and whose space is too densely populated to permit palaeotechnic time-binding. This is to say, neotechnic fossil-fuel technology is time-binding on a geologic scale; it makes possible the dedication of immature neotechnic ecosystems to output rather than to maintenance. The concentration of the unabsorbable products of time also causes the ecosystemic distortions that we know as environmental problems. The palaeotechnic Bomagai-Angoiang, on the other hand, proceed more closely along the lines of natural ecosystems and use time-bound products and conditions on a small scale as an aid to self-maintenance within a matrix of maturity. Such a process ensures permanence in comparison with the neotechnic operation. As Margalef (1968, p. 29) put it in writing on the concept of succession, "The structures that endure through time are those most able to influence the future with the least expense of energy."

Five, the energy moving through the Bomagai-Angoiang ecosystem is fairly evenly spread among the human population. Within the acephalous Bomagai-Angoiang community, control of resources is widely dispersed, and their palaeotechnic method of production is predominantly land- or labour-dependent. They have few alternatives to the use of their labour, but in many respects individuals are autonomous. Little energy is required to preserve social or economic coherence because the socio-economic structure is lateral rather than hierarchical. In less egalitarian societies, which have created specialized channels for high energy flows from outside the system and which have shifted their purpose from production for maintenance to consumption, there is a loss of autonomy at both the individual and national levels as the coherence of systems and subsystems increases. Rappaport, in a paper that has stimulated my chain of thought here, elaborates of the relationship.

> With loss of local self-sufficiency there is also loss of local regulatory autonomy, and the homeostatic capacity lost from the local system is not adequately replaced by increasingly remote centralized regulators responding to increasingly aggregated and simplified variables through operations increasingly subject to cybernetic impedances and time aberrations. Moreover, the responses of the distant regulators are often to factors extraneous to some of the local systems affected by them. For instance, changes in oil prices threaten to cause starvation in India by reducing the production of Japanese fertilizer upon which Indian agriculture depends. The coherence of the world system increases to dangerous levels as the self-sufficiency of local systems is reduced and their autonomy destroyed and replaced by more centralized agencies whose operations are inadequate to the regulation of the complex systems over which they preside. Hypercoherence is, of course, encouraged by advances in high energy technologies of production, transport, processing and communication, but money also abets it by imposing upon the diversity of the world the specious simplicity of a single metric which forces all things into apparent commensurability. (Rappaport, 1947)

Flannery (1972) in a paper on the cultural evolution of civilizations has evoked hypercoherence as one of the universal "pathologies" that can lead to the collapse and devolution of civilizations. Approaching from the direction of present-day economic development, Brookfield reaches a related conclusion

> As society and economy are enlarged in the course of development, as communities trade autarky for access to a wider range of goods and services, new and coarser patterns of resource evaluation and selection replace the older, finer patterns. Specialization replaces diversity; economic risk is added to natural risk. (Brookfield, 1975, p. 208)

Six, especially before European contact, the Bomagai-Angoiang looked on their resources as productive capital to be preserved. They saw secondary forest regrowth as a "garden mother", that is, as something out of which would issue later sustenance. In their garden management they practiced a selective weeding that gave tree seedlings a head start in plant succession, for they knew the benefits that came from rapid regrowth of forest (Figures 1–4). They preserved for their children a habitat and set of resources only slightly modified from what they had inherited themselves and they foresaw their children carrying on the same tradition. Except for what was probably a gradual shift toward grassland,* the Bomagai-Angoiang bore immedi-

---

* Clarke (1966) outlines the increased labour input that comes in New Guinea with a shift from forest- to grass-dominated spontaneous vegetation.

ately or within their shallow time-binding operations the whole cost of production rather than passing it on to "... those conveniently voiceless unfortunates, the future generations ..." (Anderson, 1974, p. 268). Of course, short-term profit at the expense of the future had little meaning to the Bomagai-Angoiang because they had no backflow of money to stimulate output. Once their basic needs for food and shelter were satisfied, wants having to do with prestige, social relations, and entertainment were constricted by the limited variety and productive capacity of their palaeotechnic life. What they wanted they could make or get by local trade without borrowing from their descendants' resources.

Seven, Bomagai-Angoiang subsistence is based on poly-culture and diversity. Their gardens and household plantings contain over three dozen species of food-producing plants, and many of the species contain a number of varieties. Wild forest and planted orchards provide other foods as well as a habitat for wild animals. As is typical of forest-dwelling shifting cultivators, the Bomagai-Angoiang plant their many crops in an intricately mixed, several-layered arrangement; segregated stands of a single species are unknown (Figures 2 and 3). The gardens too are separated from each other within a spontaneous mixture of primary forest and secondary vegetation in various stages of regrowth. The advantages of such poly-cultural diversity as an agricultural strategy are well known: protection against the epidemic spread of crop diseases and pests; fuller utilization of solar radiation and soil nutrients; a variety of foods, providing better nutrition and a more interesting diet than that obtained from a single staple; and a phased harvest of different crops over several months or longer. In ecosystemic terms, diversity is another way of saying maturity, which—according to many authorities—implies stability and resistance to perturbation. Economic disadvantages listed for poly-cultural agriculture are that its destandardized variety prevents or makes less effective the use of machinery and some other neotechnic inputs and that it is unsuitable for cash cropping. Consequently, reduction of diversity generally accompanies economic development (Janzen, 1973). In the case of peoples as remote from modern transport as the Bomagai-Angoiang, the use of machinery is an unlikely effect of Western influence, but cash cropping can penetrate. Indeed, its introduction to such peoples is encouraged as a way to tie their previously self-sufficient system to the putative benefits of the economically developed world. Because cash moves into the ecosystem in return for only one or two particular crops, these often come to dominate the agricultural system. Poly-cultural diversity is replaced by a trend toward the mono-culture that brings the cash necessary to meet at least in part the demand for extra-system goods and for foods produced elsewhere with an energy subsidy. The resilience imparted by local diversity gives way to an extenuated structure that is liable to breakage at several points.

IV. THE STRUCTURE OF PERMANENCE

It is the argument of this essay that the principles of permanence manifest in the Bomagai-Angoiang's ecosystem can contribute towards solutions of present-day ecological problems, but obviously not on the level of direct imitation. Even if practically possible, few persons now caught up in the neotechnic world would want to become palaeotechnic shifting cultivators; and when palaeotechnic man learns of the neotechnic world, he generally wants to join—a warning to us not to romanticize the palaeotechnic. As poets or philosophers we commend the intimate links between man, place and artifact in the palaeotechnic world; as ecologists we admire the resilient permanence of some of its ecosystems. But it has its own set of debilitating and disabling diseases, its discomforts, its high infant mortality, its often far from ideal nutrition, its own kinds of environmental problems, and its comparatively limited opportunities. There is no reason why palaeotechnic man should hold to these in the face of neotechnic promises of a better life. The admired permanence of some palaeotechnic systems of production results from lack of power, not from the ethnical moderation of the systems' managers.

But we, as observers from the neotechnic world, always come back to that permanence, that longevity: palaeotechnic agricultural systems such as the Bomagai-Angoiang's have gone on for 10 000 years or more, neotechnic agriculture is showing signs of a breakdown after not many decades. What is the essence of palaeotechnic permanence? Is there some sort of structural difference between permanent and impermanent systems of production? We must try to find such knowledge and apply it to our future if we want to survive with dignity. Because (Beer, 1972, p. 184): "If we do not, the future will happen to us. We shall not like it".

What I see now as the essential structural difference between the two sorts of systems is represented in Figure 5. Model ecosystem A summarizes the seven principles of permanence; ecosystem B shows the processes and results of their violation. In ecosystem A the grid lines represent the only significant input of energy—an almost even income and fairly even utilization of solar radiation throughout the

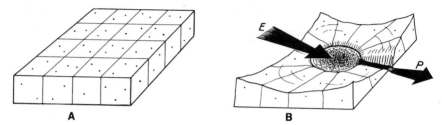

FIGURE 5. Representation of energy distribution in two ecosystems. A. Model of an ecosystem with a homogeneous distribution of energy. B. Model of an ecosystem showing the distortion and pollution (P) resulting from a large, concentrated input of energy (E) from terrestrial sources.

system. Solar energy is extra-terrestrial in origin, free, abundant but not concentrated. It is a gentle rain everywhere in the system. Because of its characteristics, there is no control necessary to import or distribute solar energy and so there is no inequality created by its use. The points in model A represent organisms or nodes of energy capture and consumption; these could be plants, animals, man or his economic activities. In accord with the even availability of energy, these nodes are fairly evenly distributed. They and the ecosystem's subsystems— represented by the cubes formed by the intersecting grid lines—are relatively autonomous, which gives the opportunity for the build up of a diversified local organization to utilize fully the local energy rain. Because the energy topography of the whole system is smooth, pooled accumulations of waste from energy use—pollution, that is—are unlikely. Some transformations of energy may be concentrated (as in the transport and subsequent burning of fuel wood) but not beyond the capacity of the system to absorb and disperse. Because there is no energy subsidy, the system must be adapted to survive on solar income, which can be considered as permanently available.

In model B a terrestrial source of neotechnic energy has been tapped and imported into the ecosystem. The result of this input is distortion and simplification. The grid lines of solar-energy use converge toward the centre of distribution of the terrestrial energy as local people together with their energy-consuming activities are attracted to the energy concentration—consider migration to cities. Put in other words, the energy topography is distorted downward toward the point of terrestrial energy input, resulting in an erosion or slippage of local energy and people toward the centre of the basin. What economists call "growth poles" can also be seen as "energy sinks". Brookfield, writing more from the point of view of economics or economic geography, clearly describes the process represented by model B

The essential fact of development has been the creation of a worldwide interconnected system, which has facilitated much higher levels of adaptation and far more complex systems of allocation and redistribution. Any redistributive system must have nodes, which can be viewed in social, economic or geographical space. The holders of these nodes have become dependent on the network and its flows, but have compensated this dependence by acquiring control over the allocation of scarce resources and production—that is, power. Among the scarce goods have been innovations of many kinds, which have been integrated into the system by entrepreneurs with such a distribution as to increase control, wealth and power in certain nodes. These 'growth poles' have become the locus of an increasing measure of control, leading to the progressive marginalization of the rest of the network. Adaptation to scarcity has thus taken the form of alleviating scarcity for some at the cost of increasing its relative impact on others. (Brookfield, 1975, p. 206)

Put in an evolutionary framework, it is clear that the process of gaining control of concentrated terrestrial energy can be seen as adaptive for particular individuals, corporations, peoples and nations. They have been able to consume energy and expand at the expense of others. As Rappaport (1974) points out, White's "basic law of cultural evolution" that "culture evolves as the amount of energy harnessed per capita per year is increased" does accord in a general way with mankind's experience—and with the history of who dominates whom. But man's experience is short in evolutionary terms, and the span of neotechnic evolution, which has so enchanted most economists, is far shorter. Some biologists and ecological anthropologists are now questioning the belief that success in competition for energy necessarily indicates the most successful mechanism of adaptation. Survival may also depend on other attributes that use little energy (Vayda and McCay, 1975). Eventually, this view will be forced on neotechnic man in the face of the high costs that more and more accompany the much praised low prices that neotechnic production has been able to bring. Economists such as Mishan (1969) have already demonstrated the harmful gap between low prices and the high cost of economic development.

To summarize the costs illustrated in model B.

a. Simplification. The energy input, which is associated with profit maximization, encourages simplification. Diversified adaptive processes and knowledge as well as actual genetic resources drain out of the ecosystem as cash flow stimulates mono-culture and other forms of standardization.

b. Accelerated entropy. Degrading energy and materials is a necessary part of life, but with neotechnic processes man carries it to extremes. Scarce, concentrated energy and materials are used at such a rate that the structure of the system is warped. If the high flow of energy is cut off, the system must contain more entropy than before and will be less able to utilize the abundant solar energy for which scarce terrestrial energy was temporarily substituted.

c. Social distortions. Along with the loss of autonomy and equality already mentioned come other social distortions such as alienation, which includes the sense of loss of control and purpose that unites individuals to their society. There is now a recognition of the need to redistribute the benefits and power that have come with high energy technology or that high energy technology has caused to be restricted to certain segments of society—witness the concern for social justice and rural improvement. But attempts to bring about redistribution require further energy inputs because the flow must be uphill against the gravity of the distorted energy topography—hence one reason for the common argument that we must use more resources to achieve a more equable world.

d. Hyper-pollution. Waste from the concentrated use of neotechnic energy and materials accumulates in a pool of pollution, which poisons both the local system and larger parts of the ecosphere. As with social distortions, so it is frequently argued with regard to hyper-pollution that we need still more energy in order to dispose of the pollution. This is like advising a fat man to lose weight by eating more so that he will have more energy to exercise more in order to lose weight.

V. FROM THE MARING TO THE WORLD

My main purpose in this essay has been to explore the structure of permanence in the hope that I could make a contribution toward creating an image to help guide neotechnic man toward a less precarious way of life. The exploration was based on the contrast of a relatively stable ecosystem inhabited by a small community of Papua New Guinean gardeners with the unstable ecosystem inhabited by neotechnic man. I argued that the first exhibited relative but not static permanence, whereas the second exhibits a trend toward breakdown because of the distorting stresses that neotechnic energy use puts on the structure of permanence. I have implied that the most valuable contribution that human ecologists may now be able to make to mankind's welfare will come from attempts to abstract from their studies of small communities principles that can be related to larger systems of human life. I used above the phrase "an image to help guide neotechnic man" because I believe there is a need for a sort of utopian purpose. By this I mean not a detailed design for an unworkably happy society but only some general goals that could be used as compass directions in a move to restructure our ideas on the relations between man and environment. The going itself is not enough—as it seems to be in societies obsessed with progress. There must be a goal, a possible and desirable destination. But at this stage to press for anything more specific than a set of principles or a general goal would be self-defeating because its implementation would require too great a diversion of energy for control and for countering resistance to changes in power relationships. Besides, I think Bateson's (1972) cautions against actions that are too purposeful must be taken seriously. As Slobodkin has written of Bateson's work

> . . . Bateson develops the distinction between 'purposeful' action (in the sense of solving a discrete problem) and 'ecological' action (in the sense of dealing with problems in their full context). Thus instead of the solution to one problem becoming a more difficult problem than the one it was meant to solve, the entire self-regulating system in its full ramification is considered. If this is done, many problems drastically change their character. (Slobodkin, 1974, p. 70)

This is to say that the first step has to do with our minds rather than with manipulation of the external world, for—as Hardin (1968) has so eloquently argued with regard to the population problem—there is no technical solution. The application of more energy will not help. A new world must begin with a new mind; if the image is strong enough, our successors will be able to work out the details as they go.

Certain necessities are already clear and have been discussed in many recent works, such as those by Taylor (1972), Odum (1969), Goldsmith *et al.* (1972) and Groth (1975). Most of the proposals point at least to some degree toward what Taylor (1972, p. 209) called "the paraprimitive society", by which he meant not an impossible return to the pure primitive but ". . . a society which tries to combine the advantages of primitive group structure with those of technology". A few of the specific necessities for the paraprimitive society are stated here.

One, a lower material standard of living than that of industrial nations. Of course, less neotechnic production means a higher standard of living in terms of unpolluted food, air and water.

Two, a slower rate of technological change, which implies a lowered energy need as well as offering several other advantages.

Three, decentralization of power and production and formation of smaller communities. Opinions vary as to optimum size of communities (Taylor, 1972, p. 212), but most authorities would agree with Rappaport (1971, p. 131) that small autonomous systems are more sensitive to ecological problems than larger, more complex organizations.

Four, changed education to develop a changed relation between man–man and man–nature. The central theme for this changed education is expressed differently by different authors but always revolves around the change from an exploitative I–It (subject–object) relationship to an I–Thou reciprocal relationship—that is, a change from man in unilinear control of nature to man within an ecosystem.

Five, limitation of population growth.

Six, moves in the direction of palaeotechnic agriculture; for example: less intensive agricultural technology, poly-culture, more diversified cropping patterns, substitution of land for artificial fertilizer, more organic fertilizer, acceptance of lower yields per unit of land, more of a live-and-let-live relationship with insects. See Dickinson (1972) and Groth (1975) for a full discussion of these and other suggested changes in neotechnic agriculture.

Seven, maintenance and deliberate creation of varied environments. Margalef (1968, p. 50) believes that the best solution to the dilemma of exploitation in opposition to conservation is ". . . a balanced mosaic, or rather a honeycomb, of exploited and protected areas". Odum (1969, p. 268) argues for a similar compartmentalization ". . . so that growth-type, steady-state, and intermediate type ecosystems can be linked with urban and industrial areas for mutual benefit". In other words, few ecologists believe that man should or successfully can "seize control of nature". We must disintensify, leave a few untended corners. Golley writes in this regard

We are a part of cybernetic systems (ecosystems) just like any other living population. Since, by definition, cybernetic systems operate by error control, we can expect that we will err in our interactions with other parts of the biosphere. If this is true, then it is illogical, indeed it is suicidal, to think that we can bring the biosphere under our control and provide the management to maintain biosphere stability. Man has always relied on the nonhuman parts of the biosphere to repair mistakes in ecosystem management and to provide control of human numbers. If we wish to live in a biosphere similar to that present today or present in the past, we must limit our control of the biosphere, so that sufficient unmanaged habitats and areas exist to provide the plants, animals, and microorganisms necessary in repair processes. We must preserve the repair processes to bring the system back to an equilibrium and permit us to start over again. (Golley, 1972, p. 89)

In conclusion, I return to my earlier remark that it is ironic that the Bomagi-Angoiang and similar palaeotechnic groups believe they have nothing to teach the neotechnic world. In studying their long-lived ecosystems, human ecologists have seen all the principles of permanence discussed or implied in this paper. Now that all over the world communities like the Bomagai-Angoiang are disappearing as "victims of progress' (Bodley, 1975), the task remaining is to apply these principles and to build into the neotechnic-dominated ecosphere a structure of permanence. If we do not, we will all—neotechnic and palaeotechnic alike—become victims of progress.

VI. REFERENCES

Anderson, E. (1974). The Life and Culture of Ecotopia. *In* "Reinventing Anthropology" (Ed. D. Hymes). Vintage Books, New York, pp. 264–283.

Bateson, G. (1972). "Steps to an Ecology of Mind". Ballantine Books, New York.

Beer, S. (1972). Management in Cybernetic Terms. *In* "Scientific Thought". UNESCO, Paris, pp. 167–185.

Bodley, J. (1975). "Victims of Progress". Cummings, Menlo Park, California.

Brookfield, H. (1973). Full Circle in Chimbu: A Study of Trends and Cycles. *In* "The Pacific in Transition: Geographical Perspectives on Adaptation and Change" (Ed. H. Brookfield). Edward Arnold, London, pp. 127–160.

Brookfield, H. (1975). "Interdependent Development". Methuen, London.

Buchbinder, G. (1973). Maring Microadaptation: A Study of Demographic, Nutritional, Genetic and Phenotypic Variation in a Highland New Guinea Population. Ph.D. Dissertation, Columbia University.

Clarke, W. (1966). From extensive to Intensive Shifting Cultivation: A Succession from New Guinea. *Ethnology* **5**, 347–359.

Clarke, W. (1971). "Place and People: An Ecology of a New Guinean Community". University of California Press, Berkeley and Los Angeles.

Dickinson, J. (1972). Alternatives to Monoculture in the Humid Tropics of Latin America. *Prof. Geog.* **24**, 217–222.

Flannery, K. (1972). The Cultural Evolution of Civilizations. *Ann. Rev. Ecol. Systematics* **3**, 399–426.

Goldsmith, E. *et al.* (1972). A Blueprint for Survival. *Ecologist* **2**, no. 1, 1–43.

Golley, F. B. (1972). Energy Flux in Ecosystems. In "Ecosystem Structure and Function" (Ed. J. A. Wiens). Oregon State University Press, pp. 69–90.

Groth, E. (1975). Increasing the Harvest. *Environment* **17**, no. 1, 28–39.

Hall, A. D. and Fagen, R. E. (1956). Definition of System. *Gen. Syst. Yearbook* **1**, 18–28. (Reprinted in W. Buckley 1968, Ed.) "Modern Systems Research for the Behavioral Scientist". Aldine, Chicago.

Hardin, G. (1968). The Tragedy of the Commons. *Science* **162**, 1243–1248.

Hewitt, K. and Hare, K. (1973). "Man and Environment: Conceptual Frameworks". (Commission of College Geography, Resource Paper No. 20). Association of American Geographers, Washington, D.C.

Hide, R. (1974). On the Dynamics of Some New Guinea Highland Pig Cycles. Unpublished Ms.

Hodder, B. W. (1973). "Economic Development in the Tropics". (Second Edn) Methuen, London.

Jackson, R. T. (1975). In Praise of Burundi, Paraguay et al. Area 7, 83–86.

Janzen, D. H. (1973). Tropical Agroecosystems. Science 182, 1212–1219.

Leighly, J., ed. (1963). "Land and Life: A Selection from the Writings of Carl Ortwin Sauer". University of California Press. Berkeley and Los Angeles.

McArthur, M. (1974). Pigs for the Ancestors: A Review Article. Oceania 45, 87–123.

Manners, I. R. (1974). The Environmental Impact of Modern Agricultural Technologies. In "Perspectives on Environment" (Eds I. R. Manners and M. W. Mikesell). Association of American Geographers, Washington, D.C., pp. 181–212.

Margalef, R. (1968). "Perspectives in Ecological Theory". University of Chicago Press.

Mishan, E. (1969). "The Costs of Economic Growth". Penguin Books, Harmondsworth.

Odum, E. P. (1969). The Strategy of Ecosystem Development. Science 164, 262–270.

Odum, H. T. (1973). Energy, Ecology, and Economics. Ambio 2, 220–227.

Pimentel, D. et al. (1973). Food Production and the Energy Crisis. Science 182, 443–449.

Rappaport, R. (1967). "Pigs for the Ancestors: Ritual in the Ecology of a New Guinean People". Yale University Press, New Haven.

Rappaport, R. (1971). The Flow of Energy in an Agricultural Society. Scient. Am. 224, no. 3, 116–132.

Rappaport, R. (1974). Energy and the Structure of Adaptation. Presented at 140th Annual Meeting of the American Association for the Advancement of Science, San Francisco.

Schumacher, E. F. (1974). "Small is Beautiful: A Study of Economics as if People Mattered". Abacus, London.

Slobodkin, L. (1974). Mind, Bind, and Ecology: A Review of Gregory Bateson's Collected Essays. Hum. Ecol. 2, 67–74.

Steinhart, J. S. and Steinhart, C. E. (1974). Energy Use in the U.S. Food System. Science 184, 307–316.

Taylor, G. (1974). "Rethink". Penguin Books, Harmondsworth.

Vayda, A. P. (1971). Phases of the Process of War and Peace among the Marings of New Guinea. Oceania 42, 1–24.

Vayda, A. P. and McCay, B. J. (1975). New Directions in Ecology and Ecological Anthropology. Ann. Rev. Anthrop. 4, 293–306.

Waddell, E. (1972). "The Mound Builders: Agricultural Practices, Environment, and Society in the Central Highlands of New Guinea". University of Washington Press, Seattle.

CHAPTER XIII

Scientific and Indigenous Papuan Conceptualizations of the Innate: A Semiotic Critique of the Ecological Perspective

ROY WAGNER

University of Virginia, Virginia, U.S.A.

I. SCIENCE AND PARADOX

Researchers in both the life sciences and the social sciences have come increasingly to face an extremely interesting dilemma. The terms in which this dilemma is perceived and negotiated are as diverse as the many particular lines of empirical inquiry and theoretical formulation that ecologists, biologists, ethologists, anthropologists and others pursue. Yet the dimensions of the problem are so nearly analogous in every specific field of inquiry that it becomes difficult to avoid or postpone the conclusion that the issue itself is of a semiotic or epistemological nature, and that it bears quite as much upon the limitations of our own scientific enterprise as upon those inherent in the subject matter.

In the most abstract terms, the problem is the old one of unity and diversity, the general or the universal as against the particular, the collective versus the individual, though it may be refracted into scarcely less abstract issues such as that of boundaries and their permeability, or that of cultural relativity. Put very crudely, the issue poses the following paradox: the more discretely and specifically we define and bound the units of our study, the more provocative, necessary, and difficult it becomes to account for the relationships among those units; conversely, the more effectively we are able to analyse and sum up the relationships among a set of units, the more provocative, necessary, and difficult it becomes to define the units.

The obvious example of this paradox within the field of biology is the issue of speciation. The acknowledged objectives (as well as the scholarly aesthetic) of taxonomy require a comprehensive and unambiguous classification of organisms according to certain pre-established parameters. But the implementation of a programme of classification invariably leads into problems involving relationships among the "types" being identified. The relationships may involve structural analogies and homologies, geographical distribution, behaviour and the criterion of viable interbreeding, and they may indeed sum all of these in a putative evolutionary reconstruction. The form, content, and significance of these relationships may vary according to the specific schema one adopts, and yet however neatly one manages to fit empirical data into taxonomic boxes, there is always a relational residuum. Indeed, we might conclude that the relationships, taxonomically registered or otherwise, are precipitated by the very attempt to demarcate and particularize species. Speciation renders evolution (as well as a whole host of other relational arrangements) visible; evolution, on the other hand, the process by which species arise from other species, or merge across specific boundaries, renders a comprehensive speciation non-viable.

The alternative (and one much favoured in ecological approaches) has been to capitalize on relationships, including the flow of evolution "in process", and speak of continua of species, intermediate types, and emergent phenomena. Although this may indeed be the preferred alternative for a scientific community whose interests have shifted in favour of integration, it should be stressed that the ecological, evolutionary interest owes much of its force and conviction to its innovative advantage over the earlier, taxonomic effort. It answers the questions and uncertainties posed by a previous stance of the discipline, but it achieves relational precision at the expense of taxonomic precision. The sacrifice appears to be less serious than it might be only because our civilization has developed an extraordinary tolerance for the generalities and ambiguities of "system" and "process". (We speak of the "omnimal", that marvellous creature that has adapted in a plastic manner to all conceivable environments; but an omnimal is precisely what any given, specific creature is not.)

The situation in present day anthropology is scarcely very different.

The tendency in traditional anthropology has been to set up units—descent groups, segments, families and ultimately cultures—and to classify and analyse these units and their interrelationships. But the experience of anthropological researchers in the last few decades has been that, as one progresses, the interrelationships come to be vastly more interesting, provocative, and significant than the units. An original concern with descent types and corporate groups, the "recruitment" of individuals to marked social collectivities, gave way to mediating constructs like "filiation" (parental ties that encompass both recruitment and relational functions) and "non-unilineal descent" (a "type" of descent that cannot, by itself, form units). Finally an interest in exchange and reciprocity has led to the conclusion, for many, that these interrelational processes are more important than the units themselves, and even that reciprocity and exchange create units, rather than vice-versa. Likewise, an earlier interest in social categorization gave way to an obsession with the creative force of liminality, the "betwixt and between", process of transforming and interrelating categories.

The parallel with the problem of speciation is evident, save that here we are dealing with social, rather than natural, species. Even the hitherto sacrosanct notion of "culture" has been involved, for cultures are simply the most obdurate of the social species. They do not, in the classic sense of their definition, interbreed. But what does the fieldworker's much celebrated "communication" with his subjects amount to, then, if not some sort of miscegenation? Phenomenologically oriented anthropologists (and I am as guilty as anyone in this regard) have challenged the viability of the culture concept itself on communicational (hence interrelational) grounds. Once again, as in biology, the force of these newer approaches owes much to innovative advantage over an earlier stance of the discipline. And again, a significant sacrifice of precision is involved: to speak of a universal, transcultural flow of symbolization is to say very little of the specific contents and orientations of particular cultures, for it is the boundaries and specificity of these cultures that the communication dissolves.

The situation in both of my examples is strikingly reminiscent of a dilemma confronted by cosmologists earlier in the century: depending upon how one used their equations and formulae, one wound up either with a universe of matter with no motion, or a universe of motion with no matter. And this, too, recalls Heisenberg's Indeterminacy Principle, the conclusion that one can either ascertain the mass of an electron or the velocity of an electron with great precision, but one cannot do both simultaneously. It would seem, then, that science has reached this particular impasse before. Let us narrow our focus to an issue of more immediate relevance: that of the ecological notion of organism and environment.

Even when stripped of its cultic and naturalistic overtones ("environment" as non-culture, as natural pristinity), the concept of environment shares the conceptual limitations of pure relation. Defined as a sum total of things in interaction, as system, process, thermodynamic balance, it maintains a certain explicational integrity, though it tends to erode and engulf the "units" that make it up. (The organisms it subsumes are themselves environments, they are significant parts of their own environments, they are, so to speak, environments of their environment. One winds up with a large pile of peelings and no onion.) Defined in a stricter etymological sense, as "that which environs" and in contrast to some particular organism or set of organisms, it fixes an arbitrary boundary purely for the sake of analysis, and one that analysis then proceeds to break down. ("Organism" becomes a rather special kind of environment separated from a more general kind of environment by a permeable boundary, across which interaction of one sort or another flows. But interaction is also environment.)

Very well, then, these are word games. And although word games is the way Wittgenstein chose to sum up semiotic activity, and this is, after all, a semiotic discussion, I have been so busy with the definition (or perhaps un-definition) of environment that I have paid scant attention to what ecologists do with this notion. What ecologists do is a subject to which I shall presently return. But first, let me explore the concept environment in a more "legitimate" way.

For any given environment, it would seem, there is one thing or element that is more important than any other, and that is the thing, or things, that it environs (though all the things it environs are simply the environment itself). This is simply because environment is defined in relation to the environed, and because environment is a relational concept. Should the environed get up on its hind legs and waddle off, it could conceivably get itself a (largely) new environment. But even if it does nothing of the sort, its own presence and actions will play a large part in determining how its environment acts upon it, "relates" to it. And since environment is a relational concept, it follows that the environed generally plays a more or less significant part in creating its environment. Likewise, if the environed should suddenly develop a new adaptive advantage, like wings, or swimmerets, or x-ray vision, it is obvious that it would have played quite as much a part as the environment itself in creating a new "ecological niche".

The relation between environed and environment is paradoxical, as any relation must be where the part is cast in a linear, one-to-one relationship with the whole that encompasses it. And this, in brief, is the difficulty with a theoretical approach that employs reflexive, dialectical concepts within the linear, causal framework that the ideological assumptions of science and scientific methodology require. And it would scarcely be fair to imply the culpability of ecology in this respect without pointing out that the paradoxes posed by speciation and evolution, or culture and communication, render biology and anthropology equally vulnerable.

Scientists, however, are seldom enough troubled by the paradoxical aspects of their conceptual underpinnings. Taxonomists exist in contented symbiosis with ecologists, and exponents of the culture concept even intermarry with radical phenomenologists (though they all have their bad days). This is because it is the business of science to "negotiate" its paradoxes, rather than to gleefully expose them, or even solve them. Established science, with its schools, its chairs, and its literatures, is a highly tentative and negotiably working "compromise", postponing the paradoxical implications of its ideas (or even contriving or subscribing to theories that deny them) so that it can get on with its work of empirically and experimentally negotiating them. The corpus of theory and knowledge that results may indeed be turgid and inconsistent, but at least there is a corpus of theory and knowledge.

None of this is intended as a condemnation or cynical dismissal of the scientific enterprise. What it portends is that this enterprise pertains, as any human semiotic activity pertains, to a particular world view or orientation, and that the world view or orientation of science has its bounding paradoxes. And if the enterprise of science should someday reform or re-orient itself, its nature as a human semiotic activity would require that the older paradoxes would simply be exchanged for new ones. Nor can I imagine any human activity or any human culture that is not so circumscribed. Paradox, though it may trouble us, is a deeply and universally human phenomenon; better: paradox is a universally human phenomenon precisely because it troubles us; and because its existence is essential to the "negotiation" that comprises human effort.

I am not oblivious to the fact that much of the scientific activity that addresses itself to these issues is carried on under the aegis of an empiricist, positivist, naturalist epistemology that would deny the significance or the existence of its paradoxes, and so deny the force of my argument. Indeed, I can scarcely imagine how it should do otherwise, for the non-recognition or downplaying of such paradoxes is essential to the task of negotiating them. Empiricism, positivism and naturalism belong to the world view of classical Western science, and its methodologies, assumptions and intentions are all in some sense derivative of them. The semiotic stance that I have taken, conversely, is a critique of world views, and although it manifests a "world view" of its own, and hence paradoxes of its own, it is forced by the very nature of its task to deal openly with paradox. It negotiates paradoxes by exposing them—even by creating them. And because this stance is committed explicitly to the negotiation of paradox through the exposure of paradox, it is imperative that we come to terms with (that we expose, in other words) the process by which the negotiation of paradox takes place also. It is true indeed that this insight has the potential of being exploited against the interests of science; but it is equally possible to employ it to the advantage of the scientific enterprise, which is what I hope to accomplish in this discussion.

II. THE ECOLOGY OF SYMBOLS

The core of the scientific paradox is a basic differentiation of semiotic modality that functions universally in meaningful construction. Every construction (and I include here acts of perception as well as expression or communication) that is realized through symbols may be analysed as the articulation of two semiotic modalities, which I shall simply contrast as "literal" and "figurative". Literal symbolization (also "indexic") denotes the combination of symbolic elements (as we combine words to make a sentence) into a total relational pattern, a "representation", that stands in a homologous and literally representational relationship to some "represented" context. This might be exemplified through the heuristic representation of natural regularities through the agency of artificially constructed ("discovered") scientific "laws". Literal constructions are relationally cohesive but contextually contrastive and dependent; like scientific laws they provide relation, but depend upon the (represented) context for substantiality and validation. Figurative symbolization (also "iconic" or "metaphorical") comprises the contrasting of symbolic elements (as we contrast the sounds or images of words, or those that make up words) as discrete entities, that combine or unite with their context but stand in a metaphorical or analogous relationship to one another. This might be exemplified by speciation: *Homo erectus* and *Homo sapiens* are (presumably) distinct species, but both belong to the genus *Homo*—they are, in this respect, analogous to one another. Figurative constructions are relationally contrastive but contextually cohesive; being self-contained, they provide substantiality, but depend upon the (incorporated) context for relation.

Literal usages denote things, objects, acts, ideas, in a conventional way, and also articulate such conventionally recognized phenomena together in terms of all manner of conventionally recognizable orders and paradigms. Thus "literal" might be used ("metonymically") in reference to the whole enterprise of conventional symbolic construction. But figurative usages necessarily contrast with literal ones, since they employ symbolic elements in non-conventional ways; by exempting themselves from conventional denominative orders, they pre-empt the representational facility and become self-representing. They "differentiate", as it were, in the most rigorous sense possible, by embodying the discreteness of individual differentiae as against conventional denomination.

It should be clear from the dependencies spelled out here that in order for any construction to be meaningful and coherent, the context of a literal expression must always be perceived as figurative, and the context of a figurative construction must always be perceived as literal. (I say "perceived" because semiotic characteristics are always imposed by human construction and are never "innate" in things.) Thus a construction is always either relating the perceptibly differentiated, or differentiating the perceptibly relational, from the standpoint of the actor. Because of the specific properties of these two modes of symbolization, a literal construction will always impose a boundary or contrast between itself (as "representor") and its context (as "represented"), whereas a figurative construction will assimilate its context.

I shall postulate that all human activity, whether it be "mental" or "physical", expressive or implementive, may be analysed into literal and figurative components, and that such analysis "contains" or "replicates" such empirical effects as "mind", "substance", and "motivation". The resolution into these components, or modalities, I shall argue, follows from the actor's conventional orientation to his world—his "world view". When the actor's intention is focussed upon "relating", he will perceive his action as a transformation of discrete phenomenal entities into a consistent relational pattern. The reflexive transformation (for every literally-oriented act has its figurative component), particularizing and differentiating the relational pattern, is perceived as emanating from sources other than the actor's intention. (It is perceived as an impinging motivation or resistance.) When the actor's intention is focussed upon differentiating, conversely, he will perceive his action as a transformation of relational continuity into differentiating distinctions, and apprehend the reflexive relational transformation—the "relating" of the context he assimilates—as emanating from sources beyond his intention. Thus all human action carries or contains its own implicit interpretation; that which the actor assumes responsibility for is intercepted by its own unacknowledged complement. Literal construction precipitates a covert figurative transformation, and figurative construction precipitates a covert literal transformation. Qualities, characteristics and motivating "forces" are invested in the context of human action quite independently of any putative properties that may be inherent in the context.

Perhaps a few lines of interpretation will help to clarify what must necessarily be a rather abstract explication. Literal symbolizations are "mere symbols", arbitrary or heuristic expressions that stand for referents other than themselves. We generally think of symbols in this way—as words, pictures, diagrams, models, etc. Figurative symbolizations correspond to things that we do not normally think of as symbols but rather perceive as pure phenomena—like individual persons, incidents, unique objects, and so forth. This is because figurative symbolizations are self-contained: they stand for themselves. As the philosopher G. Spencer Brown (1969) observes, "distinction is perfect continence". But it is also necessarily true that literal and figurative modes are completely interdependent. They "ground" each other, each being dependent upon the other for the complement to its own effect, and so each must always serve as the context for the other. Literal constructions are meaningless codings without the glossing of substantial referents, and the particular entities and events that are figurative constructions lose relatibility, and hence coherence, in the absence of a relational substratum. The precipitation of one modality by the other follows from the fact that their complementarity is essential to meaning. And the interpretive separation of one modality from the other, assuring that the actor's intention will conform to the lineaments of literal or figurative construction, but not both, or neither, or something else, emerges as a crucial factor in the construction of human experience.

This separation is always the effect of the literal component of action, whether in fact the literal mode corresponds to the deliberate intention of the actor or to the reflexive transformation that is precipitated as its context. The conventions of a culture, a people, a tradition or a discipline are always articulated literally; they build a consistent, collective ordering of things and define a set of shared associations by which this ordering becomes the meaningful centre of a common endeavour. As construction, however, they also draw a sharp distinction between the ordering they represent and its figurative complement. Thus the literal component of semiotic construction always separates itself off from the figurative, and this distinction maintains the separation of the two components. Anthropologists have taught us to call the shared, conventional ordering that pertains to a people their culture, and I shall have to add that the conventional separation entailed by a culture provides the essence of its semiotic orientation, or world view.

It provides, in other words, the determination of which semiotic component is to be conventionally understood as the province of human action and intention, and therefore also which is to be conventionally regarded as innate. To be sure, there are only two alternatives here, but they are alternatives that divide the whole world of human thought and action between them. A conventional ordering that determines its own articulation as the province of human action, like our Western notion of culture, precipitates figurative construction as the form of the innate; a conventional ordering that determines figurative symbolization as the province of human action precipitates itself and its entailed contextual distinction as the form of the innate. Both alternatives may be exemplified in existing human societies, and the implications of the semiotic inversion for human endeavour and behaviour are considerable (Wagner, 1975). But whichever modality an actor has come to regard as proper to his action, the consequences of "doing" the innate are severe, for he is obliged to work against the dictates of his own conventional orientation.

When viewed in the light of these observations, the paradox of science takes on a new significance. For it appears that this paradox is created by the aspirations of determinism to achieve knowledge and control of both components of semiotic construction and assimilate them simultaneously to a universal body of theory. If, as I have postulated, the activities of relating and defining are truly interdependent, and relative to one another, then any enterprise that aspires to pursue both of these modalities to some sort of unified, absolute and determinist conclusion is bound to reach a relativistic impasse. This is the substance of Heisenberg's Indeterminacy Principle. And it also poses the biologist's dilemma of speciation versus specific origin and interrelationship, and the anthropologist's problem of cultural discreteness and intercultural communication. The paradox of science may be apprehended in any one of a broad range of particular manifestations, but only because it derives from the invariant factor of human semiotic construction that is common to scientific endeavour in all subject areas.

Crucial as this paradox and its realization may be to certain expectations of the scientific outlook, my earlier discussion has indicated that the way in which the paradox is negotiated may be even more important. For it is this negotiation, taking one or another of the semiotic modalities as the province of one's deliberate action and responsibility, and relegating the other to the realm of the "given", that provides the potentialities and limitations of any particular scientific task. It is by subdividing in this way that science overcomes the immediate implications of its paradox, though of course this merely postpones the ultimate, universal implication. In a larger sense, then, we might expect the paradox to be negotiated for the "culture of science" in general, according to the world view of the Western society that it represents. And since the conventions that we call culture provide a centre and an orientation for symbolic construction in every human tradition, the possibility arises of drawing meaningful contrasts and comparisons between the semiotic parameters of scientific symbolization and those of symbolic construction among the peoples that scientists study.

III. THE SCIENTIFIC CONCEPTUALIZATION OF THE INNATE

The ethic and institutions of what we call Western society correspond to an ideological régime of deliberate and morally sanctioned literal construction. "Civilization", with its cities, technologies, literatures, bodies of knowledge and educated classes, is conceived and constituted as a cumulative aggregate of collective human artifice, and hence of deliberately articulated convention. We take collective responsibility for the preservation, regulation, alteration and implementation of the "culture" and social organization that gives us our orientation. Since the rise of constitutional government and the emergence of a rational and technological social order, this modality has infused our government as "democracy", and our scholarly life as "science".

One might even prefer the earlier term "natural philosophy" for this intellectual aspect of modern life, for it is addressed throughout the broad range of its conceptualization to a matrix of figurative transformation that we perceive and describe as "nature". Nature is the figurative and conventionally "innate" component of a totality of which our "culture of science" represents the literal and conventionally "artificial" component. This point may perhaps be clarified if we consider its semiotic implications. As a universal phenomenal exemplification of figurative construction (albeit a largely "precipitated" and perceived construction), natural phenomena have the spontaneous and self-contained character of standing for themselves. They merge object and event, but depend for their relational capabilities upon an assimilation of their literal context. Nature, in other words, is a flow of seemingly innate, differentiating transformation that is precipitated by our systematic and literal efforts at harnessing or understanding it.

Science, in its aspirations and experimental and theoretical formulations, provides the relational continuity that joins natural phenomena together as a palpable entity (or at least into discernible "forces", "effects", or "regularities"). Natural phenomena, for their part, appear as particular time-bound elements, though as figurative symbolizations they also assimilate the relational context that science provides for them, so that it appears that our heuristically conceived laws and formulaic descriptions are in fact replications of an innate order.

The literally conceived descriptions of science are thus necessarily "synchronic", and they effectively separate themselves off (as human artifice, "mere theory") from the allegedly innate world of precipitated differentiation that we speak of as natural phenomenon and event. The necessity of doing so, "artificializing" our theoretical formulations and hence "naturalizing" their literal complement, is the necessity of maintaining the semantic world view of our larger, rationalist civilization. Thus the illusion is maintained of an arbitrary, derivative human ordering or "coding" that is continually sustained and enveloped by its spontaneous, self-sufficient, and all-containing object. For moral and aesthetic reasons we strive to keep the artificial distinct and free from natural tendencies and temptations, but insist as we may upon the distinct character of cultural action, we are invariably forced to the conclusion that the cultural, too, is merely a part of nature. Whatever we do, we do as warm-blooded, mammalian animals, exemplifying natural effect in all of our actions. In our own terms, then, culture is nature harnessing nature, understanding nature, and coming to know itself.

But this is the paradox of environment and environed all over again: literal culture is the epitome of the environed, and figurative nature is the essence of the containing environment. The part is set against the whole that contains it, a paradox that is sustained by the perception that the nature we address embodies the relational order through which we comprehend it, and a paradox that is negotiated by the contextually isolating effect of literal construction. Positivist epistemology has generally favoured the notion of "levels", in the sense that the cultural is said to be an "abstraction from" nature—a replication of its "orders" via human artifice. I am arguing, however, that levels here are a product of the literal effect of contextual isolation, an artifact of semiotic construction, and hence inapplicable as an epistemological *a priori*. Levels are the distillate of one particular cultural world-view, assigning one semiotic component to the realm of the innate and the other to the province of human action and responsibility. The arbitration of this limit, forging a literalistic culture that continually separates itself off from a figurative nature that continually encompasses it, is the key to the "environment" problem. In fact, I shall argue that the distinction is itself non-locatable, that nature is as much abstraction from culture as the cultural is an abstraction from nature.

Just as nature "contains" every aspect of the cultural, so the semiotic construction proper to our orientation creates and contains everything that we have come to know or perceive as natural. Culture may be seen as the result of natural evolution, but nature and evolution themselves are products of cultural construction. We do not know "reality" except in symbolic terms, and the resulting shape of reality is very much a consequence of the symbolic terms through which it is conceptualized. We can, if we choose, resolve the particular tendencies and forces that have been adduced as evolutionary into properties of figurative construction. Thus the cells or organisms involved are construed as self-containing entities that "stand for" themselves, they stand in various sorts of analogous relationships to one another (various degrees of taxonomic relatedness, symbiotic arrangements, adaptational "mimicry" etc.), and "adapt" or create among themselves a homeostatic "balance of nature" by assimilating the relational context upon which their construction is predicated. Cultural (semiotic) construction and natural process completely contain or envelope one another; the "boundary" between them, and hence the determination of the innate, is negotiable—it is everywhere and nowhere. We are faced with the choice of which modality, literal or figurative, we wish to use as a basis for understanding the totality.

The ecological perspective emerges as an extremely interesting inversion of the traditional Western orientation in this regard. For ecology elects a viewpoint in which man and his culture are considered as natural, phenomenal organisms and systems in a world of other, similar organisms and systems. Especially since the work of Wynne-Edwards, the literal contextual separation between culture and nature has been abandoned in favour of a picture of analogous organism–culture complexes (of which man and his culture are one), whose collective interaction constitutes the environment. We are asked to think of ourselves as organisms, as part of the environment rather than as uniquely cultural beings distinct from it. Thus the modality of human responsibility is shifted: encouraged to act and think in figurative terms, we relegate the literal to the realm of the innate. We assimilate environment, as the relational substratum of our thoughts and actions, and yet, as precipitated literal relation, environment always manages to separate itself off as an objectified wholeness, a set of innate moral relations to be safeguarded and protected. Since I have ventured into the area of "cross-cultural" comparisons, I might suggest that environment becomes, in the ecological perspective, a kind of pan-biotic "superculture", an organic "ecumene" in which all the differentiated tribes, clans and nations have a part to play.

I have drawn this parallel self-consciously, in full awareness of the fact that collective cultures and ecumene embody explicit moral premisses, because I suspect that the ecologists' concept of environment (though not necessarily its empirical counterpart) is likewise a moral construct. In contrast to the innate differentiations (nature as discrete particularism) of the traditional rationalist orientation, the environment of the ecologists amounts to an innate moral collectivity. I shall argue that, by the terms of this inversion, the ecological perspective has come to approximate the semiotic orientation that is manifest in the world views or cosmologies of tribal peoples, including those of the Papuan area. Let us turn, then, to the indigenous Papuan conceptualization of the innate.

IV. INDIGENOUS PAPUAN CONCEPTUALIZATIONS OF THE INNATE

Elsewhere (Wagner, 1975, Chapter V) I have identified the semiotic orientation and "social self-invention" of tribal peoples with a régime of conscious and deliberate figurative construction, one that relegates the literal component of action to the realm of the innate. I realize, of course, that such a sweeping generalization can only touch upon the broadest parameters of cultural difference, ignoring many specific details of local symbolization, yet it is only on this broad basis that the sorts of comparisons I wish to make will emerge clearly. The innate world of Papuan peoples amounts to a transcendental image or realization of man and the conventional social order, one that "flows" more or less spontaneously in the world (as "time" and "event" flow for Westerners). It is immanent in man, other creatures and in the cosmos itself, and may not be "created" by human agency, but only tempered, constrained and invoked. It constitutes the thread, or strain of similarity and contiguity among all the diverse classes of beings that inhabit the world. What we are disposed to call "humanity" or "social relationship" is for Papuans the very ground of being; it is not a distinct property of man, but rather man's greatest resource.

The differentiated beings that inhabit this world are interrelated as analogous types, as the various taxa of biology are interrelated. They are, in other words, both similar to and different from one another, the similarities being considered as innate properties of being, and the differences being constituted as man's particular area of concern and responsibility. It is by maintaining a precise awareness of these differences, by differentiating himself and by differentiating the various beings in an appropriate manner, that man precipitates (or from the actor's viewpoint, invokes) a beneficent relational flow. Social life is a matter of maintaining such a flow between men and women, by cultivating and pursuing discrete sexual "lifestyles", and often a matter of pursuing the implications of age-grading and initiatory distinctions as well. Ritual life is a task of sustaining and renewing the differentiations between man and the other sorts of beings that inhabit the cosmos. The flow in the first instance is the thing that we recognize as human sociality, and in the second it is fertility, spiritual "power" and the "knowledge" of the diviner of shaman.

For the interior Papuan peoples whose cosmologies have been studied in recent years, the anthropomorphic innate is perceived as a flow of human potential across the physical diversity of the landscape. Adjacent space, above, below or laterally distinct from that of man and his gardens, is populated by spirit-beings, who are analogous to man but differ from him in bizarre though complementary ways. The discretion and ritual solicitude with which these personified aspects of man's physical surroundings are approached is strongly suggestive of the ecologist's attitude toward organisms other than man, in deference to the needs and qualities of the environment. Indeed, this parallel has been very successfully exploited in Rappaport's (1968) excellent study of the ritual and ecology of the Tsembaga Maring, a people living as swidden horticulturalists in the Simbai valley of the Bismarck range.

In one of the few studies that explores the cosmology of a central Highlands people in some detail, Rappaport discloses symbolic polarities that closely resemble those discovered by Salisbury among the Siane (Salisbury, 1965), and suggests a paradigm that may be widespread among speakers of the Eastern New Guinea Highlands stock of languages. The Tsembaga occupy land that ranges from 670 to 2200 metres above sea level, and that includes the adjacent spaces of *wora*, or low ground, and *kamungga*, or high ground in their terminology. Each of these spaces is seen as the abode of a distinct set of spirit-beings (*rawa*), of which the *rawa mai* belong to the *wora*, and the *rawa mugi* (red spirits) dwell in the *kamungga*. Each type of spirit embodies a vital and complementary principle. The *rawa mai* are said to be *kinim*, cold and wet, they are associated with femaleness and the lower part of the body, and are, in Rappaport's words, ". . . the spirits of a cycle in which life both terminates in and arises out of death" (Rappaport, 1968, p. 39). The *rawa mugi* are *romba nda*, "hot", and are associated with dryness, maleness and the upper part of the body—

indeed, they are the "ancestors", the spirits of Tsembaga who have been killed in warfare (Rappaport, 1968, pp. 39–40).

The sum of human vital and assertive potency is thus divided among the capacities and interests of two adjacent spirit peoples. Birth, fertility, death and illness are the province of the *rawa mai*, whereas the *rawa mugi* deal with the context of warfare and relations with other groups. But both sets of spirits are conceived anthropomorphically, as peoples to be dealt with morally in various ritual ways. Thus eels are said to be the "pigs" of the *rawa mai*, and marsupials and other upland game (*ma*) are the "pigs" of the *rawa mugi*. The trapping of eels and upland game that takes place before a pig-kill is conceived, in each case, as an "exchange of pigs" with the respective set of spirits: the Tsembaga take the "pigs" of the spirit people and offer the latter a chance to partake of the pork they have prepared. Human ability and potency originates as a flow across the boundaries that differentiate the complementary aspects of the cosmological whole. Ritual precautions in many cases involve taboos that seal off one kind of flow so as to facilitate the other. Men preparing for battle, for instance, must not eat cold, wet (low ground) foods, and fighting is not carried out in the rain, because otherwise the entailed principle of *kinim* would destroy the efficacy of the *rawa mugi*. (Rappaport, 1968, p. 136). Tsembaga use an idiom of assimilation to express the communion engendered by ritual action: eating pandanus is said to be like taking spirits of the low ground inside of one, and fighting men who put on battle dress (*ringgi*) are said to take red spirits into their heads (to have "a fire in the head") (Rappaport, 1968, p. 179).

We might conclude that man himself, in his ideal of "humanness", embodies and expresses the sum total of the relational flow among the complementary being of the world, much as man's life is realized in temporal–spatial movements between the adjacent spaces of *wora* and *kamungga*. The Tsembaga term for this moral totality is *nomane*, which can be used in the sense of "the moral soul" or in that of "tradition" (Rappaport, 1968, p. 169). Humanity is a totality or completeness, a relation that is precipitated and evoked by the differentiation of ritual and the surrounding world.

Spirits of the dead and of the shamanistic trance, the anthropomorphism of human affliction, are encompassed within the larger polarity of Tsembaga cosmology. Those who die of illness or accident persist as *rawa tukump*, "spirits of rot", in the low country, and we have seen that those who die in warfare persist as *rawa mugi* (Rappaport, 1968, pp. 38–39). Shamanistic divination, communing with the dead, occurs through the agency of the *kun kaze ambra*, the "smoke woman", who lives on high ground, and who is concerned, according to

Rappaport, ". . . with relationships among the spirits themselves and between the spirits and the Tsembaga" (Rappaport, 1968, p. 41). Although a (somewhat anomalous) part of the cosmological duality, the smoke woman emphasizes a distinction that cross-cuts it: that of the living and the dead.

Thus she makes a good point of transition from the world of the Tsembaga to that of the Daribi people of the Karimui area, who have been the subjects of my own research. For just as the Tsembaga cosmology subordinates the living–dead distinction to that of *wora–kamungga* (*kinim–romba nda*), so the Daribi emphasizes the anthropomorphism of human affliction, and subordinates that of adjacent cosmological spaces. Yet the Daribi, like the Tsembaga, are swidden horticulturalists, and both peoples live in local communities of about 200. The Tsembaga garden between 900 and 1600 m, the Daribi slightly lower (between 750 and 1350 m), and the Tsembaga occupy "razorback" ridge country, whereas the Daribi inhabit largely the lava plateau surrounding an extinct Pleistocene volcano (see Map 1).

Daribi mythology emphasizes a "curse of mortality" through which man came to live in his present state. Elaborate mourning practices and the doings, whims and depredations of ghosts (especially as mirrored in human affliction) are central conceptual and emotional foci in Daribi life. The Daribi pig-feast and the *habu* ceremonial ("bringing the ghost to the house") are rites of propitiating the *izibidi*, ghosts of the dead, collectively or individually. In addition, Daribi communities maintain an ongoing communion with spirits of the recently departed through the offices of (largely female) spirit mediums and *sogoyezibidi* ("tobacco-spirits"), or shamans.

Daribi cosmology might best be approached through the spatial distinction *oboba–iba*, which separates (among other things) the realm of the living from that of the dead. Like the Tsembaga polarity of *wora–kamungga*, it has an almost universal range of application, but unlike its Tsembaga counterpart it is never explicitly treated as an opposition of effective or potent principles. Nevertheless, the contents of the respective Tsembaga and Daribi symbolic divisions are remarkably similar. *Oboba* is the relative eastward or upward direction, with the connotations of life, maleness, beneficent influences and the source of things. *Iba* is the relative westward or downward direction, with connotations of death, femaleness, maleficent influences and the conclusion of things. Water is thought to rise in the east and flow westward and downward, to a lake situated somewhere to the west where the spirits of the dead dwell. Its flow prefigures the course of human mortality, and ghosts, who follow the network of streams as their "roads", are obsessed with a need for it. The sun likewise prefigures human mortality in its movement from east to west, and sunset, when the sun stands in the baleful *iba* direction, is the hour when ghosts are abroad. Thus the world may be thought of as an extensional interval separating the living from the dead (Wagner, 1972; Chapter V).

But the distinction also incorporates the vertical dimension. The men's quarters (*bidigibe'*) should always be *oboba* in relation to the women's quarters (*aribe'*) in a Daribi longhouse; if it is a single-storey dwelling, the men live to the east (Figure 1), and if it is a two-storey house, the men live on the second floor (Figure 2). In addition to its longitudinal dichotomy, the Daribi world is likewise resolved into vertically and laterally adjacent spaces. As the flow across the former is that of human mortality and the moral and spiritual essence (*noma'*) that survives death, so the flow across the latter is that of human complementarity. The spaces "above" human habitation are generally thought of as inhabited by male beings, who are neutral and sometimes beneficent, and those "below" human habitation are thought of as inhabited by female beings with a malevolent capability. The *takaru-bidi*, who live in the sky, are generally regarded as neutral to human affairs. The *buru kawai bidi* ("place spirits"), who live on mountain peaks, ridge escarpments, and in the tops of trees, are often given attributes that parody the lifestyle of Daribi men, where the *tǫ page bidi* ("ground-base people") are typically exemplified by the *izara we*, sexually jealous and meat-hungry women who live beneath the ground.

Significantly, however, mediation with these vertically and laterally differentiated beings is of a secondary, or peripheral character. Like the "little people" of Ireland, people encounter them occasionally and give fascinated accounts of the encounters. The *buru kawai bidi* are known to have their own male initiations, and can be heard playing initiation flutes around the time of the Daribi intiations. The *izara we* are thought to take the souls of children who stumble in gardens, or men who foolishly enter swampy areas after eating meat or having coitus, and are propitiated by the sacrifice of a small pig or chicken, or a "presentation" of wealth, and a small ritual. Both kinds of spirit beings add the complementarity of their particular differentiated status to human enterprise: the *buru kawai bidi* are said to have given human beings a certain kind of mourning lament, and the *izara we*, encountered in dreams, teach women how to weave net bags.

But this lateral flow of human complementarity is a far cry from the concerted ritual through which the Tsembaga mediate anthropomorphized vertical space, and it is definitely subsidiary to the major cultural preoccupation with the dead. Although the Tsembaga and

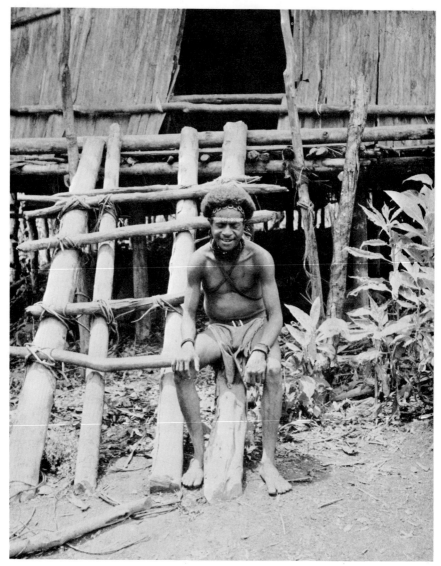

FIGURE 1. Entrance to the men's quarters (*bidigibe'*) of a large, single-storey Daribi longhouse (*kerobe'*) at Dogwaro-Hagani, Karimui, in 1965. The men's quarters occupy the forward (*oboba*) and eastward section of the house, the women's quarters occupy the rear (*iba*) and westward section.

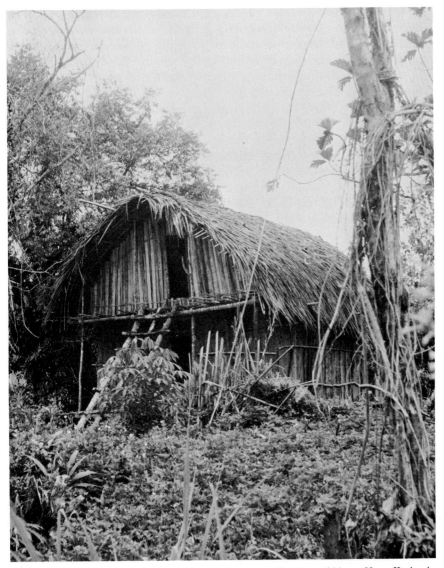

FIGURE 2. A small Daribi two-storey longhouse (*sigibe'*) standing in a swidden at Noru, Karimui, in 1965. The men's quarters (*bidigibe'*) occupy the upper (*oboba*) storey, the women's quarters (*aribe'*) occupy the lower (*iba*).

the Daribi both mediate ritually with anthropomorphized vertical extension as well as with the anthropomorphism of human affliction, the former mediation takes precedence among the Tsembaga and the latter among the Daribi. Tsembaga perceive their mediation with the dead as a part of the complementarity existing between themselves and the spirits of low and high ground; Daribi perceive their mediation with the spirits inhabiting adjacent spaces as a trivial aspect, at best, of their all-important mediation with the ghosts of the dead.

The peoples of the Papuan interior present a veritable kaleidoscope of variations on these themes. As I have remarked, the Tsembaga concern with dualities of hot and cold, and male and female, appears to be typical of the central Highlanders to whom they bear a close linguistic relationship. On the other hand, the Kaluli of Mt. Bosavi, studied by E. L. Schieffelin, perceive a bizarre cosmology of distinct but completely co-terminous and simultaneous world-spaces, "mirror-worlds", in which the inhabitants of each see one another as human, but perceive those of the other as wild creatures. Human passage and mediation between these worlds occurs at death and in the shamanistic trance, and the major ceremonials of the Kaluli, exemplified by the *gisaro*, involve the metaphorical evocation of human affliction in agonistic singing and dancing performances (Schieffelin, 1976). Although bush spirits seem to be somewhat more important to the Kaluli than to the Daribi, the Kaluli religion is generally similar to the Daribi in its emphasis on the anthropomorphism of human affliction. There are even indications of peoples in transition between "bush spirit" and "human affliction" orientations. The traditional ritual of the Anggor people in the West Sepik area is based on mediation with favourably disposed bush spirits, or *sanind* (Huber, 1973). P. Huber reports, however, that spirit mediums, who commune with the dead, have recently begun to supplant the older emphasis (Huber, 1974).

Over and above their particular cosmologies, rituals and forms of mediation, each one of these peoples locates mankind in a world of differentiated, though basically analogous, anthropomorphic entities. All recognize a kind of immanent human essence as the object and sustaining force of their mediation. It is the "moral soul" of the individual, the "tradition" or "sociality" of the community, and also the binding force of the cosmos. And it is "tapped", tempered, and constrained in rituals that emphasize the solicitude and concern of the various sets of anthropomorphic beings for one another. In effect, the forms of reciprocal expectation and interaction that characterize these human societies are applied in an analogous ritual fashion to relations between man and his (anthropomorphized) circumstances. Thus human relationships of all kinds come to be "two-sided" and dialectical, rather than "one-sided", linear and crudely exploitive. We have only to substitute ecological terms like "breeding population" for the various types of beings, and "ecosystem" or "environment" for the immanent human essence to transform these cultures into nicely construed realizations of the ecological perspective.

This, indeed, is the point of Rappaport's ecological analysis of the Tsembaga, for his methodology has been that of performing just such a substitution.

> The Tsembaga, designated a 'local population', have been regarded as a population in the animal ecologist's sense: a unit composed of an aggregate of organisms having in common certain distinctive means whereby they maintain a set of shared trophic relations with other living and non-living components of the biotic community in which they exist together. (Rappaport, 1968, p. 224)

Moreover, the fact that the "cognized model" of Tsembaga spirit beings and principles is not isomorphic with the "operational model" of the ecologist's naturalistic materialism, does not pose a serious drawback for Rappaport

> ... the important question concerning the cognized model, since it serves as a guide to action, is not the extent to which it conforms to 'reality' (i.e. is identical with the operational model), but the extent to which it elicits behavior that is appropriate to the material situation of the actors, and it is against this functional and adaptive criterion that we may assess it. (Rappaport, 1968, p. 239)

This might be paraphrased by saying that it is the kind and quality of the relationships, rather than the things related, that matters.

It is not difficult, even from a semiotic perspective, to agree with Rappaport's conclusion. In the light of my earlier observation, to the effect that semiotic construction and natural process completely contain or envelope one another, however, the question arises of why the ethnocentric concept of nature must be retained at all. Is it not sufficient, in other words, to consider the "kind and quality of the relationships" alone, as a semiotic modality, and dismiss the trappings of naturalistic materialism together with the Tsembaga bush spirits and principles as symbolic illusions of the respective cultures? The issue is a difficult, if not to say controversial one, for nature, though a symbolically "loaded" aspect of our world view, permits the application of a broad range of natural science expertise, whereas the semiotic approach, although a product of Western social science, is comparatively free of broader symbolic associations, and deals with symbolic form rather than symbolic content. Yet both are means of negotiating the paradox of science, and the issue of choosing between them ultimately devolves upon the significance of the ecological perspective within our own symbolic universe, what I shall term "the ecology of ecology".

V. THE ECOLOGY OF ECOLOGY

The semiotic constitution of ecological theory and the peculiar attractiveness of this theory for scientific as well as lay members of Western society is very much the result of the way in which ecology answers certain questions. For the semiotic environment in which ecology has grown and flourished, and to which it has adapted with surprising facility and success, is that of the traditional Western literalistic world-view. The very form of Western civilization, as I have observed earlier, embodies and asserts human responsibility for the literal component of human activity, and relegates the figurative component, including our perception of human circumstance, to the realm of the innate. By the very quality of literal construction, the distinction between culture and nature (an integral result of that construction), is likewise seen as human artifice. This is the sense of Rousseau's *contrat social,* that man's collective society is the result of a previous human charter, or agreement. And the spirit of Rousseau's thesis, which gave impetus to the American and French Revolutions, was that man, having entered into the agreement by his own will, has the right to abrogate, negotiate, and re-establish it.

But the whole enterprise, for Rousseau and his revolutionary disciples, was fostered and underwritten by the pre-eminent and self-sufficient presence of nature. Pre-cultural man lived in a regime of autonomous nurturance, what we might like to call a primordial ecological bliss, and what Rousseau's contemporaries termed the "state of nature". It is, indeed, but a step from the Jacobin call to re-establish the demarcation of culture and nature on rational grounds, and the modern tendency to transcend this "man-made" obstacle to man's "brotherhood" with other species, but it is a step that has taken 200 years to accomplish. And it is hardly accidental that these intervening centuries have witnessed an increasingly problematic attitude toward human responsibility and culture, and an increasingly sophisticated scientific grasp of "the natural". The development of a "science of culture" parallels a massive revolutionary, democratic, diplomatic and at times quite violent effort to arbitrate and define man's responsibility for the cultural. At the same time, culture's "opposite", the matrix of natural phenomena that seemingly underlies and fuels the whole enterprise, has become less and less problematic. The ecological perspective, which inverts the semiotic orientation of Western civilization, emerges as a radical "solution" to a whole host of political, economic, ethical and not least scientific questions posed by man's responsibility for the cultural. It tells us, in a rather different way to the semiotics, that we have been looking at things wrongly.

As a figurative solution to a literal problem, however, the ecological perspective is locked into a dialectical interdependence with that problem. Without the problem, the solution is meaningless, for it is the Western literal world view that gives us the concepts of nature and culture as ecologists have come to depend upon them. Like all well-adapted organisms, ecology needs the environment to which it has adapted if it is to survive. It is, indeed, the consummate means of negotiating the paradox of science. But it is equally true that an environment is not the same environment without the organisms that have adapted to it, and that without a solution a problem becomes more pressing than ever. As the ecological perspective gains in academic currency and general popularity, the institutionalized aspects of our literalist civilization (including especially its base of credibility among the populace) will come to depend more and more upon its support as a means of validating (and transcending) the culture–nature distinction. Because nature is indispensable to ecology, the ecological perspective cannot transcend this distinction without reiterating its basic premisses.

Let me be more specific in this matter of dialectical interdependence. By shifting the focus of human responsibility to the figurative sphere of nature, ecology automatically relegates the literal component to the realm of the innate. Since the literal orientation represents an inversion of this order, ecology and the orthodox Western viewpoint each recognize the innate of the other as a field of human responsibility, and they each perceive the other's field of responsibility as a "given". This explains the annoyance of traditionalists at the ecological claim to "do" nature (something that one should not ordinarily "do"), and the ecologists' resentment of those who "pollute the environment" for individual gain. But what is the literal component of the ecologist's universe, then, if not an identification of collectively formulated scientific law (understood as autonomic "ordering", as "ecosystem" or "natural balance") with the innate? Instead of ghosts, bush spirits, and the animating morality of the soul, a morality of scientifically formulated natural order flows through the universe of ecological speculation.

This permits a dialectical negotiation (or even "solution") of the paradox of science through a sort of semiotic "division of labour".

Heuristic, scientific law, the literal component, with its formulaic replication of a putative "natural order", provides the relational matrix, and the perspective of ecology, the figurative component, with its emphasis on man's immersion in nature and on the sanctity of the environment, provides the ethic. The dialectic may be operationalized in scholarly terms, to fit the evolution (cultural and natural "speciation") and specific traits of life-forms into the universe of scientifically ascribed order, or in social terms, to fit the concerns and aspirations of consuming citizens into a world view that sanctifies Western science, its workings and its world view. Ecology can be seen in many ways; as a breakthrough into explanatory sophistication, as an "adaptation" of Western science to its own predicated natural order, or (as I would choose to view it), as an adaptation to the semiotic necessity imposed by the complementary of literal and figurative symbolization.

As a way of having nature and "doing" it too, ecology provides a means of accommodating sophisticated dialectical operations within the established culture–nature world view. It is, indeed, a technique for the continual "re-invention" of that world view, and hence is indispensable to those whose personal, professional, or institutional interests and aspirations remain anchored to it. A strictly "ecological–environmental" (i.e. naturalistic) discussion of the issues I have examined here would have negotiated the whole range of questions and topics within the confines of the nature concept—that is, without questioning the existence of what we call nature. But by deliberately addressing my discussion, for the purposes of a critique, to an "ecology of symbols", and by tracing out the implications of semiotic construction, I have approached nature with scepticism, as an allegedly innate construct of a regime of symbolic invention.

There are, of course, many forms of semiotic analysis, and I do not pretend that the one I have employed here is necessarily definitive of the genre. It is, if anything, rather unusual. I have advocated and used it, nevertheless, to demonstrate that the problems and concepts dealt with by ecology are capable of another sort of analysis and resolution. Such semiotic analysis is as vulnerable to questions posed from within the naturalistic world view as naturalism is vulnerable to semiotic dissection. For instance, one might ask that if our perceived world of natural phenomena is merely a function of semiotic construction, what phenomenal orders should we regard as "given"? Does semiotics not oppose a purely "mentalistic" universe to the materialism of natural science? These questions belong to the literal orientation of Western rationalism and its Cartesian duality of mind and body. The arbitration of a boundary between innate and artificial, or between the mental and the physical (since "mind" is a derivative quantity in naturalist epistemology), is part of a game of setting up and entering a particular world view. But the assertion of ascriptive symbolic content is not a game that a conscientious semioticist might wish to, or even need to play. If the worlds of nature and semiotics are completely and mutually continent of one another, then no boundary of any sort can be established between them. And this implies that the Cartesian duality is at once completely insoluble and largely irrelevant.

What does all of this mean in practical terms? The realization that indigenous Papuans and ecologists perceive and relate to (I would say "invent") the world of experience in much the same way indicates that ecological studies will find many striking examples of environmental adaptation in the South West Pacific. Many ecologists will want to claim, of course, that such examples offer conclusive proof of the adaptive evolution of human society, and it would be very difficult to contest such a claim on its own grounds. The fact that Papuans conceptualize their innate in explicitly anthropomorphic terms, as "moral soul" or human resource, need not trouble these ecologists any more than it troubled Rappaport, for, as I have observed earlier, it is the kind and quality of the relationships that matters, not the identity of the things related.

But it is precisely for this reason that I choose to differ from the ecological conclusion. For if it is the kind and quality of the relationships, rather than the things related, that matters, a deft turn of Occam's Razor should excise our own concept of "nature" as well as the natives' ghosts and bush spirits. The semiotic analysis I have adopted here is a formal study of relationships, not a heuristic explication of social phenomena through Western man's conceptual categories. Elsewhere I have shown (Wagner, 1975; Chapter V) that the evolution of human society can be understood in purely semiotic terms. Ecologists might want to defend their adherence to nature on communicational grounds, but the dangers of working out our own problems on the soils and in the hearts and minds of other peoples should not be overlooked. They, too, are a part of our environment—a most significant part.

VI. REFERENCES

Brown, G. S. (1969). "Laws of Form". Allen and Unwin, London.
Huber, P. (1973). "Defending the Cosmos: Violence and Social Order among the Anggor of New Guinea". Presented at the ninth ICAES Congress, Chicago.
Rappaport, R. (1968). "Pigs for the Ancestors". Yale University Press, New Haven.
Salisbury, R. F. (1965). The Siane of the Eastern Highlands. *In* "Gods, Ghosts and Men

CHAPTER XIV

Problems in the Identification of Environmental Problems

ANDREW P. VAYDA AND BONNIE J. MCCAY
Cook College, Rutgers University, U.S.A.

In a recent review article (Vayda and McCay, 1975), our framework for indicating promising new directions in ecological inquiry was provided by consideration of four main criticisms of the ecological research and theory that have developed in anthropology and biology during recent decades. In the present contribution, we shall consider again one of the four criticisms and thus comment on some aspects of the past and future of human ecology in Melanesia as reflected in some preceding chapters of this volume.

Underlying our discussion is a belief in the desirability of focusing on environmental problems and how people respond to them. The kind of environmental problems with which we are especially concerned are those constituting hazards to the lives of the organisms experiencing them. In other words, we are particularly (although not exclusively) concerned with problems that carry the risk of morbidity or mortality, the risk of loosing an "existential game" in which success consists simply in staying in the game (Slobodkin, 1968; Slobodkin and Rappaport, 1974).

Examples of environmental problems and hazards and of the responses to them will be mentioned later. At this point it can be said simply that any event or property of the environment which poses a threat to the health and ultimately the survival of organisms, including people, may be regarded a hazard for them and that responding adaptively to such hazards involves in our view—as in Bateson's (1963, 1972) and Slobodkin's (1968)—not only deploying resources to cope with the immediate problem but also leaving reserves for future contingencies. It might also be noted here that we advocate a focus upon hazards and responses not out of any fundamental concern for traditional disciplinary objectives—such as the anthropologists' goal of understanding or explaining culture or the sociologists' goal of explaining groups—but rather because we think that gaining understanding of what is involved in successful or adaptive responses to environmental problems is itself an important objective. Thus we recognize that responses to environmental problems may include processes whereby the unit of action shifts from individuals to various forms (and degrees of inclusiveness) of groups and perhaps back to individuals in accord with the magnitude, persistence and other characteristics of the hazards in question; a possible illustration is Down's (1965) study of how a large extended family formed and dissolved in the Navajo Indian Reservation as changes occurred in the availability of water. We are interested in looking at such processes because they are (or may be) responses to environmental problems—in Melanesia (cf. Lowman, 1975; Watson, 1970) as elsewhere—and not because we hold to the sociological objective of accounting for changes in the characteristics of groups.

A main criticism of the work of human ecologists is that they have tended to concentrate their inquiries upon the production and consumption of food to a degree that amounts to the sin of "nutritional reductionism" (Cook, 1973, pp. 45–46) or to what Brookfield (1972, p. 46), in a discussion of Pacific agriculture, called a "calorific obsession". This is the criticism that we shall consider here.

Making the basic assumptions that all living organisms compete ultimately for energy and, therefore, that adapted organisms will be energetically efficient ones, biologists and human ecologists have spent much time, effort and money in studying the transformation of energy by plants and animals and in measuring and simulating flows of energy through ecosystems (see Odum, 1971, part 1; attempts to include man in the study of these systems in Melanesia are presented in Little and Morren, 1976, pp. 69–83; Rappaport, 1971; and Chapters IX–XI). Some biologists, however, are now questioning the assumptions underlying much of this work. Slobodkin, for example, distinguishes effectiveness from energetic efficiency

> . . . an animal may be effective at hiding or effective at searching for food in the sense that it does these acts well and in the way that is appropriate to whatever environmental problems it may face. The energetic cost or lack of energetic cost associated with these acts may prove of interest if energy is, as a matter of fact, limiting. The conditions under which energy is limiting can also be specified, but there is not any formal necessity for a connection between effectiveness and efficiency. Effectiveness may or may not involve optimization or maximation of some function relating to energy. (Slobodkin, 1972, p. 294)

Similar points are made repeatedly by Colinvaux in his introductory textbook, as, for example, in the following passage.

It is a mistake to believe that animals and plants have all evolved primarily as efficient converters of energy. The pressures of natural selection are pressures for survival, and survival may sometimes be more concerned with the efficient use of nutrients, ensuring that individuals mate, safe over-wintering, or swift growth and dispersal than with the efficient use, or even collection, of energy. (Colinvaux, 1973, p. 233)

The implication of this for research is that studying the efficiency of energy capture and use by an individual organism or population can be valuable for understanding the strategies employed by that unit if, as Slobodkin says, energy is limiting. If it is not, and if other problems such as floods or water shortages or predation are threats to the survival of an organism, then the effectiveness of the organism's response to those problems and not the energy expended in making the responses is the important subject matter.

These implications have as much pertinence in human ecology as in studies of non-human organisms. In the case of people for whom energy and its translation into food and fuel calories do appear to be major limiting factors, energy flow studies can be expected to contribute significantly to our understanding of how the existential game is played. Opportunities for research among such people certainly exist: shortages of calories, sometimes escalating to widespread famines (as happened recently in Ethiopia, Bangladesh, Afghanistan and the Sahel), are major hazards for many people in the modern world. With respect to Melanesia, it is clear that this is sometimes the case in parts of the region, for example, after severe frosts in the New Guinea Highlands (Sinnett, Chapter IV). Careful studies might show it to be also the case in some Melanesian urban areas, where, as in other parts of the world (e.g. see the Peruvian study by Frisancho *et al.*, 1973), the poverty of migrants from the hinterlands may make them more subject to the hazards of limited energy availability than they were as farmers and/or hunters in their homelands.

But what about cases in which the energy available is not a limiting factor for the people? The Gadio Enga as described by Dornstreich (Chapter IX), the Bomagai-Angoiang Marings as described by Clarke (Chapter XII), and the Tsembaga Marings as described by Rappaport (1968, 1971) seem to be examples. It may be noted incidentally that Buchbinder's (1973) study, to which Morren and Clarke refer in this volume, in no way suggests that energy availability is a problem for any Maring groups, although the study does raise some questions, to be discussed shortly, about the significance of the limited availability of protein. Vayda, who has done research among the Marings, also does not see energy availability as a problem for the people except in special circumstances such as being in refuge after defeat in warfare (Vayda, 1976, pp. 24–30).

Research on energetic efficiency among such people as the Gadio Enga and the Marings can provide answers to some questions. It is as a result of such research that, for example, the old notions about the grinding, unremitting nature of the food quest in "low energy" farming and hunting societies are being laid to rest. The research bears also on the kinds of questions which Clarke (Chapter XII) raises about the likelihood that a system under consideration will or will not run out of energy for maintaining itself.

But how much can such research tell us about how effectively the hazards actually confronting people in their environments—for example, malaria-transmitting anopheles mosquitoes in the case of some Marings—are dealt with? If (as, in fact, is the case) Marings respond to many deaths from malaria by moving from the locations where the deaths have occurred, assessment of the effectiveness of the response would have to be based on such procedures as comparison of morbidity and mortality rates from malaria in the new and old locations rather than on measurements of the energetic cost of actually making the moves. In saying this, we are agreeing with Morren's proposal (Chapter X) for testing "response effectiveness" by means of measuring changes in the intensity of problems and in their effects on the "biological attributes" of groups. At the same time, we are disagreeing with such proposals as Dornstreich's (Chapter IX) for using studies of time apportionment and energy expenditure to determine the relative importance of activities. If by "importance" is meant importance for health and survival, then how effectively an activity meets the problems actually at hand counts for more than how much time and energy are expended on it. It is true, as Morren suggests in his chapter, that expending energy in responding to one problem (or one set of problems) may impair the ability to respond to others, but, contrary to what he suggests, it seems doubtful to us that this effect should always appreciably obtain. Whether it does or not must surely depend on such factors as how soon after response is made to one problem do other problems occur; how much energy is required for the responses; and how much energy is available at particular times. Thus, having to deploy labour or energy for dealing with some new environmental problems is likely to be less difficult or consequential at times other than those of peak agricultural labour demands, such as forest clearing time among New Guinea swidden cultivators or rice harvesting time among peasants of monsoon Asia.

While he attributes greater general utility to energy flow studies than we would, Morren, insofar as he recognizes that energy itself is not always "a significant problem", cannot be said to be suffering from the calorific obsession. Indeed, the plea, made by us in the original version of our review article (Vayda and McCay, 1975), for paying attention to many possible hazards or problems in addition to caloric ones is echoed by Morren in his chapter, which is concerned with various health hazards in montane New Guinea and with the so-called protein problem. The attention devoted by Morren and also by Dornstreich to protein must make one wonder, however, whether there is danger that some human ecologists will replace the calorific obsession with a protein one (see also Gross, 1975, alleging that limitations on the availability of protein constitute a problem throughout the Amazon region). The fact is that nowhere in the present volume is there any clear evidence given to show that protein shortages or limitations are indeed an important problem for any New Guinea people. Morren's assertion of the primacy of the protein problem among montane New Guinea people in general certainly seems difficult to reconcile with his report that the Miyanmin, whose life-support system he himself studied, are getting 65 g protein per capita per day and show no clinical signs of protein malnutrition. While he presents this as evidence that the Miyanmin are responding effectively with their hunting and gathering activities to the protein problem, it makes more sense to us to regard it as evidence that the protein problem does not obtain among them. Let us not be misunderstood on this point: it may indeed be at least partly because of their hunting and gathering activities that the Miyanmin do not have a protein problem, but, on the basis of the evidence given, it seems to us no more legitimate to say that the Miyanmin do have the problem and that their activities are a response to it than to say that Catholic priests and nuns have a venereal disease problem and that their celibacy is a response to that.

Furthermore, even with respect to New Guineans whose protein intakes are much lower than those of the Miyanmin and, in some cases, much lower than the "safe levels" set forth by FAO/WHO in 1973 (Norgan et al., 1974), the evidence presented in the chapters by Hornabrook, Sinnett, and McArthur (Chapters III, IV and V) shows that adults, in spite of having experienced growth retardation, are well built, physically fit, effective in their environments, and without clear symptoms of protein insufficiency. It is possible that this is, as suggested by the three authors, the result of past adaptations to low levels of intake. However, regardless of whether protein shortages were an important problem for New Guinea people in the past, we find no compelling evidence for arguing that such shortages are a general and primary problem for present New Guinea populations, although we recognize, along with Sinnett, that further research on such matters as the relation between protein intakes and childhood morbidity and mortality is needed.

In choosing to focus upon environmental problems and responses to them, one is of course faced with problems in the identification of environmental problems. *Prima facie*, the protein may have seemed a likely candidate for being a major problem in New Guinea simply because New Guinea protein intakes are so far below the intakes of healthy Western subjects studied by nutritionists in the past. Provisional identification of environmental problems on such bases is a justifiable part of the research process, and there is no cause to regard the ensuing research effort as wasted if it shows that something which we had reasonable grounds for expecting to be a major problem is not one for the people under study. If this is indeed what is shown by the research in New Guinea on the so-called protein problem, the finding has broad significance for indicating that the range and variety of diets which can sustain healthy human beings are greater than had been generally thought. But, in light of such a finding, those concerned with environmental problems and responses to them might be well advised to turn their research efforts in New Guinea to something other than protein shortages as problems with which people need to cope. Some specific directions for research in this regard are, in fact, indicated by Hornabrook in his discussion and advocacy of case studies of "disorders which arise from disturbances", for example, the endemic cretinism that developed in the Jimi valley after the recent substitution of iodine-deficient commercial salt for indigenously produced, iodine-rich distillates from mineral pools.

In connection with problems in the identification of environmental problems, it may be noted that Hornabrook's preference for specific case studies and his doubts about the fruitfulness of "formal complex multi-disciplinary investigation" accord with our own view of the difficulties of using general models, however sophisticated, for identifying or predicting problems in particular communities and responses by members of those communities. Hornabrook himself puts his finger on some sources of the difficulties when he notes the enormous variability among Papua New Guinea people in demographic patterns, genetics and history. Because of such variability, environmental hazards which may be similar in terms of some physical measurements will have different impacts on different groups and individuals and will evoke different responses (cf. Burton and Hewitt, 1974). As Feachem suggests in his introductory chapter, predictions about these impacts and responses need to be based on micro-level data.

Readers with nomothetic inclinations should be reassured, however, that such considerations do not necessarily mean that no broad generalizations about responses to hazards can be developed in human ecology. A hope that one of us has expressed elsewhere is that it will be possible to elucidate general features of hazards and of successful or adaptive responses to them and to develop generalizations in terms of such variables as the magnitude, duration and novelty of hazards, the magnitude and reversibility of responses to them, the temporal order in which responses of different magnitudes occur, and the persistence or non-persistence of response processes (Vayda, 1974, 1976). A good example of the kinds of studies needed for developing these generalizations is provided from the New Guinea Highlands by Waddell's recent (1975) analysis, showing how the sequence and other temporal properties of the Fringe Enga's adaptive responses to frost—responses ranging from agricultural mounding to mass movement down to lower altitudes —relate to the timing, recurrence and severity of the frost problem. The fact that Waddell's analysis shows also that various interventions may have the effect of disrupting traditional coping mechanisms in Melanesia is a reason for assigning high priority to research on them at the present time.

REFERENCES

Bateson, G. (1963). "The Role of Somatic Change in Evolution". *Evolution* **17**, 529–539.

Bateson, G. (1972). "Ecology and Flexibility in Urban Civilization". *In* "Steps to an Ecology of Mind" (Ed. G. Bateson). Ballantine, New York, pp. 494–505.

Brookfield, H. C. (1972). "Intensification and Disintensification in Pacific Agriculture: A Theoretical Approach". *Pac. Viewpoint* **13**, 30–48.

Buchbinder, G. (1973). "Maring Microadaptation: A Study of Demographic, Nutritional, Genetic, and Phenotypic Variation in a Highland New Guinea Population". Unpublished Ph.D. Dissertation, Columbia University.

Burton, I. and Hewitt, K. (1974). "Ecological Dimensions of Environmental Hazards". *In* "Human Ecology" (Ed. F. Sargent II). North-Holland Co., Amsterdam, pp. 253–283.

Clarke, W. C. (1971). "Place and People: An Ecology of a New Guinean Community". University of California Press, Berkeley and Los Angeles.

Colinvaux, P. A. (1973). "Introduction to Ecology". John Wiley and Sons, New York and London.

Cook, S. (1973). "Production, Ecology, and Economic Anthropology: Notes Toward an Integrated Frame of Reference". *Soc. Sci. Inform.* **12**, 25–52.

Downs, J. R. (1965). "The Social Consequences of a Dry Well". *Am. Anthrop.* **67**, 1388–1416.

Food and Agriculture Organization/World Health Organization (1973). *Energy and Protein Requirements, Report of a Joint FAO/WHO Ad Hoc Expert Committee.* FAO, Rome.

Frisancho, A. R., Sanchez, J., Pallardel, D. and Yanez, L. (1973). "Adaptive Significance of Small Body Size Under Poor Socio-economic Conditions in Southern
Peru". *Am. J. phys. Anthrop.* **39**, 255–260.

Gross, D. R. (1975). "Protein Capture and Cultural Development in the Amazon
Basin". *Am. Anthrop.* **77**, 526–549.

Little, M. A. and Morren, G. E. B., Jr (1976). "Ecology, Energetics, and Human
Variability". Wm C. Brown, Dubuque, Iowa.

Lowman, C. (1975). "Cultural Behavior, Environmental Management, and Individual
Adaptation in the Maring Region of Papua New Guinea". Paper read at Annual
Meeting of Am. Anthropol. Assoc., San Francisco, Dec. 5, 1975.

Norgan, N. G., Ferro-Luzzi, A. and Durnin, J. V. G. A. (1974). "The Energy and
Nutrient Intake and the Energy Expenditure of 204 New Guinean Adults". *Phil.
Trans. R. Soc.* Ser B **268**, 309–348.

Odum, E. P. (1971). "Fundamentals of Ecology" (Third Edn). Saunders, Philadelphia.

Rappaport, R. A. (1968). "Pigs for the Ancestors". Yale University Press, New Haven.

Rappaport, R. A. (1971). "The Flow of Energy in an Agricultural Society". *Scient.
Am.* **225**, 116–132.

Slobodkin, L. B. (1968). "Toward a Predictive Theory of Evolution". *In* "Population
Biology and Evolution" (Ed. R. C. Lewontin). Syracuse University Press, pp. 187–
205.

Slobodkin, L. B. (1972). "On the Inconstancy of Ecological Efficiency and the Form
of Ecological Theories". *In* "Growth by Intussesception: Ecological Essays in
Honor of G. Evelyn Hutchinson", *Trans. Connecticut Acad. Arts Sci.* **44**, 293–305.

Slobodkin, L. B. and Rapoport, A. (1974). "An Optimal Strategy of Evolution".
Q. Rev. Biol. **49**, 181–200.

Vayda, A. P. (1974). "Warfare in Ecological Perspective". *Ann. Rev. Ecol. Systematics* **5**,
183–193.

Vayda, A. P. (1976). "War in Ecological Perspective: Persistence, Change, and Adaptive Processes in Three Oceanian Societies". Plenum Press, New York.

Vayda, A. P. and McCay, B. J. (1975). "New Directions in Ecology and Ecological
Anthropology". *Ann. Rev. Anthrop.* **4**, 293–306.

Waddell, E. (1975). "How the Enga Cope with Frost: Responses to Climatic Perturbations in the Central Highlands of New Guinea". *Hum. Ecol.* **3**, 249–273.

Watson, J. B. (1970). "Society as Organized Flow: The Tairora Case". *SWest J.
Anthrop.* **26**, 107–124.

Index

Note. This is an Index which also contains (1) *all place names mentioned in the text;* (2) *those authors' names whose work is quoted at length;* (3) *plants, animals and diseases, but Latin names are only included for the most important species.*